Understanding Intracardiac EGMs

A Patient Centered Guide

To Howard and Sumiko Kusumoto

Understanding Intracardiac EGMs

A Patient Centered Guide

Fred Kusumoto MD

Professor of Medicine
Mayo Clinic College of Medicine
Jacksonville, Fl, USA

WILEY Blackwell

Library of Congress Cataloging-in-Publication Data

Kusumoto, Fred, author.
    Understanding intracardiac EGMs : a patient centered guide / Fred Kusumoto,.
        p. ; cm.
    Includes index.
        ISBN 978-1-118-72136-0 (paperback)
    I. Title.
    [DNLM: 1. Electrophysiologic Techniques, Cardiac–methods–Problems and Exercises.
2. Electrocardiography–methods–Problems and Exercises. WG 18.2]
    RC683.5.E5
    616.1'207547—dc23

                                                    2015012078

A catalogue record for this book is available from the British Library.

Contents

Preface

The field of electrophysiology has evolved rapidly over the past three decades from a niche field with minimal clinical impact to an essential part of cardiology that warrants specialized training for two years and has a separate board certification from the American Board of Internal Medicine. This evolution in knowledge and clinical applicability has been accompanied by the development of many specialized tools that have facilitated procedures in the electrophysiology laboratory. Although these new tools that allow reproducible mapping of arrhythmias in the heart, mapping with computerized algorithms, and advanced imaging, among other capabilities have become almost essential for any fully functioning electrophysiology laboratory, it remains just as important for the clinician to have a clear understanding of arrhythmias using the most fundamental electrophysiologic technique–direct mapping of the myocardium with electrode catheters and evaluating the response of cardiac tissue to electrical stimulation.

This book is designed as a series of cases that illustrate the process of evaluation of arrhythmias using standard electrophysiologic techniques. Although patients may come to the electrophysiology laboratory with a tentative diagnosis, all experienced electrophysiologists know that these only represent "best guesses" and more often than not the guesses are partially or completely wrong. Like any good puzzle (and perhaps to our frustration), there can be many twists and turns during an electrophysiology study due to misinterpretation of data and conflicting or confusing pieces of data that must be cobbled together into a coherent (and accurate!) diagnosis. The cases in this book go in sequence from initial presentation of the patient, strategies for comprehensive evaluation in the electrophysiology laboratory, and where appropriate, therapeutic options for ablation.

It is important to note that there are many different approaches and styles to electrophysiology studies, so there will be some disagreement on the best method for the electrophysiologic evaluation of the patient. Where applicable, I have tried to provide the reader with insight with situations where different tactics for the diagnostic evaluation of tachyarrhythmias in the electrophysiology laboratory might be pursued. I will be the first to acknowledge that evaluation of intracardiac electrograms is an art that is often subjective and that experienced clinicians will have different interpretations of the same set of recordings. If the text provides a flashpoint for arguments and discussion at your laboratories, then my overarching goal of getting people to appreciate the importance of electrogram interpretation even with today's technology has been accomplished.

This book can be read alone, but it also references concepts illustrated from *Understanding the ECG and EGM* (Wiley-Blackwell 2010). That first book takes the traditional approach of sequentially discussing a known type of arrhythmia, for example, atrial flutter or atrioventricular node reentry. In addition, it starts with basic but fundamental concepts such as filtering and evaluation of basic intervals and refractory periods, which are subjects that are not addressed or only cursorily discussed in this book. In contrast, this book starts from clinical presentation of an individual patient where the exact type of arrhythmia is not known a priori, the usual situation that confronts the clinical electrophysiologist. Although the book will be more easily read by the health professional that already understands some of the basics of electrophysiology, I am hopeful that the book will appeal to a wide audience including experienced staff in the electrophysiology laboratory, cardiology and electrophysiology fellows, and electrophysiologists who are taking care of patients with complex arrhythmias or are studying for their electrophysiology boards.

I would like to thank Mel Scheinman, who, over two decades ago, first taught me the fundamentals of electrogram interpretation but more importantly instilled an appreciation of the nuances of intracardiac recordings and the importance of curiosity, patience, and always putting the patient first during an electrophysiology study. I can still fondly recall late evenings when Mel would find me at the end of the day and take time to review the day's cases (does the man ever tire of thinking about electrophysiology?). Putting a book together like this takes many long hours, and as I am hunched over my computer tapping out these last words in the late evening, I know that I am indebted to my daughters Miya, Hana, and Aya for putting up with an occasionally distracted father and to my wife Laura for her understanding and patience over 25 wonderful years.

Glossary

Common abbreviations/terms in the electrophysiology.

Tachycardia types

SVT	Supraventricular tachycardia
PSVT	Paroxysmal supraventricular tachycardia
AF	Atrial fibrillation
MAT	Multifocal atrial tachycardia
AT	Atrial tachycardia
AVNRT	AV node reentrant tachycardia
AVRT	Atrioventricular reentrant tachycardia
ORT	Orthodromic reciprocating tachycardia
ART	Antridromic reciprocating tachycardia
NPJT	Nonparoxysmal junctional tachycardia
PJRT	Permanent junctional reciprocating tachycardia
VT	Ventricular tachycardia
VF	Ventricular Fibrillation

Refractory periods

AERP	Atrial effective refractory period
AVNERP	AV node effective refractory period
VERP	Ventricular effective refractory period
VAERP	Ventriculoatrial effective refractory period
APERP	Accessory pathway effective refractory period

Pacing nomenclature

BCL	Basic cycle length
AVBCL	Atrioventricular blocked cycle length
VABCL	Ventriculoatrial blocked cycle length
S1S2	Coupling interval of the first premature beat
S2S3	Coupling interval of the second premature beat
"Singles"	Single premature stimulus
"Doubles"	Two premature extrastimuli
"Triples"	Three premature extrastimuli

Intervals

PR	Interval from the beginning of the P wave to the beginning of the QRS
QRS	Interval from the beginning of the QRS to the end of the QRS
QT	Interval from the beginning of the QRS to the end of the T wave
AH	Interval between the atrial signal and the His bundle recording measured from a catheter straddling the tricuspid valve
HV	Interval between the His bundle recording and the initial ventricular activation (usually identified by the first deflection on a surface lead)
RR	Interval between two QRS complexes

(continued overleaf)

Common abbreviations/terms in the electrophysiology (*continued*).

Anatomic locations	
CS	Coronary Sinus
CTI	Cavotricuspid Isthmus
LVOT	Left Ventricular Outflow Tract
RVOT	Right Ventricular Outflow tract
Miscellaneous	
PVC	Premature Ventricular Contraction
PAC	Premature Atrial Contraction
AP	Accessory pathway

CHAPTER 1

Basic electrophysiology

For our discussion, electrophysiology is a general term used to describe the "electrical" characteristics of the heart. The fundamental diagnostic tools used by electrophysiologists are small catheters that are placed in the heart most commonly via the vascular system. The catheters are essentially plastic-coated wires with metal electrodes at the tip that have two functions: measurement of the electrical activity of the heart and provision of a conductive pathway to allow stimulation of the heart. Often, multiple catheters are placed in different parts of the heart, which when evaluated together can provide clues into possible mechanisms for bradycardia or tachycardia in an individual patient. Bradycardia is a far less common reason for performing an electrophysiology study and is often evaluated in the context of a patient with syncope (Chapter 26).

Most commonly, electrophysiology studies are often performed in patients with known tachycardia or patients who are at risk for tachycardia. Practical use and performance of the electrophysiology study in the evaluation of tachycardias will be the focus of all but one of the subsequent cases. Before we go through the cases, it is instructive to review the basic methods for classifying tachycardias. Clinically, tachycardias are usually classified by QRS complex width, because a narrow QRS complex suggests that the ventricles are being activated normally, while a wide QRS complex is a sign of abnormal activation of the ventricles. Although supraventricular tachycardias can be associated with profound symptoms such as shortness of breath or chest pain, they are generally not life-threatening, while a wide QRS tachycardia may signify the presence of ventricular tachycardia that can be life-threatening due to ineffective cardiac contraction. In the electrophysiology laboratory, more detailed evaluation of tachycardias is possible and, because it is often possible to treat the tachycardia

by identifying and eliminating critical components, it is important to consider both anatomic location and mechanism. Unfortunately, electrophysiology can use specialized jargon or phrases that are hard to "keep straight" particularly for the novice. Some common abbreviations used in electrophysiology are defined in Table A1 in Appendix.

Mechanistic tachycardia classification

From a mechanistic standpoint, there are two basic types of tachycardias. The most common tachycardia mechanism is reentry. In reentry, there are two parallel pathways that are electrically separate and with different electrophysiologic properties (differences in conduction and refractoriness). An electrical impulse (generally an early beat) conducts "down" only one pathway and is able to enter the other pathway in a retrograde direction. The most well-studied example of this phenomenon are tachycardias that use an accessory pathway (Figure 1.1). In this case, the accessory pathway and the atrioventricular (AV) node provide anatomically separate connections between the atria and the ventricles. The accessory pathway and the AV node/His bundle axis are anatomically discrete, and the atria and the ventricles are electrically separated by the mitral and tricuspid annuli. Reentry can also occur in the setting of a scar that has a slowly conducting pathway through it. In this case, the slowly conducting pathway and normal tissue represent the two pathways that form the substrate for development of reentry. Traditionally, scar is described in ventricular tissue because of a myocardial infarction but could also be present in atrial tissue in the setting of atrial fibrosis from natural processes or prior ablations. It is not surprising that reentry generally is more common around "holes"

Understanding Intracardiac EGMs: A Patient Centered Guide, First Edition. Fred Kusumoto.
© 2015 John Wiley & Sons, Ltd. Published 2015 by John Wiley & Sons, Ltd.

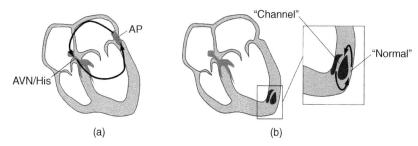

(a)   (b)

Figure 1.1 For most types of reentry, two separate pathways have different electrophysiologic properties, and with a carefully timed impulse, depolarization can occur in one pathway and "turn around" to depolarize the parallel pathway. The most well-described and the best clinical example of this is a patient with an accessory pathway (a). Normally, the AV node forms the only electrical connection between the atria and the ventricles, but in patients with an accessory pathway, the second electrical connection between the atria and ventricles can allow a reentrant circuit to develop. Another common scenario for reentrant arrhythmias is ventricular tachycardia in the setting of a prior myocardial infarction (b). In this case, a "patchy" myocardial scar forms an alternate pathway along with normal myocardium to activate one side of a scar to the other side of the scar.

in the heart, because these "holes" increase the likelihood that two separate pathways of electrical activation exist. For example, in the most common form of atrial flutter, the reentrant circuit uses a critical isthmus formed by the inferior vena cava and the tricuspid valve. The inferior vena cava and the tricuspid valve act as natural barriers that allow perpetuation of a reentrant circuit. In this case, the inferior cavotricuspid isthmus serves as one pathway, and the superior portion of the right atrium serves as the second pathway (Figure 1.2).

The second type of tachycardia is a focal source of rapid activation. This tachycardia mechanism is easier to conceptualize and can be thought of as outward spreading of electrical activation similar to a series of waves from repetitive drips into a pool of still water. Often, rapid activation is due to abnormal automaticity from a nest of cells, but in some cases, very small reentrant circuits can appear as focal activation. This type of reentry is often called microreentry to differentiate it from larger circuits of reentry that are called

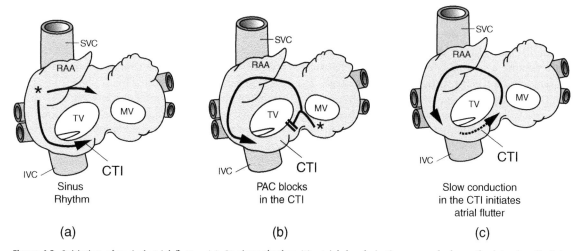

(a)   (b)   (c)

Figure 1.2 Initiation of typical atrial flutter. (a): In sinus rhythm (*), atrial depolarization proceeds down the lateral wall of the right atrium (RA) and superiorly toward the septum. (b): With a premature atrial contraction from the left atrium (*), inferior atrial depolarization blocks in the cavotricuspid isthmus (CTI), but the wave of depolarization travels superiorly to activate the superior and lateral portions of the right atrium and enters the CTI from the other direction. (c): Slow conduction through the CTI initiates atrial flutter.

macroreentry. The actual reentrant circuit cannot be visualized unless specialized techniques are used, and often, the reentrant mechanism must be inferred by the behavior of the tachycardia. For example, termination of a tachycardia with a premature extrastimulus suggests the possibility of reentry. While reentrant circuits can be extinguished by a single early depolarization causing refractoriness, a tachycardia due to automaticity generally does not terminate, instead the usual response is transient suppression of the tachycardia.

The reason that tachycardia mechanism is so important is that it will dictate the therapeutic plan, particularly if ablation will be an option. In patients with reentry, effective ablation targets a critical pathway, isthmus, or "channel" that is essential for maintaining the tachycardia (often called "substrate"). Successful ablation is characterized by producing conduction block that can be thought of as a "dam" or a "wall" that prevents electrical current from passing. In patients with a focal source of tachycardia successful ablation targets the specific "source" of the arrhythmia.

Anatomic tachycardia classification

In addition to mechanism, it is also important from an electrophysiologic standpoint to consider tachycardia using an anatomic classification. Obviously, considering the anatomic location of the tachycardia is important to effectively treat the arrhythmia with ablation. A comprehensive review of different types of tachycardia is discussed in *Understanding Intracardic EGMs and ECGs* (Wiley Blackwell 2010) and is beyond the scope of this case-based book. However, a cursory review at this point is reasonable. In general terms, there are only four basic anatomic locations for tachycardia (Figure 1.3).

Firstly, a tachycardia can arise solely within the atrium. This could be due to a stable reentrant circuit within the atrium, continuous irregular activation of the atrium (perhaps due to unstable reentrant circuits), or one or more abnormal foci of automaticity. The way to consider this is that in atrial flutter or atrial fibrillation, there is activation of the atrium somewhere all the time. In contrast, in focal or multifocal atrial tachycardias, a site(s) leads to depolarization of the atria, and the atria are quiescent until the next depolarization. Perhaps, another analogy distinguishing between reentry and automaticity is useful. Automaticity or repetitive focal firing is similar to a blinking light(s): when the light goes "off" there is no light. Reentry can be compared to the spinning earth, where as the earth spins, different areas of the earth are in the dark and "lights are turned on." In the latter case, there is always somewhere where the lights are on (the Pacific Ocean, with very few lights from ships and islands could be thought of as a region of "slow conduction"). Regardless of whether automaticity or reentry is the cause of the arrhythmia, the entire abnormal focus or circuit is located within atrial tissue. To further confuse things, all of these arrhythmias are often collectively called atrial tachycardias. The second "anatomic" type of tachycardia is an abnormal focus or small reentrant circuit localized within the AV junction. Although the most common cause of tachycardia arising from the junction is due to small reentrant circuits within the AV node and perinodal atrial tissues, rapid automatic rhythms can be observed from the AV junction in certain situations. The most commonly encountered automatic junctional tachycardia is called nonparoxysmal junctional tachycardia (NPJT) and can be seen after cardiac surgery, particularly surgeries that involve the aortic or mitral valve. An example of NPJT is shown in Figure 1.4. Notice the AV dissociation and underlying sinus bradycardia. In NPJT, AV conduction is intact, and properly timed P wave will conduct to the ventricles and result in a shorter R-R interval or a subtle change in the QRS morphology as shown in this example. In this case, a "blinking light" in the AV junction is competing with a slower "blinking light" in the sinus node. The third anatomic classification of tachycardia arises solely from ventricular tissue and includes ventricular tachycardia and ventricular fibrillation (again differentiated by whether there is relatively repetitive depolarization of ventricular tissue vs irregular chaotic depolarization of ventricular tissue). The fourth anatomical classification is a tachycardia that uses an accessory pathway. Tachycardias using accessory pathways will be the subject of several of the cases in this book, and the reader should refer back to Figure 1.3 as required. Identification of the tachycardia mechanism (reentry vs automaticity) and the critical anatomic sites necessary for initiating or for sustaining tachycardia is the principal goal of electrophysiology studies and will be the principal subject for all of the cases covered throughout this book.

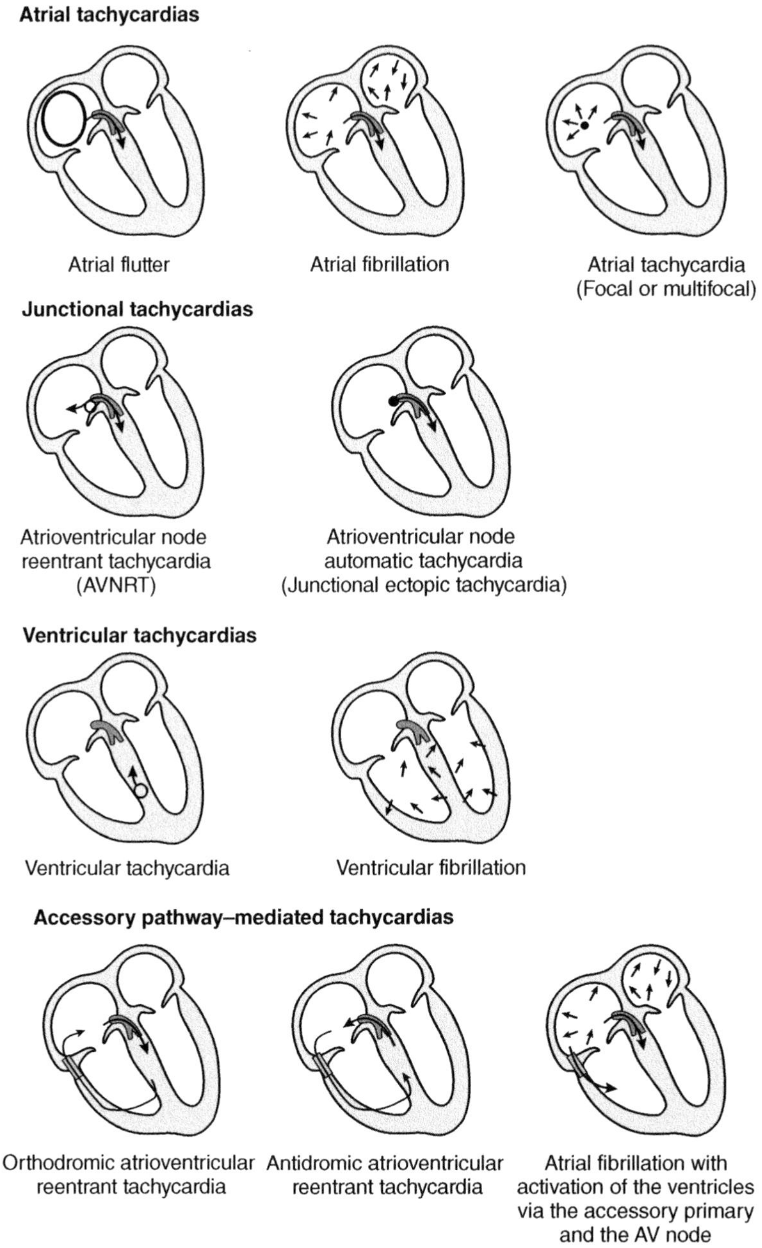

Atrial tachycardias

Atrial flutter   Atrial fibrillation   Atrial tachycardia
                                                   (Focal or multifocal)

Junctional tachycardias

Atrioventricular node   Atrioventricular node
reentrant tachycardia   automatic tachycardia
(AVNRT)   (Junctional ectopic tachycardia)

Ventricular tachycardias

Ventricular tachycardia   Ventricular fibrillation

Accessory pathway–mediated tachycardias

Orthodromic atrioventricular Antidromic atrioventricular   Atrial fibrillation with
reentrant tachycardia   reentrant tachycardia   activation of the ventricles
                                                            via the accessory primary
                                                                and the AV node

Figure 1.3 Anatomic classification of tachycardias (adapted with permission from Kusumoto F, Cardiovascular Pathophysiology, Harris Barton Press 1999).

Electophysiology basics

From a simplistic standpoint, an electrophysiology study involves measuring the baseline electrical characteristics of the heart, "stressing" the heart by pacing, and then evaluating whatever arrhythmias are induced by the "stress." Once catheters are in position, all electrophysiology studies begin by measuring baseline parameters. Even in an electrophysiology study,

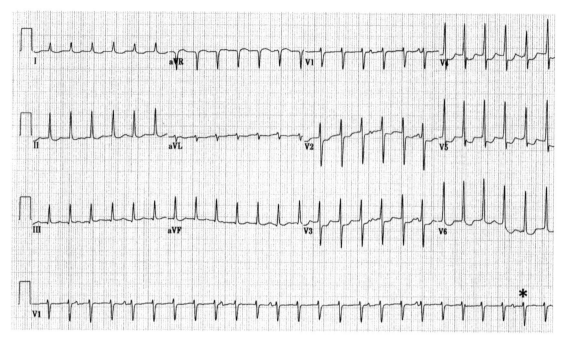

Figure 1.4 Patient with an automatic tachycardia from the AV node region observed in the first few hours after aortic valve surgery. This arrhythmia, called nonparoxysmal junctional tachycardia (NPJT), usually resolves after 1 or 2 days. Intermittent intrinsic AV conduction can sometimes be observed when a properly timed P wave results in an early QRS complex or a subtle change in the QRS morphology (*).

standard electrocardiogram (ECG) measurements such as the PR interval, QRS width, and QT interval are important to document. It is important to reemphasize that intracardiac recordings are simply electrodes within the heart and simply provide more accurate and complete evaluation of timing and direction of depolarization for both atrial and ventricular tissues.

For example, we infer that the sinus node is driving the atrium by the shape of the P wave from the surface ECG. If the P wave is negative in lead AVR and positive in lead II, we know that the atria are being depolarized from right to left, and "High-Low." However, by placing electrodes in different regions of the atria, we can confirm this by direct recording of electrical activity. For most electrophysiology studies, catheters will be placed in the high right atrium (HRA), straddling the tricuspid valve, in the right ventricle, and in the coronary sinus (Figure 1.5 and Table A2 in Appendix). These initial catheter positions are chosen because they all can be placed via venous puncture (generally the two femoral veins, although the internal jugular and subclavian veins can also be used), and together they can evaluate

electrical activity in the critical regions of the heart. The HRA is near the location of the sinus node; the right septal region straddles the tricuspid valve and allows identification of septal atrial activation, His bundle depolarization, and depolarization of the septal portion of the right ventricle, and the right ventricle records depolarization of the right ventricular apex. The coronary sinus travels in or near the left AV groove separating the left atrium and the left ventricle and is accessible from the right atrium via the coronary sinus os located in the inferior portion of the tight atrial septum near the triscuspid valve, an additional catheter is often placed here when evaluation of left atrial and left ventricle depolarization would be helpful.

Baseline electrograms from a patient undergoing an electrophysiology study for supraventricular tachycardia are shown in Figure 1.6. The general strategy for evaluating electrograms is shown in Figure 1.7. Although laboratories vary, all will generally place several ECG recordings at the top of the page. In our laboratory, we usually use three leads – I, II, and V1. This set provides a lateral lead (lead I), an inferior lead (lead II), and a

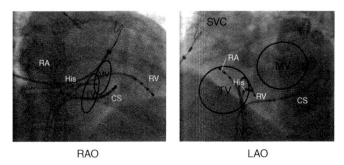

RAO   LAO

Figure 1.5 Basic catheter positions for electrophysiology study in the right anterior oblique (RAO) and the left anterior oblique (LAO) projections. Quadripolar catheters are located in the right atrium (RA), His bundle region (His) straddling the tricuspid valve, and the right ventricle (RV). A decapolar catheter is placed in the coronary sinus (CS). For orientation, the approximate locations of the mitral valve (MV), tricuspid valve (TV), inferior vena cava (IVC), and superior vena cava (SVC) are shown (reprinted with permission from Kusumoto FM, Understanding EGMs and ECGs, Wiley 2010).

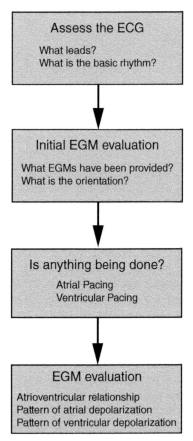

Figure 1.6 Flow sheet for the evaluation of electrograms during a typical electrophysiology study.

precordial lead (lead V1). We use lead II for the inferior lead, as the P waves are generally most easily seen in this lead particularly during sinus rhythm, and lead V1 as our precordial lead, as the QRS morphology in the setting of bundle branch block has been very well described. The ECG leads are placed "on top" because they serve as basic landmarks and should always be the *first* signals to be assessed when evaluating intracardiac electrograms.

Electrograms are usually grouped by catheter and by personal preference. In Figure 1.6, atrial signals are placed above ventricular signals, right-sided structures above left-sided structures, and with distal electrodes "on top" and proximal electrodes "below." This setup is personal preference and dates back to my initial training at the University of California, San Francisco. Preferences for electrogram display will vary from operator to operator usually depending on training (you can often guess where an electrophysiologist trained by their electrogram display and their approach to electrophysiology studies). How many electrograms displayed for a particular catheter will be dependent on the number of electrodes on a specific catheter. Traditionally, quadripolar catheters with four electrodes have been used, and recordings between the distal electrode pairs and the proximal pairs are depolarized. If a catheter has more electrodes, then more electrogram pairs can be displayed. All of this emphasizes that once the ECG is evaluated, the next step in evaluating electrograms is to first look at the anatomic location and

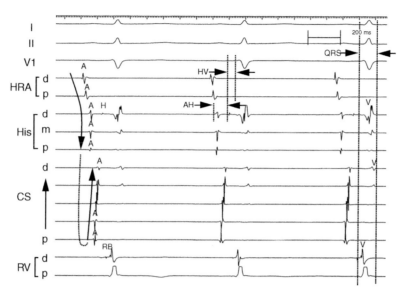

Figure 1.7 Electrograms recorded from catheter positions in Figure 1.5. The AV relationship is 1:1 with atrial activation (both P waves and atrial EGMs) preceding or "driving" ventricular activation (both QRS complexes and ventricular EGMs). Atrial activation is seen first in the high right atrium (HRA), followed by the His bundle, and last in the coronary sinus (vertical arrows). A His bundle deflection (H) and a right bundle (RB) potential can be seen during the isoelectric period of the PR interval. AV conduction is usually divided into two parts: the AH interval (first septal atrial activation to the His deflection) that represents conduction through the AV node and the HV interval (His deflection to first ventricular depolarization) that represents His bundle, bundle branch, and Purkinje fiber depolarization. Ventricular (V) activation is seen first in catheters located in the septum (His and RV) and later in the coronary sinus.

number of electrograms that have been provided and in what orientation they are displayed.

In our patient, the basic cycle length is 775 ms, and the PR interval is normal (160 ms), with the QRS interval being normal as well (106 ms). The electrograms from four catheters are provided, from superior to inferior: the HRA, the His bundle, the coronary sinus, and the right ventricle. The electrodes are recorded as discrete pairs except for the His bundle where overlapping signals from the four electrodes are recorded – distal: first and second; mid: second and third; proximal: third and fourth. There is a 1:1 relationship between atrial and ventricular electrograms (as would be predicted by the normal PR interval on the surface ECG). Closer inspection of the atrial electrograms shows that atrial depolarizarion occurs from right to left and superior to inferior (first in the HRA, then the His, and last atrial signals in the left atrium). After atrial depolarization, the sharp deflection of the His bundle can be seen followed by a sharp deflection from the right bundle.

Ventricular activation is first identified in the septum (the His and RV catheters) and later in the left ventricle (low amplitude potentials recorded in the coronary sinus catheter). As mentioned previously, the coronary sinus straddles the left atrium and left ventricle, so electrograms from both structures are recorded, but generally the atrial signal is of higher amplitude and higher frequency ("sharp and spikey").

For AV conduction via the AV node and His Purkinje system, the AH interval (measured from the atrial electrogram to the His bundle electrogram) represents conduction time through the AV node proper, and the HV interval (measured from the His bundle to first sign of ventricular depolarization) represents depolarization of the His bundle, the right and left bundles, and the Purkinje fibers. This is the reason why the right bundle potential is located within the HV interval. As the AV node conduction is slow and has innervation from the autonomic nervous system, the normal range for the AH interval is quite wide from 50 to 140 ms.

The HV interval measures conduction via the His Purkinje system, and because these structures have rapid conduction properties and do not have significant innervation by the autonomic system, the normal range is shorter with less variation (35–55 ms).

Baseline atrial pacing

Atrial pacing is performed for the evaluation of any changes in the QRS complex with higher atrial rates and of AV conduction and for the induction of tachycardia. There are two forms of atrial pacing: (i) atrial overdrive pacing where the atria are paced from a single location at progressively faster rates and (ii) delivery of premature extrastimuli, where after consistent capture of the atria occurs (usually 8 beats), one, two, or three premature atrial stimuli are introduced.

Atrial overdrive pacing is shown in Figures 1.8 and 1.9. Normally, as the atria are paced at progressively faster and faster rates, delay begins to develop in the AV node (think of the AV node as a "regulator" that limits ventricular depolarization; this characteristic is important for "protecting" the ventricle from rapid stimulation in the setting of rapid atrial activity, e.g., in

atrial fibrillation, ventricular depolarization, although fast, is often limited to 120–180 beats per minute depending on the patient's age). The cycle length in which 1:1 AV conduction stops (in other words there are more "A's" than "V's") is called the AV blocked cycle length (AVBCL). The AVBCL is a measure for AV conduction, with a shorter AVBCL associated with more "slick" AV node conduction.

In patients with an accessory pathway, delay in the AV node due to atrial pacing can lead to more of the ventricles being depolarized by the accessory pathway. Delay in the AV node is characterized by prolongation of the AH interval, and more ventricular depolarization due to the accessory pathway leads to a more abnormal-looking QRS complex. We will discuss these changes extensively in the cases that involve patients with accessory pathways.

For premature atrial extrastimuli, after a drive of 8–10 stimuli at a constant drive cycle length, a premature atrial stimulus is delivered. This premature beat is programmed to earlier and earlier values, and the response of the AV node and His bundle are assessed. The usual response is shown in Figures 1.10 and 1.11. In Figure 1.10, after pacing

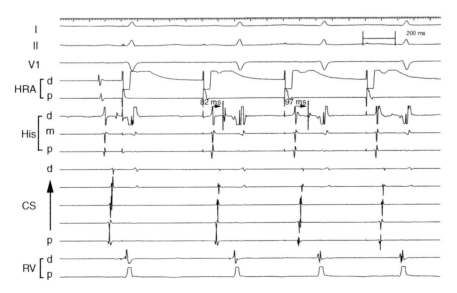

Figure 1.8 Initiation of atrial pacing at a cycle length of 500 ms. The first atrial pacing stimulus does not capture the atria, because depolarization via the sinus node has just occurred. However, the second and third atrial stimuli capture the atrium (the atrial stimuli are followed by atrial electrograms). The AH interval of the third stimulus is prolonged (from 82 to 97 ms) because of decremental conduction in the AV node.

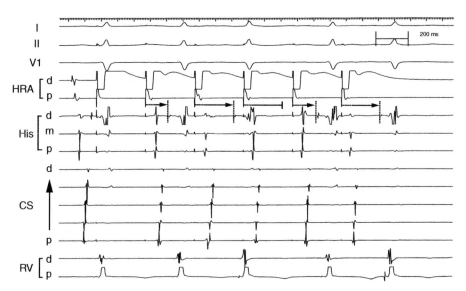

Figure 1.9 More rapid atrial pacing leads to AV Wenckebach behavior. Pacing associated with gradual prolongation of the AH interval is observed until a dropped "H" and QRS complex. This response is characteristic of block within the AV node.

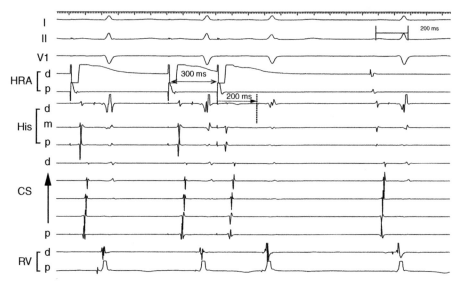

Figure 1.10 After a basic cycle length of 600 ms, a premature atrial stimulus at a coupling interval of 300 ms, the AH interval prolongs to 200 ms because of delayed conduction in the AV node.

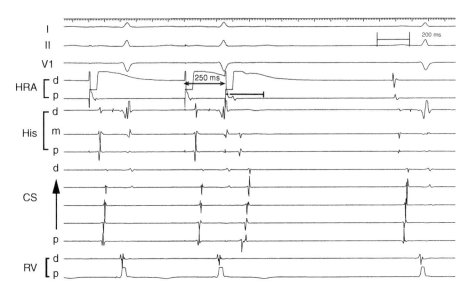

Figure 1.11 Continuation of Figure 1.10. When the coupling interval is shortened to 250 ms, the atrial electrogram is not followed by a His bundle signal and QRS complex due to block in the AV node. The coupling interval of the two atrial electrograms recorded on the His catheter (270 ms) defines the AV node effective refractory period (AVNERP).

from the HRA at a basic cycle length of 600 ms, a premature extrastimulus at a coupling interval of 300 ms is delivered. In response to this premature atrial stimulus, there is prolongation of the AH interval due to delay within the AV node. In Figure 1.11, when the coupling interval is shortened to 250 ms, an atrial electrogram is observed, but there is no subsequent His bundle recording and QRS because of block in the AV node. The AV node effective refractory period (AVNERP) would be defined as 250 ms (usually measured as the interval between atrial signals in the His catheter).

Sometimes, atrial pacing will induce an arrhythmia of interest. Initiation of different arrhythmias with atrial pacing will be described in detail in later chapters.

Baseline ventricular pacing

Just as in atrial pacing, ventricular pacing is performed by pacing at shorter and shorter cycle lengths and assessing retrograde VA conduction (ventricular overdrive pacing) or by delivering earlier premature ventricular beats (premature ventricular stimulation). In Figure 1.12, baseline ventricular pacing at a cycle length of 500 ms is not associated with VA conduction.

The atria continue to be depolarized by the sinus node with first atrial activation recorded in the HRA. Figure 1.13 shows the response to ventricular pacing in the setting of sympathetic activation with isoproterenol. Isoproterenol is a synthetic amine related to epinephrine but exclusively acts on beta-receptors causing both an increase in heart rate (β1 receptors) and hypotension (β2 receptors). It is generally started as an intravenous infusion at 0.5–1 mcg/min and titrated up until the desired clinical effect is achieved (generally initiation of sustained tachycardia – usually 2–5 mcg/min). Isoproterenol is useful in the electrophysiology laboratory because of its rapid onset of action and short half-life (<1.5 min). In this case, low-dose isoproterenol infusion improves VA conduction, and now stable VA conduction is observed. VA conduction can be identified by a change in the pattern of atrial depolarization and an increase in the atrial rate to the paced ventricular rate (450 ms). The typical response to ventricular premature stimulation is shown in Figure 1.14. In this case, after pacing at a basic cycle length of 400 ms (notice the 1:1 VA conduction since the patient is on isoproterenol), a premature ventricular stimulus at a coupling interval of 200 ms is associated with a delay in VA conduction. Prolongation of VA conduction can be due to delay in intraventricular conduction, the bundle branches, the

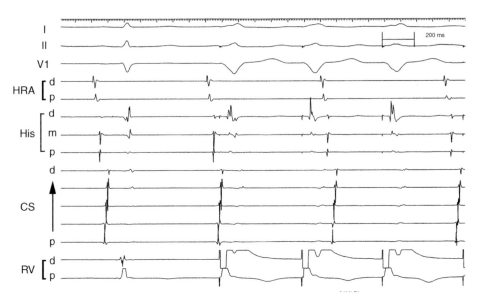

Figure 1.12 Baseline ventricular pacing is not associated with VA conduction. Notice the pattern of atrial depolarization remains "high-low" with first atrial depolarization noted in the HRA.

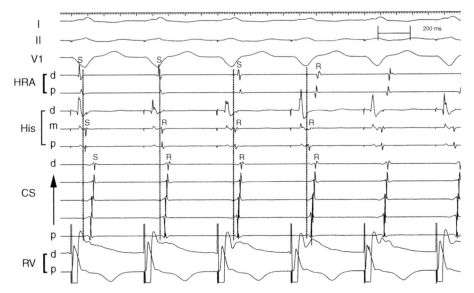

Figure 1.13 Continuation of Figure 1.12. Infusion of isoproterenol and sympathetic activation facilitates development of VA conduction. Notice that in response to the pacing stimulus, the pattern of atrial depolarization switches from "high-low" to "low-high" due to retrograde VA conduction via the AV node. The atrial rate now increases to the ventricular paced rate. Notice the subtle changes in the timing of atrial depolarization as activation progressively switches from being "sinus node driven" (S) to "AV node driven" (R). Although one could quibble about whether atrial activation recorded in the His bundle region (S*) for the first paced beat is actually from retrograde activation, it is likely from the sinus node, as the coronary sinus depolarization remains relatively late. Similarly, one could argue whether coronary sinus depolarization from the third paced beat is actually due to depolarization from the sinus node, but it is likely due to retrograde depolarization because of the shortened interval between atrial depolarization recorded in the His bundle and the proximal coronary sinus. It is instructive to note that as a separate but important point, the pattern of coronary sinus depolarization (from proximal to distal) is the same in this case regardless of whether atrial depolarization is "sinus node driven" or "AV node driven."

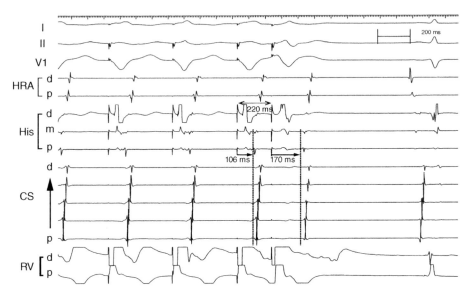

Figure 1.14 Normal retrograde AV node response to ventricular extrastimulation. A ventricular extrastimulus at a coupling interval of 220 ms is associated with prolongation of the stimulus to atrium interval from 106 to 170 ms. Earliest atrial activation is still observed in the His bundle catheter. This response is consistent with delayed retrograde conduction in the AV node.

His bundle, or in the AV node. Although a retrograde His bundle can often be difficult to identify, the absence of an identifiable His bundle suggests that most of the VA conduction delay is due to delay in the AV node. Just as in atrial pacing, ventricular pacing may lead to induction of arrhythmias.

Electrograms during tachycardia

The most common reason for patients to be referred for electrophysiologic testing is for the evaluation (and possibly definitive treatment) of tachycardia. Once the baseline electrophysiologic characteristics for a patient have been determined, pacing is generally performed in hopes of inducing the patient's clinical tachycardia. If the clinical tachycardia can be induced, the tachycardia can be studied and the critical anatomic components can be defined with a sense for the critical tissues involved.

When tachycardia is induced, the electrophysiology study can help define the relationship between atrial and ventricular electrograms. For example, if there are more atrial signals than ventricular signals, then an atrial tachycardia driving ventricular activation is the most likely possibility. Conversely, if there are more ventricular signals than atrial signals, ventricular

tachycardia becomes the likely diagnosis. In fact, the greatest benefit of intracardiac electrograms is definitive information on the timing of atrial depolarization. Remember that the most difficult thing about analyzing the ECG of a patient in tachycardia is identifying the P waves that are often obscured by the QRS complexes or the T waves.

In patients with supraventricular tachycardia, ventricular activation is normal, so generally evaluation of a supraventricular tachycardia initially focuses on the timing and pattern of atrial activation (Figures 1.15–1.17 and Table 1.1). Generally, supraventricular tachycardias are classified first by the relative number of atrial and ventricular electrograms. If there are more atrial electrograms than ventricular electrograms, it is likely that atrial activation is "driving" ventricular activation and increases the likelihood that an atrial tachycardia is present. If there are more ventricular electrograms than atrial electrograms during a supraventricular tachycardia, both atrial tachycardia and accessory pathway-mediated tachycardia are very unlikely and essentially rules in a tachycardia focus from the junctional region. When a 1:1 relationship between atrial electrograms and ventricular electrograms is present, any of the three anatomic types of tachycardia may be present, and the clinician must focus on the timing

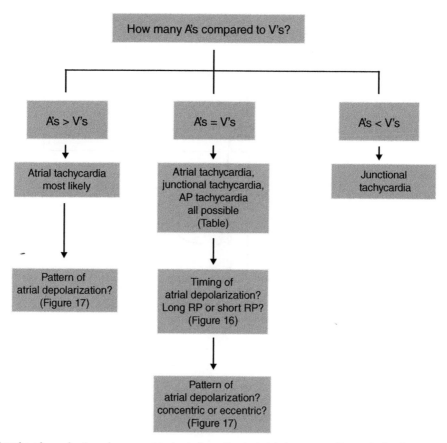

Figure 1.15 Flowchart for evaluation of supraventricular tachycardia. A: Atrial electrogram; V: ventricular electrogram.

between atrial activation and ventricular activation and the pattern of atrial activation. Firstly, the timing of atrial activation and ventricular activation is assessed: is atrial activation present in the first half of the interval between QRS complexes ("short RP" tachycardia) or in the second half of the interval between QRS complexes ("long-RP" tachycardia)? The likely causes of tachycardia vary by the relationship between ventricular and atrial activation, although this can be difficult (Figure 1.16). In addition to the timing of atrial activation, the direction of atrial activation is evaluated (Figure 1.17). The direction of atrial activation can be evaluated in the plane of the tricuspid and mitral valves (left to right, right to left, or from the center outward) and the perpendicular plane – anterior to posterior or posterior to anterior. In supraventricular tachycardia, it is important to decide whether retrograde activation is present – in other words, is it likely that ventricular

depolarization "drives" atrial depolarization? If atrial activation is high-low, then the ventricles are generally not responsible for atrial depolarization. When atrial depolarization appears to be coming from the mitral or tricuspid annulus, atrial depolarization is further classified as "concentric" or beginning from the septum and extending to the left and right (and thus the AV node could be responsible for retrograde activation), or "eccentric," where initial atrial activation is identified more laterally away from the septum in either the left or the right atria.

The tachycardia can be carefully evaluated to determine whether changes in the atrial cycle lengths precede and predict those in the AV node or His bundle cycle lengths (making atrial tachycardia more likely), or whether AV node conduction is essential for continuation of tachycardia (AV node dependent), which would "rule out" atrial tachycadia.

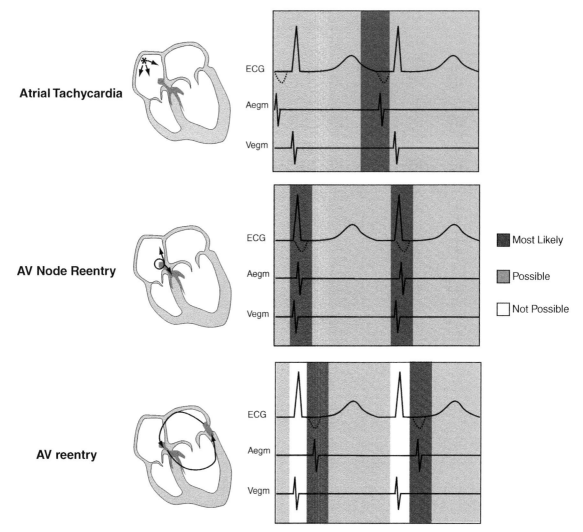

Figure 1.16 Usual relationship between atrial and ventricular depolarization in patients with supraventricular tachycardia and 1:1 atrial and ventricular relationships. However, many exceptions exist and will be explored throughout the first portion of the book.

Pacing during tachycardia

Once a tachycardia is induced, after initial inspection of the electrograms (and confirmation of hemodynamic stability!), the electrophysiologist can study the response of the tachycardia to different stimuli.

For example, as we have covered, in a patient with supraventricular tachycardia, there are only three basic anatomic possibilities: atrial tachycardia, junctional tachycardia, and tachycardias that use an accessory pathway. Once a supraventricular tachycardia is induced and the patient is stable, the best course of action is delivery of ventricular stimuli (either single, double, or as a pacing train). Regardless of how ventricular stimuli are delivered, the stimuli are most likely to interact with a tachycardia using an accessory pathway, less likely with a tachycardia within the junction, and least likely with an atrial tachycardia (Figure 1.18).

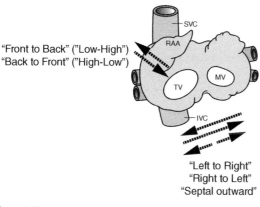

"Front to Back" ("Low-High")
"Back to Front" ("High-Low")

"Left to Right"
"Right to Left"
"Septal outward"

Figure 1.17 Determining the direction of atrial activation during supraventricular tachycardia. The focus of investigation should be whether "High to Low" or "Low to High" and whether "Left to Right," "Right to Left," or "Septal Outward."

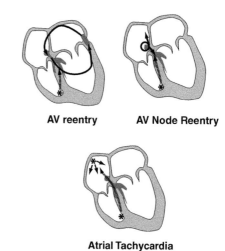

AV reentry   AV Node Reentry

Atrial Tachycardia

Figure 1.18 Schematic of the likelihood of a ventricular stimulus interacting with different types of supraventricular tachycardias. Because AV reentrant tachycardia (AVRT) using an AV accessory pathway encompasses such a large circuit, it is relatively easy for a ventricular stimulation to "get into" the circuit or interact with the tachycardia. At the other end of the spectrum, in atrial tachycardia, the reentrant circuit or focus is "guarded" by the bundle branches, His bundle, and AV node.

Understanding this graded response rate can help differentiate between these tachycardias. Although the response of the tachycardia to atrial pacing can also be evaluated, it is generally less helpful because it will interact "early" with both atrial tachycardias and accessory pathway-mediated tachycardias. Table 1.1 shows the general characteristics of the three different anatomic types of supraventricular tachycardia.

Table 1.1 Findings that are *generally* associated with the most common forms of specific supraventricular tachycardia types.

Tachycardia type	Characteristics
Atrial tachycardia	• "Long-RP" tachycardias (VA interval $> \frac{1}{2}$ RR) • Continuation of the tachycardia despite AV block (AV node independent) • Variable VA intervals • Requires very early V's to interact with the tachycardia (sometimes not at all)
AVNRT	• Very "short-RP" tachycardia (VA interval <65 ms) • Usually AV node dependent • Fixed VA intervals • Early V's can interact with the tachycardia
AVRT	• "Short-RP" tachycardia (VA interval >65 ms, but $< \frac{1}{2}$ RR) • AV node dependent • Fixed VA intervals • Late V's can interact with the circuit

AVNRT, AV node reentrant tachycardia; AVRT, AV reentrant tachycardia; RR, Interval between QRS complexes; VA, Ventriculoatrial; V, Ventricular stimulation.

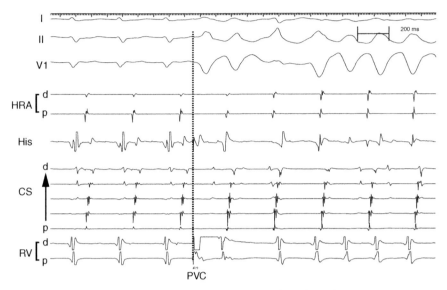

Figure 1.19 A premature ventricular stimulus delivered during supraventricular tachycardia initiates a wide complex tachycardia at a more rapid rate than the underlying tachycardia (which is unaffected by the PVC). Ventricular tachycardia can be identified immediately, because there are more QRS complexes than atrial activity during the stable wide QRS tachycardia (the last four QRS complexes).

Likewise, in patients with wide complex tachycardia, it becomes very important to distinguish between ventricular tachycardia and supraventricular tachycardia with aberrant conduction. In this case, pacing from the atrium is extremely helpful, because it will interact with the different types of supraventricular tachycardia before interacting with ventricular tachycardia. Obviously, if a wide complex tachycardia is induced, it is even more important to confirm that the patient is stable from a clinical standpoint before embarking on the electrophysiologic analysis of the arrhythmia.

Figure 1.19 emphasizes the importance of continuous evaluation of the patient during electrophysiology studies. In this case, the patient has supraventricular tachycardia, and timed premature ventricular stimuli are being delivered. Although generally safe in patients with structurally normal hearts, a premature ventricular stimulus delivered on the T wave results in the initiation of ventricular tachycardia.

KEY POINTS

- Anatomically, there are only four types of tachycardia.

- In an electrophysiology study, baseline conduction intervals are measured and pacing protocols are performed to evaluate the electrical characteristics of different cardiac tissues and to induce tachycardias.

- If a tachycardia is induced/observed during the evaluation, the response to pacing during tachycardia can help define the mechanism of the tachycardia.

- Generally, in patients with supraventricular tachycardia, response to ventricular pacing is most useful for determining the type of tachycardia present.

CHAPTER 2

Supraventricular tachycardia case 1

A 34-year-old woman was seen in the emergency room 2 weeks ago with a rapid heart rate. She was treated with adenosine with conversion to sinus rhythm and was started on a beta-blocker (metoprolol 25 mg twice daily). She has not had any recurrent episodes but notes some tiredness since she was started on the medication. Her past medical history is unremarkable, and her physical examination is normal. Her ECG during tachycardia and her baseline ECG are shown in Figure 2.1. What is her prognosis and next steps?

Whenever possible, it is extremely useful to compare tachycardia and baseline ECGs. Subtle differences in the ST segment, T wave, and QRS complex can represent atrial activity and provide an important clue for the underlying mechanism of tachycardia. In this case, during tachycardia, the terminal positive deflection in the QRS complex in lead V1 is not present in sinus rhythm and probably represents a P wave. As reviewed in Figure 1.16, this P wave location is most consistent with AV node reentrant tachycardia (AVNRT) due to near-simultaneous activation of the atria and ventricles. Evaluation of the QRS complex shows no evidence of preexcitation (which will be reviewed more extensively in subsequent chapters) that would signal the presence of an atrioventricular (AV) accessory pathway.

Given the different underlying mechanisms, it is not surprising that the natural history of supraventricular without preexcitation is varied. In addition, even patients with the same arrhythmia mechanism can have very different clinical courses. For example, some patients with documented AVNRT will have frequent recurrent arrhythmias, while others have only rare and infrequent episodes. The decision on treatment options should account for the fact that the supraventricular tachycardia (SVT), although sometimes uncomfortable, is not life-threatening. However, it is important to acknowledge that some patients with SVT can have significant reduction in quality-of-life when compared to age-matched controls.

Case (continued): after a discussion about the diagnosis and management of SVT (and probable AVNRT), she is taught vagal maneuvers and her beta-blockers are stopped. She does well off beta-blockade for several years but returns to your office after a recent episode that required an emergency room visit when vagal maneuvers performed at home failed to terminate the tachycardia. She notes that over the last year she has short episodes of rapid heart rate every month, and once every 2–3 months, she has a longer episode that she can generally terminate with a Valsalva maneuver.

At this point, the patient is having more frequent episodes, and it is reasonable to consider electrophysiologic testing and possible catheter ablation. As in the initial discussion, a frank discussion of the treatment options and associated risks and benefits is required. Fortunately, the success rate of ablation for SVT is extremely high (>95%) and the risk of severe complications is low, probably <1%. The current accepted guidelines for catheter ablation of SVT are listed in Table A7 of the Appendix. Given her continued episodes of tachycardia, the patient chooses to undergo electrophysiologic testing with ablation if appropriate.

There are many strategies to electrophysiology studies, and specific issues such as number and location of venous access sites and number and type of catheters placed will vary by likely diagnosis, operator preference, and institution. The catheter position and type used at Mayo Clinic Florida vary and are summarized in the Table A2 of Appendix. For SVT, generally four catheters are reasonable, with two catheters in the right femoral vein and two catheters in the left femoral

Understanding Intracardiac EGMs: A Patient Centered Guide, First Edition. Fred Kusumoto.
© 2015 John Wiley & Sons, Ltd. Published 2015 by John Wiley & Sons, Ltd.

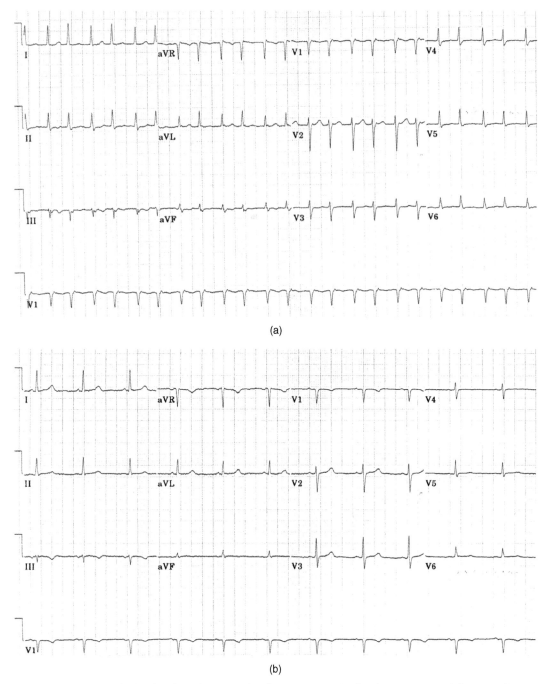

(a)

(b)

Figure 2.1 ECG in SVT (a) and at baseline (b). When comparing the two ECGs, notice that there is a positive deflection in the terminal portion of the QRS complex in lead V1 that is present during SVT but not during sinus rhythm. This deflection probably represents atrial depolarization, and this position for atrial depolarization is most commonly associated with AVNRT in a patient with paroxysmal SVT that is responsive to adenosine or a vagal maneuver.

vein. Although venous access from the internal jugular vein allows relatively easy cannulation of the coronary sinus, given the advent of steerable catheters and the discomfort and the small risk of pneumothorax associated with central venous access via either the internal jugular vein or the subclavian vein, I abandoned this approach over a decade ago. However, given the ease of cannulation of the coronary sinus, the right internal jugular vein remains a reasonable venous access point and is still used by many operators.

At baseline, a decapolar catheter is placed in the coronary sinus, and quadripolar catheters are positioned in the high right atrium (HRA) (generally at the SVC-RA junction), straddling the tricuspid valve between the right atrium and right ventricle for His bundle recording and in the right ventricle (Figure 1.3). Certainly, some operators will put catheters with more electrodes in the His bundle region that allows for evaluation of multiple components of the His bundle and the right bundle potential and has the added benefit of allowing ventricular pacing (thus obviating the need for a fourth venous access point). Again, there are multiple clinically reasonable approaches, but it is important for individual operators to continuously evaluate their practice and decide what approach provides the best combination of efficiency and quality.

Evaluation of baseline electrograms

Baseline electrograms for our patient are shown in Figure 2.2. Evaluation of the baseline activation focuses on the pattern of atrial and ventricular depolarization and AV conduction. In this case, atrial activation is normal (from the right atrium to the left atrium as recorded by the coronary sinus) and from superior to inferior. Ventricular depolarization occurs normally, and the QRS is of normal duration and morphology. AV conduction is occurring with a 1:1 relationship, and the AH and HV intervals are normal. In a patient with SVT, the baseline electrograms can suggest the presence of an accessory pathway if the HV interval is short and/or the QRS has abnormal morphology (see Chapters 7 and 8 for a discussion of preexcitation).

Pacing protocols

For all SVT cases, my preference is to sequentially perform atrial overdrive pacing, atrial extrastimuli, ventricular overdrive pacing, and ventricular extrastimuli. For every case in a patient with an unknown type of SVT, I perform all four components in the same order. By taking a systematic approach to all studies,

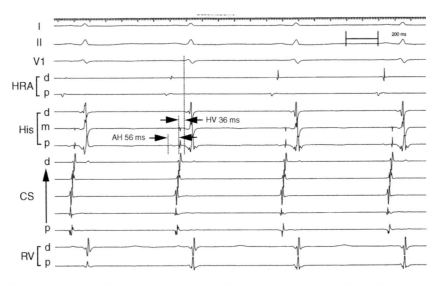

Figure 2.2 Baseline electrograms. Atrial depolarization is normal with first atrial signal observed in the HRA and the last atrial signal observed in the coronary sinus. The QRS width is normal (70 ms) and has a normal frontal axis with a monophasic R wave in lead II. AV conduction is normal with an AH interval of 56 ms and an HV interval of 36 ms.

it is less likely that an essential component of the electrophysiology study will be forgotten in "the heat of battle." Although it is reasonable to start with ventricular pacing to evaluate for initial eccentric activation suggestive of an accessory pathway, I prefer to perform atrial pacing protocols first, so that I don't get overly excited about identifying the presence of an accessory pathway that could "color" my judgment later.

For our case, atrial pacing is shown in Figures 2.3 and 2.4. When pacing from the atria, the clinician must assess atrial capture, intraatrial conduction, and AV conduction. In Figure 2.3, with pacing at 500 ms, every pacing stimulus is associated with an atrial electrogram and every atrial electrogram is associated with a ventricular electrogram; thus every atrial stimulus captures atrial tissue and every atrial depolarization leads to ventricular depolarization. Notice that compared to baseline, the interval between atrial and ventricular activity remains similar and that AV conduction can be assessed by evaluating the interval between the atrial signal and the His bundle signal and between the His bundle and the ventricular activation. As shown in Chapter 1, for most patients, progressive shortening of

the pacing cycle length leads to prolongation of the AH interval due to slower conduction within the AV node. However, in this case, AH lengthening is not observed, and instead more rapid atrial pacing results in loss of atrial capture (Figure 2.4).

Once atrial overdrive pacing is performed, then atrial extrasimuli are given. In this case, a drive train of atrial stimuli are given at a constant drive cycle length, and an atrial premature stimulus is delivered at progressively shorter coupling intervals (Figures 2.5 and 2.6). With shortening of the coupling interval, an atrial stimulus does not lead to capture of atrial tissue due to atrial refractoriness. This interval defines the atrial refractory period or AERP. A full discussion of refractory periods can be found in Chapter 3 of Understanding ECGs and EGMs. However, for our case, as we "run into AERP," the electrophysiologic properties of the AV node have not been fully tested, because we have been unable to define the AV node effective refractory period. In order to overcome atrial refractoriness to test the electrophysiologic properties of the AV node, the clinician has several options. First, the output of the pacing stimulus can be increased, second, the catheter

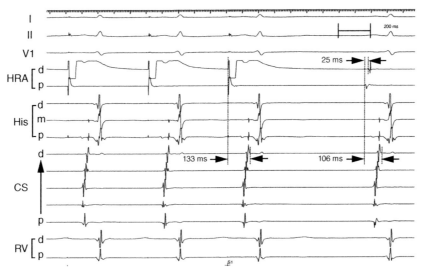

Figure 2.3 Atrial pacing at a cycle length of 500 ms. Notice the interatrial delay by comparing the interval between the pacing stimulus and the distal coronary sinus electrogram (140 ms) to sinus rhythm (109 ms). This delay is not due to intrinsic atrial conduction slowing but rather is because of the position of the high right atrial catheter within the right atrial appendage. Notice that adding the sum of the interval measured from proximal to distal electrodes in the HRA catheter almost fully accounts for the interatrial conduction delay observed during pacing. As an aside, this is the reason that generally the Asense–Vpace interval is programmed to shorter intervals than the Apace–Vpace interval in dual chamber pacing. Importantly, the AV relationship remains 1:1, and the AH interval remains essentially unchanged.

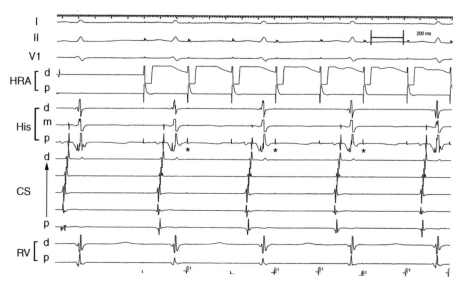

Figure 2.4 With shortening of the atrial pacing cycle length, every other atrial stimulus (*) fails to depolarize the atria. Loss of atrial capture is most easily seen in the coronary sinus electrograms.

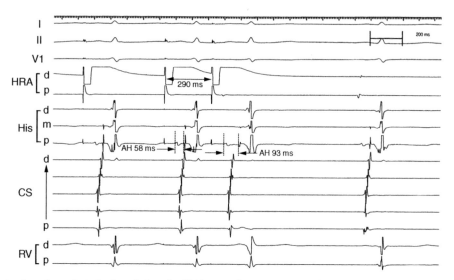

Figure 2.5 Pacing is performed at a basic cycle length of 500 ms, and a premature atrial stimulus is delivered at a coupling interval of 290 ms. In response to the premature atrial stimulus, the AH is slightly more prolonged (93 ms) when compared to sinus rhythm (58 ms) due to normal decremental conduction properties of the AV node.

can be repositioned, hopefully to an atrial site that might have a shorter AERP, third, use isoproterenol to shorten the atrial refractoriness, fourthly, pace at a faster base cycle length (because atrial refractoriness is dependent on the preceding cycle lengths), or, fifth, deliver double extrastimuli (the first extrastimulus is

used as a "conditioning" impulse to shorten the atrial refractoriness).

Of these options, it is reasonable to first confirm stable catheter position by fluoroscopy. If catheter position is stable, I will generally proceed to double extrastimuli to avoid changing electrophysiologic properties by the

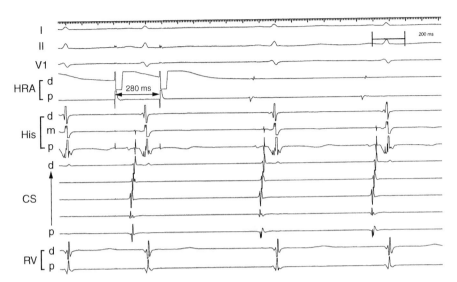

Figure 2.6 Continuation of Figure 2.5. When the coupling interval is shortened by 10–280 ms, there is loss of atrial capture because of atrial refractoriness (AERP or atrial effective refractory period).

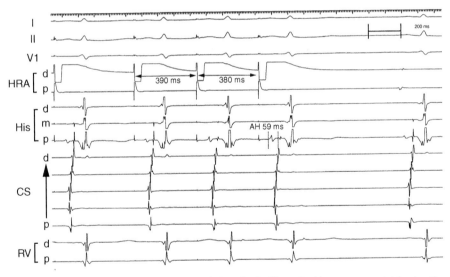

Figure 2.7 Double atrial extrastimuli. With a basic pacing cycle length of 500 ms, double premature atrial extrastimuli at coupling intervals of 390 ms and 380 ms is associated with an AH interval of 59 ms.

use of isoproterenol. To perform double extrastimuli, the first extrastimulus is delivered at an intermediate coupling interval and the second extrastimulus is delivered at a slightly shorter coupling interval (Figures 2.7–2.10). The coupling interval for the second extrastimulus is progressively shortened until AERP is reached, and then the coupling interval for the first extrastimulus is shortened. In Figure 2.7, the basic cycle

length remains 500 ms, and two extrastimuli at coupling intervals of 390 and 380 ms are delivered. The coupling interval of the second extrastimulus is progressively shortened, and gradual prolongation of the AH interval is observed (Figure 2.8). When the second extrastimulus does not result in atrial capture, it is shortened, and although operators will vary on exact steps, after shortening the first extrastimulus by 10 ms, the second

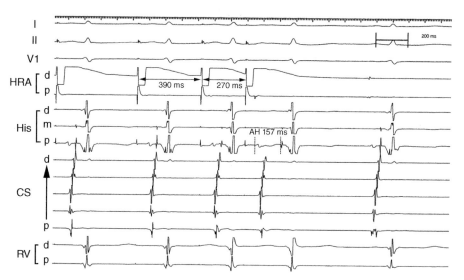

Figure 2.8 Double atrial extrastimuli. Continuing from Figure 2.7, the coupling interval of the second extrastimulus is progressively shortened, and progressive AH interval prolongation is observed. When the coupling interval of the second extrastimulus has been shortened to 270 ms, the AH interval has prolonged to 157 ms. When the coupling interval is further shortened to 260 ms, loss of atrial caprure is observed (not shown).

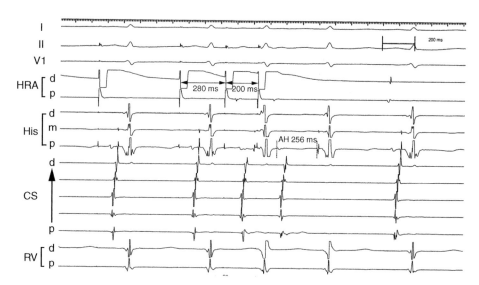

Figure 2.9 Double extrastimuli. Continuing from Figure 2.8, the coupling interval of both the first and the second extrastimuli are shortened, and at coupling intervals of 280 and 200 ms, the AH interval is 256 ms.

extrastimulus is further shortened until AERP is again reached. At this point, the first extrastimulus is shortened by 10 ms, and the entire process is repeated again and the second extrastimulus is shortened until AERP. In our patient, at coupling intervals of 280 and 200 ms, the AH interval has been gradually prolonging and is currently 256 ms (Figure 2.9), and further shortening of either the first or the second extrastimulus leads to loss of atrial capture (Figure 2.10) again precluding full evaluation of the AV node.

The most common cause of adenosine responsive paroxysmal SVT is AVNRT where a localized reentrant

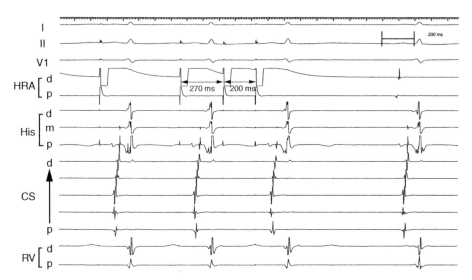

Figure 2.10 Double extrastimuli. Continuing from Figure 2.8, when the coupling interval of the first extrastimulus is shortened further to 270 ms, atrial capture does not occur.

circuit can develop in the AV node and adjacent atrial tissues due to functional separation of two or more "pathways." In many patients with AVNRT, a sudden change in the AH interval will be observed with a small decrease in the coupling interval. This change is due to a sudden shift in the anterograde conduction from a rapidly conducting pathway or input into the AV node to a slower conducting pathway. Generally, the refractory period of the fast conducting pathway is longer than that of the slowly conducting pathway, and a "jump" has been arbitrarily defined as a 50-ms increase in conduction time with a 10-ms decrease in the coupling interval. Obviously, whether a "jump" will be observed depends on the electrophysiologic properties of the AV node. In our patient, there has been prolongation of the AH interval with double extrastimuli but no "jump" using the conventional definition, although we still have yet to truly test the AV node refractoriness. Although further evaluation of the baseline anterograde properties of the AV node could be explored with triple extrastimuli or stimuli from other atrial tissue (such as the coronary sinus), at this point, it is reasonable to evaluate retrograde conduction before returning to further evaluation of anterograde conduction (which may require the use of isoproterenol to shorten the AERP effectively).

Figure 2.11 shows baseline ventricular pacing at a cycle length of 500 ms. One-to-one retrograde conduction is present with earliest atrial activation observed in the midcoronary sinus. Ventricular pacing at a faster cycle length leads to retrograde block first with gradual prolongation of the ventriculoatrial (VA) conduction time and block until stable 2:1 block (Figure 2.12). Ventricular premature stimulation demonstrates that the retrograde conduction pathway has decremental properties with gradual ventriculoatrial conduction with earlier coupling intervals (Figure 2.13). As premature ventricular stimuli are given at shorter coupling intervals, the ventricular effective refractory period (VERP) is reached (Figure 2.14).

Initiation of tachycardia and evaluation

After baseline pacing maneuvers, we are left with no evidence of abnormal electrophysiologic properties either in atrial or ventricular tissues or in AV or VA conduction, but we have not been able to fully test either anterograde or retrograde AV conduction properties because of prolonged AERPs and VERPs. At this juncture, it is critical to induce the clinically relevant

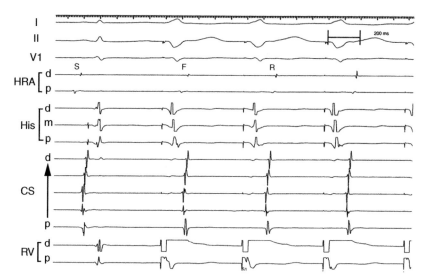

Figure 2.11 Ventricular pacing at a constant cycle length of 500 ms. The astute reader will notice that there are three forms of atrial depolarization: from sinus node activation (S), from retrograde activation via the AV node (R), and a fusion beat (F) where the coronary sinus atrial electrograms are due to retrograde conduction, and the HRA electrograms from the sinus node.

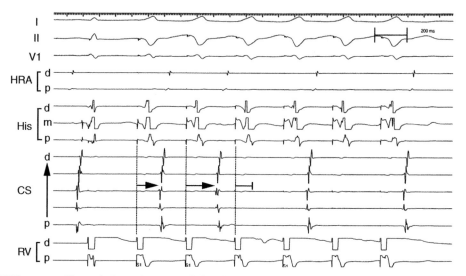

Figure 2.12 With more rapid ventricular pacing at a cycle length of 350 ms, retrograde activation via the AV node initially exhibits Wenckebach behavior with gradual prolongation of the V-A interval and subsequent block and then later develops 2:1 retrograde block.

sustained tachycardia. The first step that is generally used is to begin infusion with the beta-agonist isoproterenol. Isoproterenol is helpful because it shortens the refractoriness of tissues and, in particular, differential tissue effects on the electrophysiologic properties can facilitate induction of sustained arrhythmias. This is often particularly important in AVNRT. In patients with AV reentrant tachycardia (AVRT), the two parallel pathways are anatomically discrete entities (the accessory pathway and the AV node) that usually have

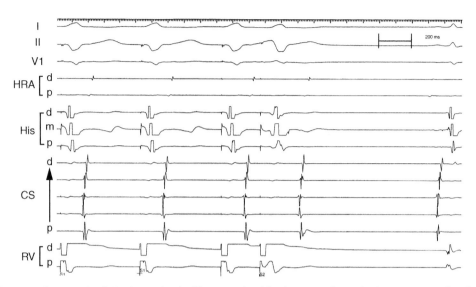

Figure 2.13 Ventricular extrastimulation is associated with progressive delay in retrograde conduction, suggesting that this pathway has decremental conduction properties and because depolarization is midline, likely represents retrograde conduction via the AV node.

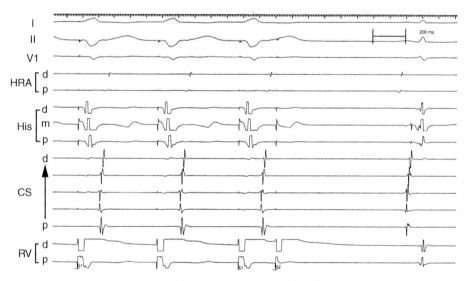

Figure 2.14 Earlier ventricular stimulation again leads to VERP (a pacing stimulus without ventricular capture).

very different properties (accessory pathways usually conduct rapidly and the AV node has slow conduction). For AVNRT, recent work by Effimov and colleagues has shown the existence of discrete compartments within the AV node that could facilitate the development of reentry, but often the pathways must be "functionally separated," often with the use of a drug such as isoproterenol.

With isoproterenol started, pacing maneuvers are again performed. Another option to facilitate arrhythmia induction is to pace from different regions of the atria. In some cases, tachycardia will be more easily induced from a left atrial site (by pacing the coronary sinus) when compared to pacing from the right atrium. Finally, pacing from the coronary sinus at a cycle length of 250 ms leads to initiation of tachycardia with a cycle

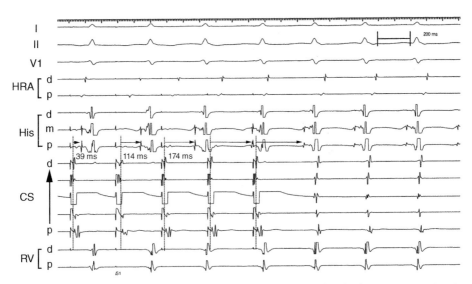

Figure 2.15 Rapid pacing from the coronary sinus initiates tachycardia with a cycle length of 275 ms. Notice that the tachycardia initiation is associated with a series of dramatic increases in the AH interval. Once tachycardia is initiated, the ECG and electrograms show almost simultaneous depolarization of the atria and the ventricles. This finding cannot be associated with AVRT using an accessory pathway. In addition, with the initiation of tachycardia, the HA interval remains constant despite changes in the cycle length, thus making AVNRT a much more likely diagnosis than atrial tachycardia.

length of 275 ms (Figure 2.15). Careful inspection of the electrograms during initiation shows relatively sudden increases in the AH interval. Although not a "jump" as defined by conventional terms, sudden changes in AH interval before initiation of tachycardia should arouse suspicion that AVNRT is the likely diagnosis.

Once tachycardia is initiated, there are several findings identified either during the tachycardia, at spontaneous termination, or during ventricular stimulation that can help differentiate between different tachycardia mechanisms (Table 2.1). It is interesting to note that there are no specific criteria that "rule in" the diagnosis of AVNRT. Unfortunately, as shown in Table 2.2, there are far fewer findings that are "definitive" for a specific diagnosis. I acknowledge that one can argue on the threshold of "definitive" and that for any finding exceptions can exist (as will be shown in later cases). Once SVT has been initiated, a flowsheet for the general evaluation is shown in Figure 2.16.

Initial inspection of the ECG and electrograms during tachycardia shows that atrial activation and ventricular activation occur almost simultaneously with a VA interval of 15 ms and an HA interval of 52 ms. Atrial activity in the coronary sinus electrograms is earliest

in the mid-portion and right atrial activation is "late." Atrial electrograms cannot be specifically identified in the His bundle catheter. The short VA interval rules out an orthodromic reciprocating tachycardia using an AV accessory pathway, because in this tachycardia, obligatory ventricular activation (and thus sequential ventricular and atrial contraction) leads to temporally separate atrial and ventricular activation. It is generally accepted that a VA interval of <65 ms (measured from the beginning of the QRS complex to the earliest atrial electrogram) rules out retrograde conduction via an accessory pathway. Another way to consider this is to compare the HA interval during tachycardia and the VA interval during pacing (as the His bundle signal is often difficult to identify during ventricular pacing). In AVNRT, as the HA interval is not a true interval (because anterograde activation via the His bundle is occurring at the same time as retrograde activation is occurring via the "fast" pathway; Figure 2.17), the HA interval will be significantly shorter than the VA interval (usually >50 ms). In contrast, in AVRT, as there is sequential activation of the His bundle, ventricular tissue, and the accessory pathway, the HA will usually be longer than the VA interval (see Figures 4.12 and 4.13).

Table 2.1 Observations that provide clues for the diagnosis of SVT.

	Observation		
	During tachycardia	**Termination**	**During ventricular stimulation**
"Rules in" atrial tachycardia	• Variability of VA intervals during tachycardia	?	• V-A-A-V response to ventricular pacing*§

"Rules out" atrial tachycardia	• V-A intervals are linked despite changes in cycle length	• Spontaneous termination with an atrial signal in the absence of preceding AV block	• PVC response
			  ○ PVC terminates the tachycardia without resetting the atrium
			  ○ PVC resets the tachycardia with atrial delay
			• V-A-V response to ventricular pacing*§

"Rules in" AVRT	• Tachycardia cycle length changes with bundle branch block	?	• PVC on His
			  ○ His refractory PVC terminates the tachycardia
			  ○ His refractory PVC resets the atrial signal with the same atrial activation pattern (either earlier or later)

"Rules out" AVRT	• Tachycardia continues despite AV block† • Very short HA interval or VA interval‡ • Variability of VA intervals during tachycardia	?	• V-A-A-V response to ventricular pacing*§
"Rules in" AVNRT	?	?	?
"Rules out" AVNRT	• Variability of VA intervals during tachycardia • Eccentric atrial activation	?	• V-A-A-V response to ventricular pacing*§

PVC, premature ventricular complex.

*Ventricular capture and subsequent atrial depolarization.

†A tachycardia using a nodoventricular AP may continue despite the presence of AV block.

‡A tachycardia that uses an atrial-Hisian accessory pathway may have a very short VA or HA interval.

§There are several exceptions to the response to the Morady maneuver that are reviewed in Table 3.1.

At this point, from an anatomic and clinical perspective, the clinician must simply distinguish between an atrial tachycardia and AVNRT (Table 3.1). Of the catheters in place, earliest atrial activation is identified in electrode pair 5,6 of the coronary sinus catheter. Once stable catheter positions have been confirmed, the tachycardia could represent an atrial tachycardia from a left atrial site that is not being evaluated or AV node reentry in with earliest activation of the mid-portion of the coronary sinus (Figure 2.18). Although multiple techniques and electrophysiologic responses have been described, they all generally depend on determining whether the tachycardia is AV node dependent (thus "ruling out" an atrial tachycardia) or showing that the tachycardia is AV node independent (making AVNRT far less likely).

Several spontaneous findings confirm that the tachycardia is AV node independent and make atrial tachycardia far more likely. The most obvious is continuation of the tachycardia despite blocked AV conduction. However, this finding does not completely rule out AVNRT, because in some cases, the reentrant circuit in the AV nodal region involves more proximal tissue and AV block develops more distally (Figure 2.19). Another finding that suggests the tachycardia is AV node dependent is a fixed HA interval despite cycle length changes.

Table 2.2 *"Definitive"* Findings for Identifying the Mechanism of SVT.

	Observation
"Rules in" atrial tachycardia	• V-A-A-V response to ventricular pacing*

"Rules out" atrial tachycardia	• Spontaneous termination with an atrial signal in the absence of preceding AV block
	• V-A intervals are linked despite changes in cycle length
	• PVC response
	  ∘ PVC terminates the tachycardia without resetting the atrium
	  ∘ PVC resets the tachycardia with atrial delay
	• V-A-V response to ventricular pacing*

"Rules in" AVRT	• Tachycardia cycle length changes with bundle branch block
	• PVC on His
	  ∘ His refractory PVC terminates the tachycardia
	  ∘ His refractory PVC resets the atrial signal with the same atrial activation pattern (either earlier or later)

"Rules out" AVRT	• Tachycardia continues despite AV block† • Very short HA interval or VA interval‡
"Rules in" AVNRT	• ?
"Rules out" AVNRT	• ?

*Rare exceptions do exist.
†A tachycardia using a nodoventricular AP may continue despite the presence of AV block.
‡A tachycardia that uses an atrial-Hisian accessory pathway may have a very short VA or HA interval.

A fixed HA interval suggests that atrial depolarization is dependent on the preceding activation of the His bundle ("V drives the A"). In a patient with AVRT, this could represent retrograde conduction via an accessory pathway, but in this case where AVRT cannot be possible, a fixed HA implies the tachycardia is dependent on retrograde conduction via the AV node. An atrial tachycardia would "not care" about the preceding HA interval (the "A drives the V"). In our patient, the fixed HA interval at initiation of tachycardia, despite cycle length changes, makes AVNRT much more likely than atrial tachycardia (Figure 2.15). Finally, a less intuitive sign of AV node dependence is spontaneous termination of the tachycardia with an atrial electrogram. In a patient with an atrial tachycardia, AV conduction

follows passively, and if the atrial tachycardia were to spontaneously stop, it would be followed by a ventricular signal if the tachycardia is characterized by a 1:1 atrial–ventricular relationship. Tachycardia ending on an atrial electrogram suggests that termination was due to block in anterograde conduction within the AV node (Figure 2.20). Unfortunately, in our case, the tachycardia terminates spontaneously with a ventricular signal (Figure 2.21). This type of termination could occur with either atrial tachycardia or AVNRT.

To further evaluate between the two possibilities, tachycardia must be reinduced and studied by observing the behavior of the tachycardia to ventricular stimulation. Recall from Chapter 1 that in the setting of a SVT, ventricular stimulation will generally first interact with an AVRT, then AVNRT, and finally an atrial tachycardia. In addition, ventricular stimulation can be used to cause block in the AV node and prove AV node dependence of a tachycardia. Ventricular stimulation can be performed by delivering either a train of ventricular stimuli at a cycle length slightly shorter than the tachycardia cycle length or progressively premature ventricular stimuli (often referred to as "scanning diastole").

Tachycardia is reinduced, and, when compared to the original tachycardia, notice the subtle change in coronary sinus activation with the earliest signal identified in electrode pair 7, 8. This change does not represent a truly different atrial activation pattern and is a consequence of deeper placement of the catheter within the coronary sinus. In this case, scanning ventricular stimuli are chosen (Figures 2.22–2.24). Traditionally, longer coupling intervals are initially used so that the ventricular stimulus is delivered at the end of diastole. For example, in our case for a tachycardia with a cycle length of 275 ms, the first stimulus is delivered 260 ms after the prior QRS complex. The coupling interval of the stimulus is gradually shortened until the premature stimulus does not capture the ventricle (VERP). In this case, single premature ventricular stimuli do not interact with the tachycardia. This often occurs because of retrograde block in the right bundle and His bundle. To overcome refractoriness in these structures, double ventricular stimuli can be given (Figure 2.24). Double ventricular stimuli interact with the tachycardia, and shortening of the cycle length of the coronary sinus electrograms is noted. Even with the change in the cycle length, the HA interval remains constant, again providing evidence that the patient has AVNRT. Although

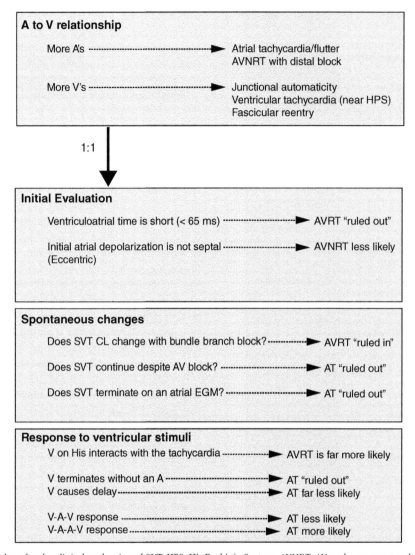

Figure 2.16 Flowsheet for the clinical evaluation of SVT. HPS, His Purkinje System; AVNRT, AV node reentrant tachycardia; AT, Atrial tachycardia; AVRT, AV reentrant tachycardia.

this finding provides supporting evidence for AVNRT, the most specific response would be termination of the tachycardia without resetting the atrium or without an atrial signal (Figure 2.25 and Figure 3.9), either of which confirms AV node dependence of the tachycardia and thus "rules out" atrial tachycardia. Another way to consider this concept is that the only way an atrial tachycardia can be terminated by a premature ventricular stimulus is if the ventricular stimulus produces early atrial depolarization.

Instead of delivering single or double extrastimuli at varying coupling intervals, another option is to pace the ventricle at a rate just faster than the tachycardia (Figure 2.26). Once the tachycardia has been entrained (usually identified by a shortening of the atrial to atrial cycle length from the tachycardia cycle length to the pacing cycle length), pacing is stopped and the subsequent response is evaluated. This technique is often called the "Morady Maneuver" named for Fred Morady from the University of Michigan where this

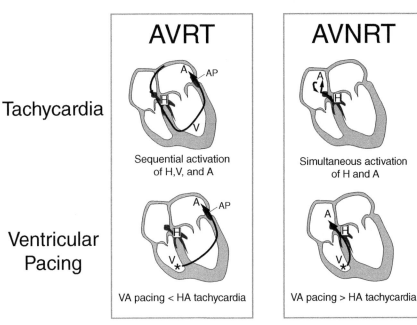

Figure 2.17 Schematic showing the differences between HA intervals during tachycardia and VA intervals during ventricular pacing for both AVNRT and AVRT.

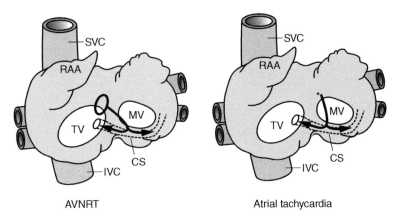

Figure 2.18 Schematic of possible tachycardia mechanisms. The near simultaneous ventricular and atrial depolarization "rules out" AVRT. As the earliest atrial signal is located in the midportion of the coronary sinus (CS), the tachycardia could represent AVNRT from a reentrant circuit within the atrial septal region, or an atrial tachycardia (*) somewhere within the left atrium (because right atrial depolarization is so late) with first-degree AV block.

technique was first described. When ventricular pacing is stopped, AVNRT will have a V-A-V response as shown in Figure 2.27 (from a different patient). In contrast, Figure 2.28 shows the response to a Morady maneuver in a patient with an atrial tachycardia arising near the coronary sinus os. In this case, ventricular pacing entrains the atrium (the A-A interval is equal to the pacing interval, but when pacing is stopped, an atrial signal is seen before the ventricular signal). This occurs because during ventricular pacing, retrograde conduction leads to atrial depolarization, and on cessation of pacing, an atrial signal is observed from the last paced beat, and continuation of atrial tachycardia leads to a second consecutive atrial signal.

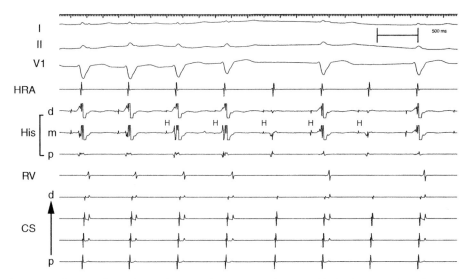

Figure 2.19 Electrograms from another patient with AVNRT that continues despite AV block. The patient has left bundle branch block (see lead V1) and a long HV interval. During AVNRT, tachycardia continues despite AV block because block is occurring distal to the His bundle (H).

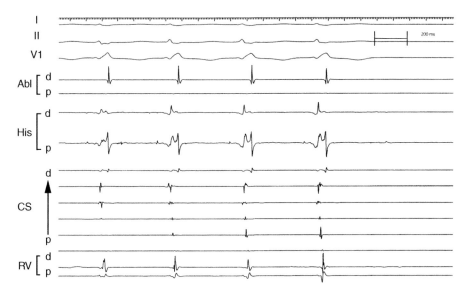

Figure 2.20 Electrograms from another patient with spontaneous termination of the tachycardia ending with an atrial electrogram. This termination implies the tachycardia is AV node dependent with anterograde block within the AV node and rules out atrial tachycardia.

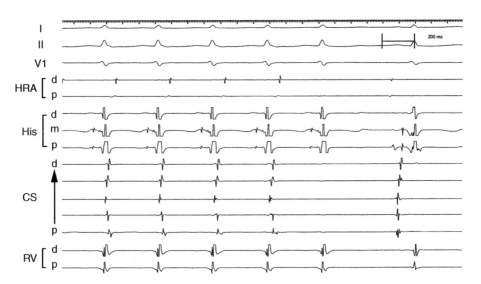

Figure 2.21 Termination of tachycardia in this patient ends on a ventricular signal. Before termination, both the AH and HA intervals remain constant. Termination could be due to either cessation of an atrial tachycardia (with passive AV conduction) or retrograde block in an AV node pathway in AVNRT.

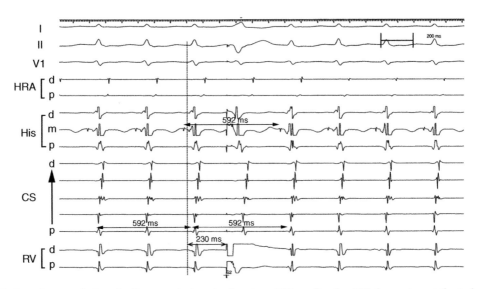

Figure 2.22 Scanning ventricular stimuli: a ventricular stimulus given 230 ms after the QRS does not reset the tachycardia (2 CL = 592 ms in all EGMs).

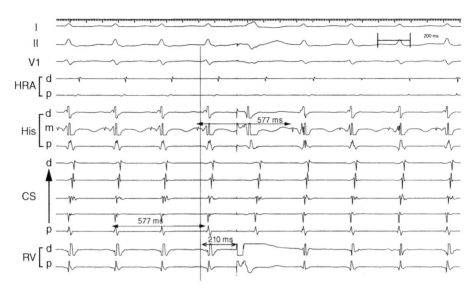

Figure 2.23 Continuation of scanning ventricular stimuli: a ventricular stimulus is given earlier (210 ms after the QRS) and the tachycardia is not reset. Notice that the tachycardia rate has increased slightly (2 CL = 577 ms).

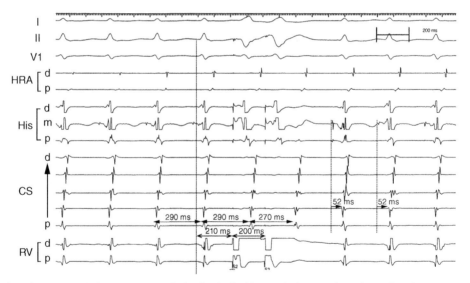

Figure 2.24 If single extrastimuli do not interact with the circuit, double ventricular stimuli can be used. In this case, two premature ventricular contractions at coupling intervals of 210 and 200 ms, the second premature ventricular stimulus shortens the interval between electrograms recorded from the proximal CS from 290 to 270 ms. Despite the change in the tachycardia interval, the HA interval remains constant (52 ms), making AVNRT the likely diagnosis.

In our patient, response to ventricular pacing is shown in Figure 2.29. Although the atria are not entrained by ventricular pacing, the tachycardia terminates without an atrial electrogram, confirming the presence of an AV node dependent tachycardia and "ruling out" atrial tachycardia. The response is similar to Figure 2.25 and shows that scanning ventricular stimuli and the Morady maneuver are "related" on a continuous spectrum. Scanning ventricular stimuli reset the tachycardia once, while the Morady maneuver represents repetitive resetting or entrainment of the tachycardia.

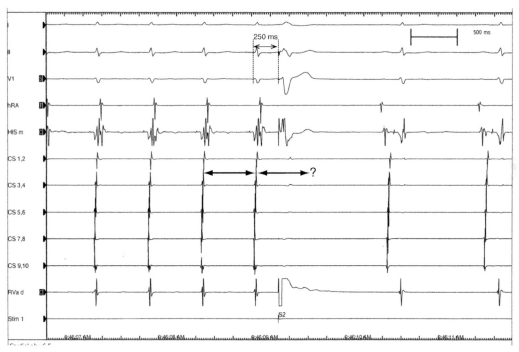

Figure 2.25 In another patient with AVNRT, a premature ventricular stimulus given 250 ms from the prior QRS terminates the tachycardia without an atrial electrogram, thus confirming the AV node dependence of the tachycardia.

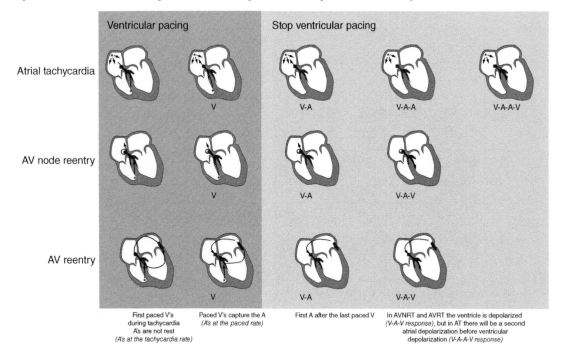

Figure 2.26 Schematic showing the electrophysiologic basis of the Morady maneuver. Ventricular pacing is performed at a rate faster than the tachycardia, and the tachycardia is entrained in the atrium when the atrial electrogram cycle length is equal to the paced cycle length. On cessation of pacing, the last atrial signal will lead to a subsequent ventricular signal (more accurately, a His bundle electrogram because there could be distal His block – but generally, a QRS complex is used, and it is referred to as a V-A-V response) in AVNRT, whereas in atrial tachycardia, the last entrained atrial electrogram will be followed by an atrial signal from the atrial tachycardia and then a ventricular signal (V-A-A-V response).

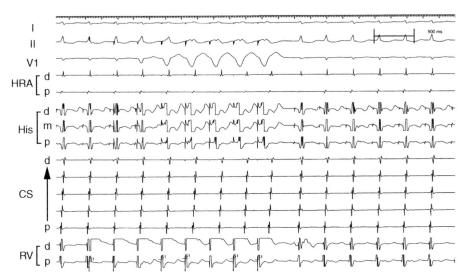

Figure 2.27 Morady maneuver from another patient with AVNRT showing a V-A-V response. Atrial capture is confirmed by shortening of the atrial electrogram cycle length to the paced cycle length. On cessation of pacing, a V-A-V response is observed.

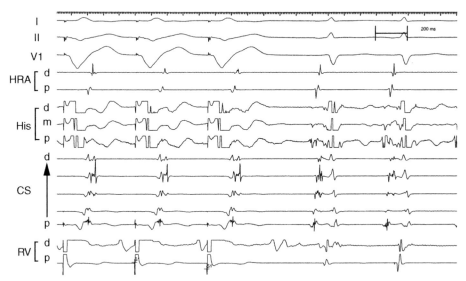

Figure 2.28 Morady maneuver in another patient with an atrial tachycardia near the coronary sinus os. With cessation of pacing, a V-A-A-V response diagnostic of an atrial tachycardia is observed.

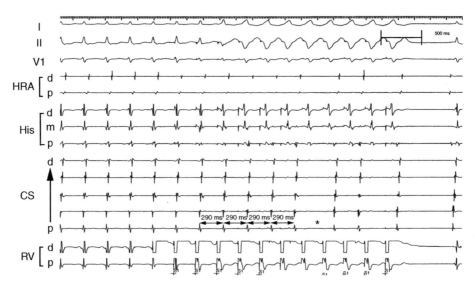

Figure 2.29 A Morady maneuver terminates the tachycardia but confirms the presence of an AV-node-dependent tachycardia because the tachycardia terminates without an early atrial electrogram (*). If the patient had an atrial tachycardia, the only way ventricular pacing could terminate the tachycardia would be by early atrial depolarization via retrograde AV node conduction.

Ablation of typical AVNRT

A discussion of the exact anatomy and pathophysiology of AVNRT is beyond the scope of this monograph, but it is generally thought that different inputs or pathways into the AV node facilitate the development of reentry. Sustained reentry occurs if two inputs can support a stable repetitive circuit, and usually a slow pathway with a relatively short refractory period and a "fast" pathway with rapid conduction but a longer refractory period are present. This electrophysiologic difference facilitates the development of a reentrant circuit, and in the typical form, a premature atrial contraction will "block" in the fast pathway due to its longer refractory period and conduct slowly in the slow pathway. The wave of depolarization can enter the distal portion of the "fast" pathway (because it is no longer refractory because of the slow conduction) and travel retrogradely with initiation of a stable reentrant circuit. In this case, as retrograde activation is "fast," the HA interval is extremely short. Although this is the "typical" form of AVNRT, there are several different "atypical" forms that will display different AV relationships because of varying conduction properties (Figure 2.30).

The anatomy of the inferior and septal portion of the right atrium in the region of the coronary sinus and tricuspid valve area is complex, and it is critical for the electrophysiologist to have an understanding of this space (Figure 2.31). Typically, the "fast" pathway is located superiorly and the slow pathway inferiorly.

There are two potential targets for ablation of typical AVNRT. Initially, the fast pathway was targeted. The fast pathway is generally located superiorly and septally. Although ablation of the fast pathway abolishes SVT in 80–90% of patients, it often led to first-degree AV block and a risk of significant worsening of AV conduction in up to 20% of patients. Ablation of the fast pathway is no longer performed except in extremely rare circumstances.

We are indebted to the seminal work performed by Sonny Jackman for the initial description of the technique for mapping and ablation of the slow pathway. A mapping catheter is used to explore the region around the coronary sinus (Figures 2.32 and 2.33). As the tricuspid valve is positioned more apically than the mitral valve, the atrial septal region on the tricuspid valve is characterized by a larger ventricular and smaller atrial signal. Several forms of "slow pathway" potentials have been described: from relatively sharp discrete spikes to lower-frequency, lower-amplitude signals. Regardless of the type of AVNRT, as a general rule,

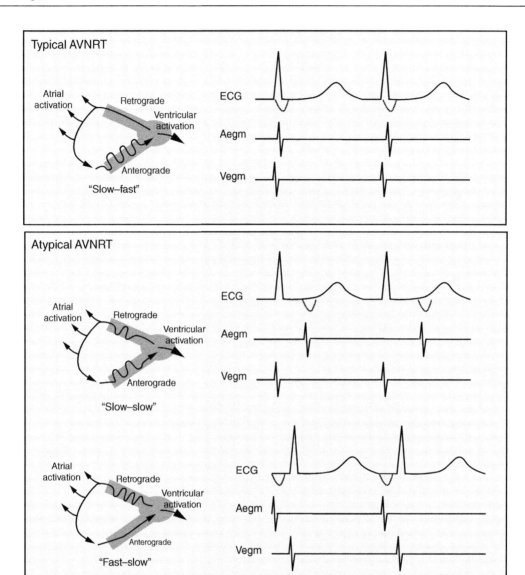

Figure 2.30 Schematics showing the different electrophysiologic patterns observed in AVNRT. The relationship between the atrial and ventricular electrograms will be dependent on the relative conduction velocities of anterograde and retrograde pathways. In typical AVNRT, anterograde conduction is much slower than retrograde conduction, leading to a short VA interval and near-simultaneous depolarization of the atria and ventricles. In the atypical forms of AVNRT, anterograde conduction is not as slow relative to retrograde conduction (either anterograde conduction is more rapid or retrograde conduction is slower), and the P wave will be observed later after the preceding QRS.

the pathway with the slowest conduction properties is generally chosen as the primary ablation target.

For ablation of the slow pathway, the ablation catheter is generally placed in a region just apical to the coronary sinus (Figure 2.33). As the tricuspid valve

is more apically displaced than the mitral valve, the electrogram recorded in this case generally has a smaller atrial electrogram. As discussed previously, slow pathway potentials are sought, but generally the region is characterized by lower-amplitude and lower-frequency

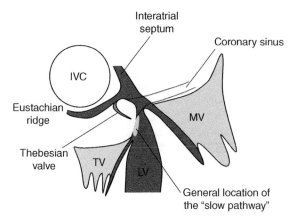

Figure 2.31 Schematic of the anatomy of the floor of the right and left atria. The slow pathway is generally anterior to the coronary sinus and posterior to the tricuspid valve (TV). Since the tricuspid valve is more apically displaced than the mitral valve (MV), the electrogram in this region is characterized by a larger ventricular signal and smaller atrial signal. IVC: inferior vena cava.

atrial electrograms (Figure 2.34). Because the coronary sinus is often contiguous to the slow pathway, too much septal torque on the ablation catheter will lead to displacement of the tip of the catheter into the coronary sinus. This often results in a sudden increase in the atrial electrogam amplitude.

Radiofrequency energy application in the region of the slow pathway can result in junctional rhythm

(Figure 2.35). The junctional beats should be carefully evaluated during ablation to ensure that retrograde fast pathway conduction continues and is uninjured. Prolongation of the HA interval or loss of retrograde conduction during ablation would suggest injury of the fast pathway and ablation should be stopped (Figure 10.20 in Understanding Intracardiac EGMs and ECGs). Other concerning finding is more rapid junctional rates during ablation that can be a marker for more extensive ablation in the AV node region. In addition, persistent junctional rhythm after ablation may also be a sign of more extensive AV nodal injury. In our laboratory, we take a "team" approach, and anyone is allowed to "stop" the ablation if they see something suspicious and voice any concerns about significant injury to AV node conduction.

Once ablation is performed, it is important to reevaluate the electrophysiologic properties of the heart (Figures 2.36–2.38). In a successful ablation, tachycardia will not be reinduced and isoproterenol is often used and required if isoproterenol infusion was necessary before ablation for the initiation of sustained tachycardia as in our patient. In our patient, after ablation, a "jump" in the AH interval is still observed just before reaching AVNERP. However, even with the "jump," no tachycardia is initiated nor is an "echo" beat present. An echo beat suggests that in addition to an anterograde "jump" in the AH interval (Figure 2.39), there are

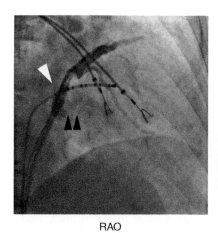

RAO

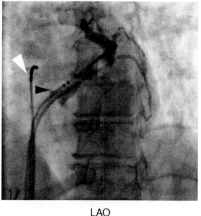

LAO

Figure 2.32 Anatomy of the proximal coronary sinus region. A decapolar catheter and a balloon-tipped catheter have been placed in the coronary sinus. A decapolar catheter is located on the superior septum straddling the right atrium and right ventricle. Contrast has been injected into the coronary sinus. The slow pathway is often located just anterior to the coronary sinus os in line with the most superior portion of the roof of the coronary sinus (black arrowheads). The fast pathway is generally superior (White arrowheads). RAO, right anterior oblique; LAO, left anterior oblique.

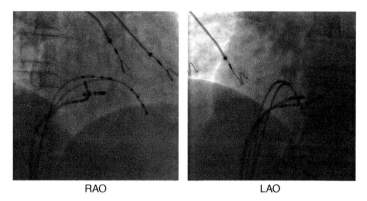

RAO   LAO

Figure 2.33 Fluoroscopic positions of catheters for slow pathway modification. Diagnostic quadripolar cathters are located at the His bundle and right ventricle, and a decapolar catheter is placed in the coronary sinus. The ablation catheter (identified by its larger distal electrode) is just anterior to the coronary sinus os. RAO, right anterior oblique; LAO, left anterior oblique.

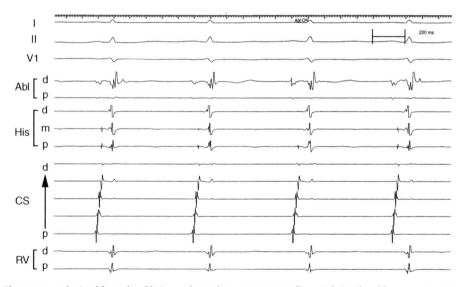

Figure 2.34 Electrograms obtained from the ablation catheter demonstrate a smaller atrial signal and larger ventricular signal.

two functionally separate pathways present in the AV node region (one anterograde, the other retrograde). Although practices vary, most electrophysiologists will "leave" a single echo in after slow pathway modification for AVNRT. There are several practical reasons for this practice. First, it is important to remember that the goal of the ablation is to "modify" the AV node to prevent the development of sustained AVNRT. Second, the original studies by Jackman and colleagues suggested that the presence of a single residual echo did not predict the recurrence of AVNRT. Finally, although the second point may be controversial, there is no question that AVNRT

is not a life-threatening arrhythmia and that significant injury to the AV node (with or without the requirement of a pacemaker) is not a good outcome, particularly in a young patient. Even if an echo is present, a high likelihood of long-term success has been described if the tachycardia window has been shortened (Figure 2.40). The concept of the tachycardia window can be most easily understood by graphing the relationship between the coupling interval of premature atrial extrastimuli and the resulting AH interval. In patients without dual AV node physiology, the AH interval will gradually lengthen without any discontinuities. In a patient with

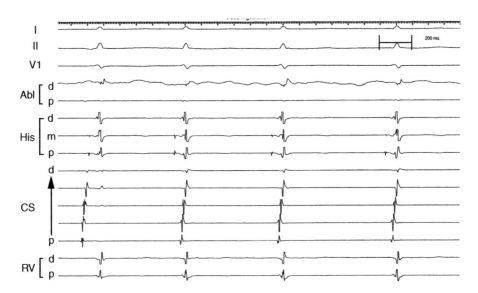

Figure 2.35 During ablation, junctional rhythm develops. Importantly, junctional rhythm is associated with retrograde conduction via the fast pathway suggesting that normal AV node conduction remains intact.

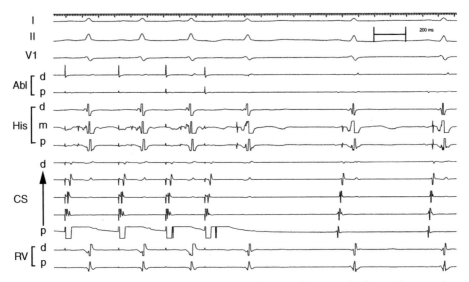

Figure 2.36 Premature atrial stimulation protocol. With two extrastimuli at coupling intervals of 290 and 240 ms, the AH interval is 157 ms.

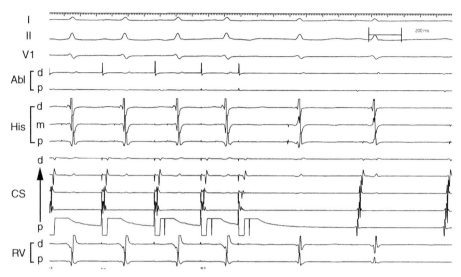

Figure 2.37 Continuation of the premature atrial stimulation protocol. With two extrastimuli at coupling intervals of 290 and 230 ms, the sudden prolongation of the AH interval is observed (301 ms), but a retrograde atrial "echo" is not observed.

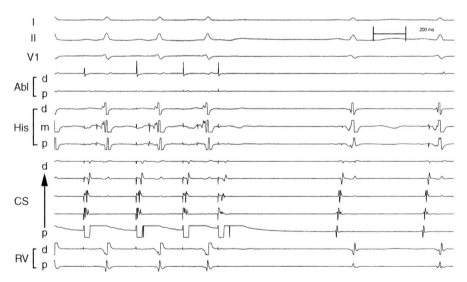

Figure 2.38 Continuation of premature atrial stimulation protocol. With two extrastimuli at coupling intervals of 290 and 220 ms, AV node refractory period (AVNERP) is reached (330 ms).

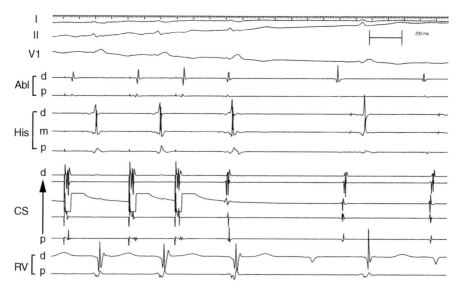

Figure 2.39 In another patient, a single echo after ablation. The patient had sustained AVNRT before the ablation, but after slow pathway modification, the slow pathway cannot be repetitively activated.

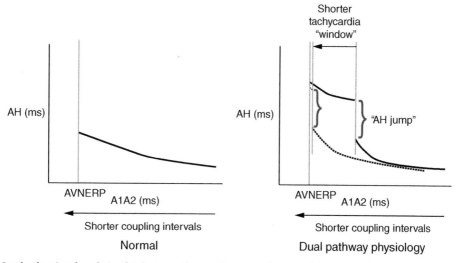

Figure 2.40 Graphs showing the relationship between the coupling interval of an atrial extrastimulus and the AH interval (delay in the AV node). *Left:* In most patients, the AH interval will gradually prolong until block develops. *Right:* In patients with dual pathway physiology, a discontinuity will be observed because of sudden prolongation of AV nodal conduction as conduction "switches" from the "fast" pathway to the "slow" pathway. In some cases, ablation shortens the tachycardia window. The initial relationship between the coupling interval and AH prolongation (solid line) shows a jump to the slow pathway at a relatively long coupling interval. After ablation (dashed line), a jump still occurs but only at very short coupling interval near the AVNERP.

AVNRT, shift from the fast pathway to the slow pathway will lead to a discontinuity in the curve. The tachycardia window is the range of coupling intervals associated with a prolonged AH interval. Recent studies have suggested that shortening of the tachycardia window is associated with a high likelihood of medium-term success.

Another marker for successful AV node modification is an increase in the AV Wenckebach cycle length that likely reflects "injury" to the slow pathway. Another commonly observed phenomenon after successful ablation is a relative sinus tachycardia that some have speculated is due to injury of the parasympathetic nervous system as it travels through the inferior portion of the interatrial septum to the sinus node.

KEY POINTS

- SVT can be associated with significant symptoms, but management must take into account the arrhythmia burden, and careful discussion about the natural history and treatment options with the patient is required.

- Electrophysiologic testing should be performed in a systematic manner and include atrial overdrive pacing, atrial extrastimulation, ventricular overdrive pacing, and ventricular extrastimulation.

- Initiation of sustained tachycardia is critical for electrophysiologic testing and may require drug infusion and multiple extrastimulation protocols.

- If a SVT with a short HA interval is initiated, evaluating the response to ventricular stimulation is the best way to identify the tachycardia mechanism.

- In typical AVNRT, the slow pathway is targeted for ablation. The slow pathway is usually located near the coronary sinus os.

- After ablation, the patient should be reassessed. The "endpoint" for ablation of AVNRT varies from operator to operator and will depend on the clinical situation.

CHAPTER 3

Supraventricular tachycardia case 2

> A 63-year-old gastroenterologist has had a 2-year history of tiredness and fatigue. He has a history of hypertension treated with hydrochlorothiazide 25 mg daily. On physical examination, he has cannon A waves, but otherwise there are no significant murmurs or other abnormalities. Two ECGs are shown in Figure 3.1.

The ECG demonstrates a junctional rhythm of 80 beats per minute. The normal junctional rate is 40–60 beats per minute. Junctional rhythm can be observed in the setting of slow sinus rates in patients with sinus node dysfunction or in those who are taking beta-blockers or other medications that suppress the sinus node. However, in this patient with a more rapid junctional rate, possibilities include increased automaticity (sometimes seen after cardiac surgery as discussed in Chapter 1) or a slow reentrant circuit within the AV node. Regardless of the cause, persistent junctional rhythms can be associated with symptoms such as tiredness and fatigue due to mistiming of atrial and ventricular contractions. Atrial and ventricular contractions occur almost simultaneously when the tricuspid valve and mitral valves are closed. Resulting regurgitant flow within the vena cavae and the pulmonary veins can lead to elevated left and right atrial pressures and is associated with cannon A waves on physical examination and in some cases overt pulmonary edema. The pathophysiology is similar to "pacemaker syndrome" in patients with ventricular pacing and (often) retrograde 1:1 ventriculoatrial (VA) conduction.

Given the patient's significant symptoms, an electrophysiology study to further explore the mechanism of his arrhythmia is reasonable. Baseline electrograms are shown in Figure 3.2 and demonstrate normal intervals. Response to premature atrial stimulation is shown in

Figures 3.3 and 3.4. With a coupling interval of 360 ms, the AH interval is 330 ms (Figure 3.3). As an aside, it is important to notice several low-amplitude signals in the intracardiac recordings. The low-frequency signals recorded in the distal His catheter electrodes are independent of cardiac activity and probably represent artifact. The low-frequency signals observed in the distal right ventricular electrograms appear to be coupled with the preceding ventricular depolarization and as they occur at the same time as the T wave represent intracardiac measurement of ventricular repolarization. Recording of low-frequency signals will depend on the filtering parameters that are chosen by the clinician. One of the skills learned with experience is differentiating low-frequency, low-amplitude signals that provide important clues to the pathophysiology of arrhythmias from spurious signals due to artifact or other causes. In Figure 3.4, the coupling interval is shortened to 350 ms, and block in the atrioventricular (AV) node occurs.

Ventricular pacing at baseline shows retrograde conduction at relatively long paced cycle lengths (Figure 3.5). With infusion of a low dose of isoproterenol, ventricular stimulation induces supraventricular tachycardia (SVT) with a cycle length of 590 ms (Figure 3.6). As in Chapter 2, the differential diagnosis in this case is either an atrial tachycardia or an AV node reentrant tachycardia (AVNRT) because AV reentrant tachycardia (AVRT) would not be associated with such a short HA or VA time (Table 3.1).

Several findings in this case confirm the presence of AVNRT. In Figure 3.7, the tachycardia spontaneously terminates on an atrial electrogram proving AV node dependence. In Figure 3.8, two premature ventricular stimuli terminate the tachycardia with minimal resetting of the atrial electrogram. This finding makes

Understanding Intracardiac EGMs: A Patient Centered Guide, First Edition. Fred Kusumoto.
© 2015 John Wiley & Sons, Ltd. Published 2015 by John Wiley & Sons, Ltd.

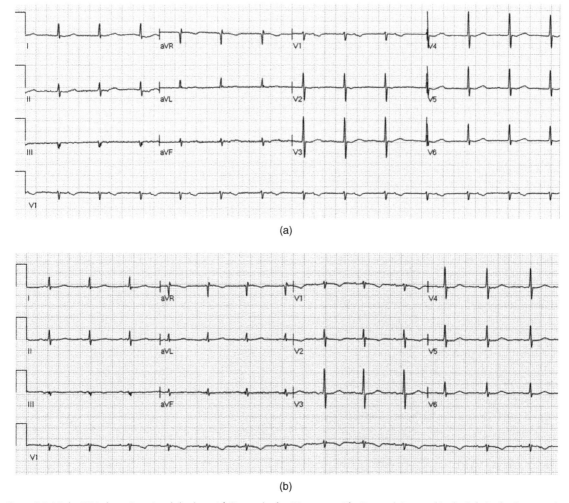

Figure 3.1 (a) the ECG shows junctional rhythm with P wave in the ST segment. The P wave is inverted in the inferior leads suggesting that it represents retrograde conduction. (b) Another ECG recorded 2 days later shows sinus rhythm.

reentry a far more likely diagnosis than automaticity and suggests the presence of AVNRT rather than a tachycardia due to increased automaticity of the junction that might be transiently suppressed but would unlikely to be terminated by one or two premature stimuli. Finally, a Morady maneuver shown in Figure 3.9 shows a V-A-V response. Any one of these three responses would be sufficient to "rule out" atrial tachycardia and confirm AVNRT as the mechanism for

the patient's tachycardia, but it is instructive to see the different techniques for identifying and corroborating the tachycardia mechanism in a single patient.

Once the diagnosis is made, an ablation catheter is positioned in the inferoseptal region between the coronary sinus os and the tricuspid valve (Figure 3.10). The associated electrograms with this catheter position are shown in Figure 3.11 and is characterized with a signal that appears to be discrete from the accompanying atrial

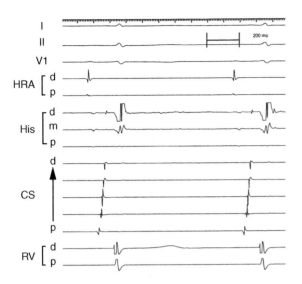

Figure 3.2 Baseline electrograms. The baseline cycle length is 871 ms. AV conduction is normal with an AH interval of 82 ms and an HV interval of 43 ms.

signal. The main concern for slow pathway modification in patients with AVNRT is inadvertent AV block during the procedure and perhaps a higher likelihood of permanent pacing in the future. Although the ablation catheter is located at a significant anatomic distance from the His bundle catheter, evaluation of the electrograms during pacing maneuvers can be helpful for distinguishing discrete slow pathway potentials from His bundle electrograms. In this case, pacing from the coronary sinus is associated with loss of the discrete potential due to either block or fusion of the electrograms. Regardless of the mechanism, separation of the signal from the His bundle electrogram provides strong evidence that the potential is not due to His bundle depolarization. Ablation was performed in this case with loss of slow pathway conduction, and the patient has been arrhythmia free with resolution of his symptoms of fatigue.

This case illustrates that in some cases, abnormal arrhythmias can be associated with relatively normal

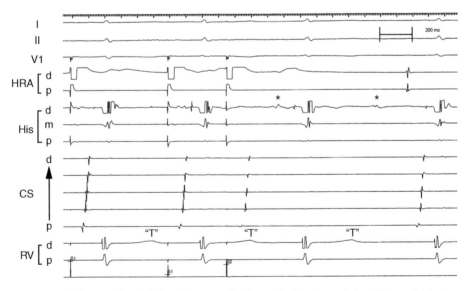

Figure 3.3 A premature atrial contraction is delivered at a coupling interval of 360 ms, and the AH interval is 330 ms as measured from the proximal coronary sinus electrodes. Notice the low-frequency, low-amplitude signals on the distal His catheter that appear to be independent of cardiac activity (*). These signals probably represent artifact. Another low-frequency, low-amplitude signal can be observed on the distal right ventricular electrograms ("T"). These signals are related to prior ventricular activation and represent ventricular repolarization and are the intracardiac electrogram equivalent of "T waves."

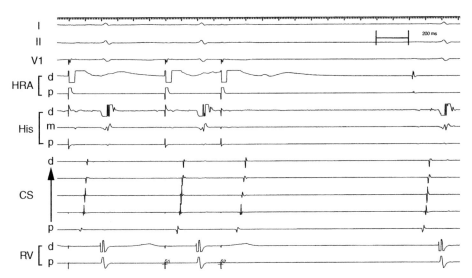

Figure 3.4 Continuation of atrial extrastimulation. At a coupling interval of 350 ms, AV block occurs because of block in the AV node. Some interatrial conduction delay can be observed with a slight increase in the interval between the stimulus and the proximal sinus electrogram.

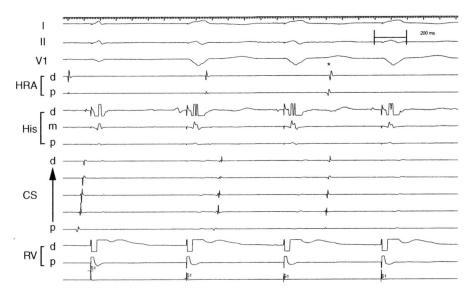

Figure 3.5 Ventricular pacing at a cycle length of 700 ms demonstrates a single retrograde atrial electrogram (*) before block.

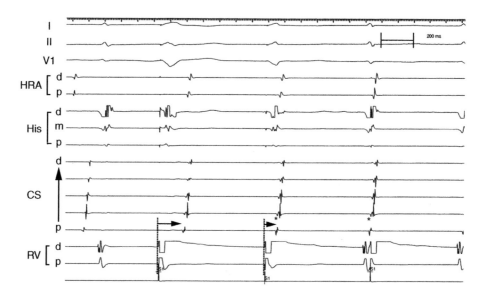

Figure 3.6 After initiation of a low dose of isoproterenol, ventricular pacing at 650 ms initiates supraventricular "tachycardia" at a cycle length of 570 ms. Notice that the first beat of tachycardia occurs after the first ventricular paced beat as shown by the early atrial electrograms observed in the proximal coronary sinus (*), as a shortened stimulation to intracardiac electrogram interval (arrows) would not be the normal behavior of the AV node from the second pacing stimulus. Although this behavior could be observed by retrograde conduction switching from the AV node to an accessory pathway, the very short VA interval observed on the next beat rules out AVRT using an AV accessory pathway. The astute reader will note that the third QRS complex is a fusion beat due to tachycardia and ventricular pacing.

Table 3.1 Differential diagnosis of a supraventricular tachycardia with a very short VA time (<65 ms).

	Favors AVNRT	**Favors AT**
During tachycardia	• Fixed VA intervals • Termination with AV block	• Variable VA intervals • Continuation with AV block
Spontaneous termination	• Termination with an atrial electrogram	

Response to ventricular stimuli	• V-A-V response to ventricular pacing
	• VPC terminates SVT:
	  ○ Without an A
	  ○ Without resetting the A
	• VPC causes delay of the next A
		• V-A-A-V response to ventricular pacing

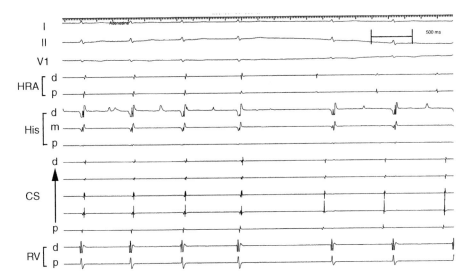

Figure 3.7 The supraventricular tachycardia has a cycle length of 590 ms, and a short HA interval terminates spontaneously on an atrial electrogram, providing strong evidence that the tachycardia is AV node dependent and ruling out atrial tachycardia.

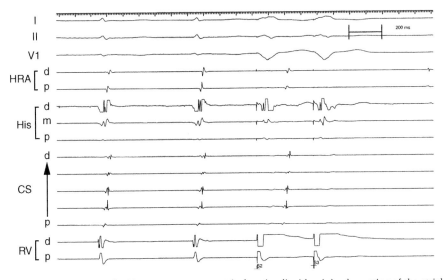

Figure 3.8 The tachycardia is terminated with two premature ventricular stimuli with minimal resetting of the atrial electrograms. This finding makes reentry the most likely mechanism for the tachycardia.

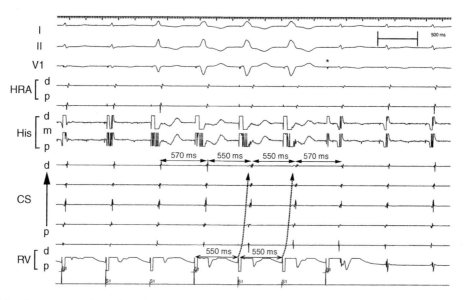

Figure 3.9 Morady maneuver. The tachycardia cycle length is 570 ms. Ventricular pacing at 550 ms entrains the tachycardia as evidenced by shortening of the atrial cycle length to 550 ms (dashed arrows). The last pacing stimulus does not capture the ventricles (*), but a V-A-V response is still observed, making AVNRT the likely diagnosis.

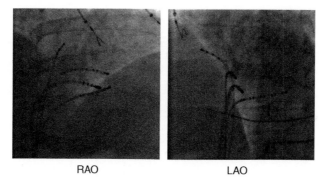

RAO   LAO

Figure 3.10 Fluoroscopic position of catheters with an ablation catheter placed inferoseptally between the coronary sinus and the tricuspid valve in the right anterior oblique (RAO) and left anterior oblique (LAO) projections.

rates. Another example is shown in Figures 3.12–3.14. Figure 3.12 shows a patient with several months of chronic fatigue. In this case, an abnormal atrial tachycardia can be identified by the inverted P wave in aVL.

The patient underwent electrophysiology study and had ablation of an atrial tachycardia focus near the os of his left superior pulmonary vein (Figure 3.13). His ECG in sinus rhythm is shown in Figure 3.14.

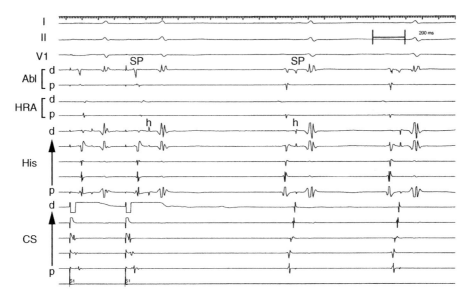

Figure 3.11 Electrograms recorded from the fluoroscopic position shown in Figure 3.10. The ablation catheter has a multicomponent atrial signal with a discrete potential (SP) that occurs just before His depolarization (h). Pacing from the coronary sinus shows dissociation of this potential from the His bundle electrogram.

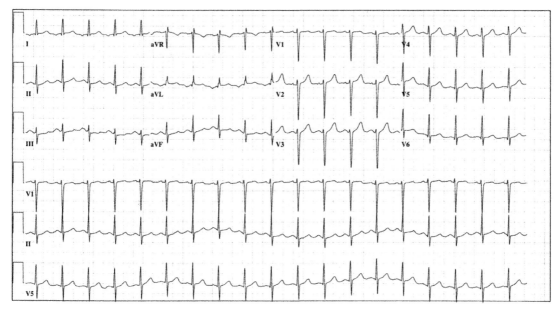

Figure 3.12 Baseline ECG of a patient complaining of chronic fatigue. The hart rate is approximately 100 bpm. The P wave is inverted in leads I and aVL and biphasic in lead aVR, suggesting that the sinus node is not initiating atrial depolarization. (Kusumoto 2009. Reproduced with permission of Springer Science + Business Media.)

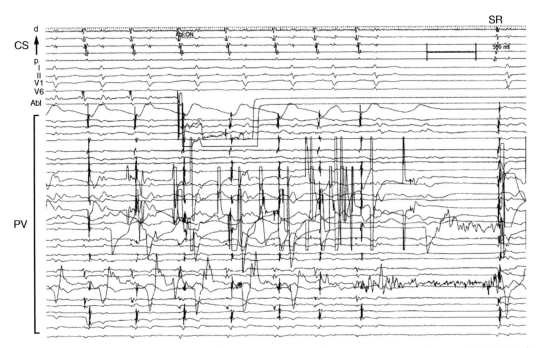

Figure 3.13 Electrograms showing an atrial tachycardia arising from the os of the pulmonary vein with prompt termination during catheter ablation. A decapolar catheter is located in the coronary sinus, and an 8 splined, 64 electrode basket catheter is located in the pulmonary vein. The ablation catheter (Abl) is located at the os of the left superior pulmonary vein and has an early atrial electrogram (*).

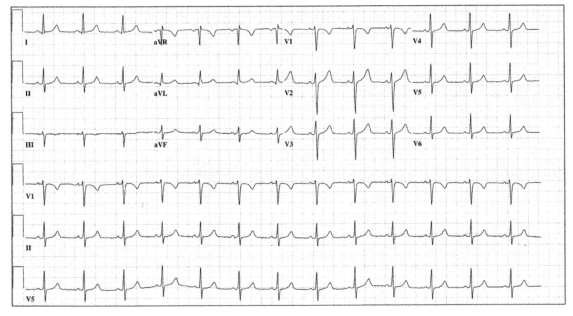

Figure 3.14 ECG after ablation showing sinus rhythm and a normal-appearing P wave, now deeply negative in lead aVR and positive in lead II. (Kusumoto 2009. Reproduced with permission of Springer Science + Business Media.)

KEY POINTS

- Abnormal heart rhythms at relatively normal heart rates can be observed, and the electrophysiologist must have an "open mind" to potential diagnoses.

- When a tachycardia with a short VA interval is present, the focus of the study is to distinguish between an arrhythmia arising from the AV junction or the atrium and whether the mechanism of the tachycardia is reentry or automaticity.

- Careful examination of electrogram behavior during pacing maneuvers can provide information on the possible anatomic source of specific components of the electrogram.

CHAPTER 4

Supraventricular tachycardia case 3

A 42-year-old woman began having episodes of rapid heart rate in her 20s. Her first documented episode was 3 years ago when she had a sudden onset of rapid heart rate (200 bpm) associated with near syncope. She went to the emergency room and was given adenosine with termination of her tachycardia. She has continued to have episodes despite the use of atenolol and has now been referred for evaluation. Her past medical history is unremarkable, and her physical examination is normal. A baseline ECG is normal without evidence of preexcitation.

Electrophysiology study is certainly reasonable in the setting of drug refractory, symptomatic supraventricular tachycardia (Table A7 in Appendix). In patients with supraventricular tachycardia, women are often more symptomatic than men, and unfortunately, their symptoms are often ascribed to anxiety. Importantly, women often have an excellent response to ablation for supraventricular tachycardia, often with a more significant improvement in many aspects of quality-of-life. The baseline electrograms for our patient are shown in Figure 4.1. The basic cycle length is 1020 ms, and the HV interval is 34 ms. Atrial pacing is unremarkable with an AVBCL of 350 ms. Representative responses to atrial premature stimuli are shown in Figures 4.2 and 4.3. As atrial coupling intervals were shortened, there is gradual prolongation of the AH interval without a "jump," and when the coupling interval was decreased to 360 ms, the AVNERP was reached. Further shortening of the coupling interval yielded an AERP of 210 ms.

Ventricular pacing was unremarkable with a VA BCL of 350 ms and a VA ERP of 290 ms. Ventricular pacing results in a retrograde activation pattern that is earliest in the septum and appears to decrement with shorter coupling intervals, suggesting that it represents

retrograde AV nodal conduction (Figures 4.4 and 4.5). In contrast, retrograde conduction via an accessory pathway generally is characterized by an "all-or-none" behavior with very little progressive increase in ventriculoatrial conduction time (accessory pathways are most commonly composed of tissues with electrophysiologic properties similar to atrial and ventricular myocytes). At this juncture in the electrophysiology study, it is imperative to induce supraventricular tachycardia, and as in the preceding two cases, isoproterenol is again used to facilitate AV node conduction and perhaps create regional changes in refractoriness and conduction to allow initiation of a stable reentrant circuit.

With isoproterenol infusion, atrial pacing now induces a sudden prolongation in the AH interval (Figures 4.6 and 4.7) and initiates a tachycardia with a cycle length of 390 ms, an HA interval of 105 ms, and a VA interval of 75 ms (Figure 4.8). The VA interval is longer than the cases discussed in Chapters 2 and 3, so all three mechanisms for supraventricular tachycardia are possible: atrial tachycardia, AVNRT, or an accessory pathway using a septal accessory pathway. Scanning single ventricular stimuli are delivered and do not engage the tachycardia circuit (Figure 4.9). This is indirect evidence that AVRT using an accessory pathway is less likely, as the ventricular stimuli should generally interact with the large AVRT circuit but does not provide definitive "proof" for mechanism. In order to interact with the circuit, double extrastimuli are delivered at very short coupling intervals and supraventricular tachycardia is terminated (Figure 4.10). Both ventricular extrastimuli interact with the circuit and "reel in the atrial electrograms." Careful review of the electrograms provides some indirect evidence for the underlying mechanism of the tachycardia by taking each possibility in turn. If the patient had an atrial tachycardia with first-degree

Understanding Intracardiac EGMs: A Patient Centered Guide, First Edition. Fred Kusumoto.
© 2015 John Wiley & Sons, Ltd. Published 2015 by John Wiley & Sons, Ltd.

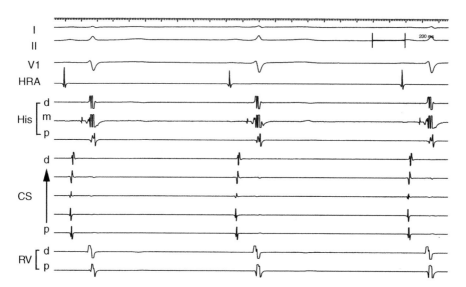

Figure 4.1 Baseline electrograms show a basic cycle length of 1022 ms with normal conduction properties and normal atrioventricular conduction (PR interval: 150 ms, AH interval: 103 ms; HV interval: 30 ms) and normal QRS morphology.

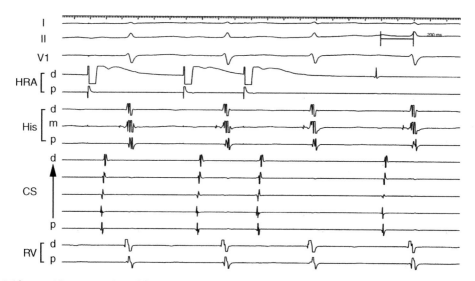

Figure 4.2 With an atrial premature beat delivered at a coupling interval of 370 ms, the AH interval is prolonged (290 ms from the earliest CS activation). As the atrial coupling interval was shortened, there was gradual prolongation of the AH interval without a "jump" (50 ms increase with a 10 ms decrease in the coupling interval).

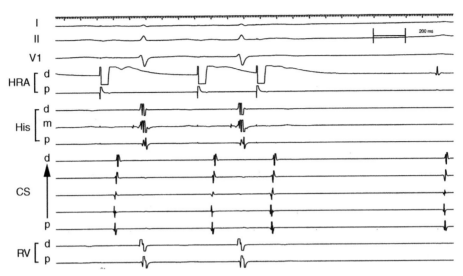

Figure 4.3 With a coupling interval of 360 ms, the premature atrial stimulus results in atrial capture but no His electrogram signifying block in the AV node and defining the AVNERP.

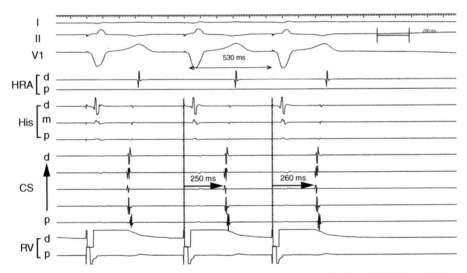

Figure 4.4 At a drive cycle length of 600 ms, a premature ventricular stimulus at a coupling interval of 530 ms leads to a stimulation to atrial electrogram of 260 ms, which is slightly longer than the stimulation to atrial electrogram interval during basic pacing 250 ms. The pattern of atrial activation is similar to the first atrial electrogram recorded in the mid-coronary sinus.

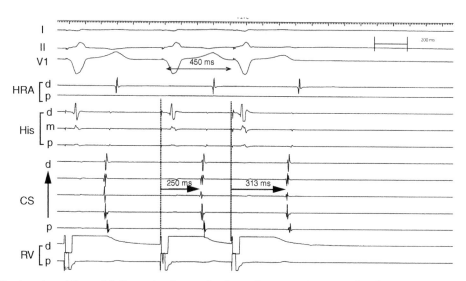

Figure 4.5 Continuation of Figure 4.4. Shortening the coupling interval to 450 ms is associated with an increase in the stimulation to electrogram interval of 313 ms with the same pattern of atrial activation observed at the longer coupling interval. This gradual decrement suggests that this pattern of retrograde activation is produced by tissue with decremental conduction properties such as the AV node.

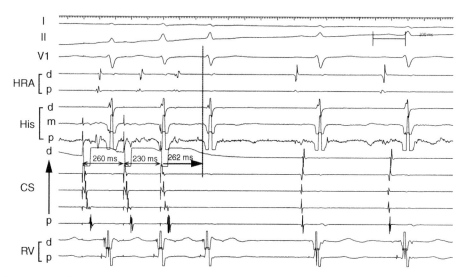

Figure 4.6 After initiation of an isoproterenol infusion, coronary sinus pacing at a baseline pacing cycle of 400 ms, with two premature beats (260 and 230 ms), the patient has an AV interval of 262 ms.

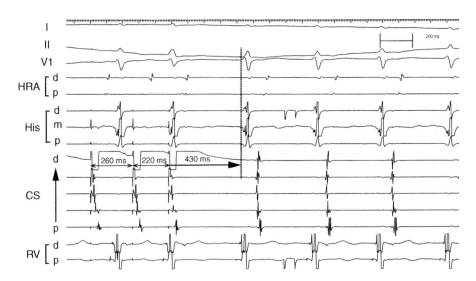

Figure 4.7 Continuation of Figure 4.6. Shortening the last coupling interval (s3) to 220 ms leads to sudden prolongation of the AV interval to 430 ms and initiation of tachycardia. Unfortunately, a His bundle electrogram is not available, but such a profound prolongation in the AV interval can only be mediated by delay in AV nodal conduction.

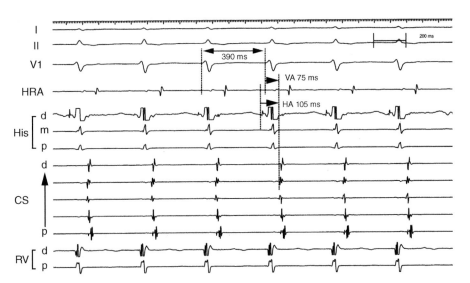

Figure 4.8 Electrograms during tachycardia reveals a tachycardia cycle length of 390 ms, an HA interval of 105 ms, and a VA interval of 75 ms, with earliest atrial activation observed in the proximal coronary sinus.

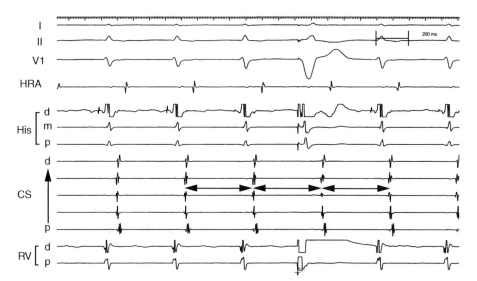

Figure 4.9 Premature ventricular stimulus at a coupling interval of 350 ms does not reset the tachycardia.

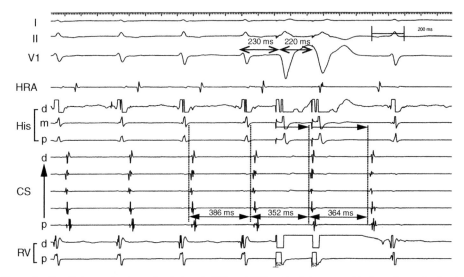

Figure 4.10 Two extrastimuli at very short coupling intervals (230 and 220 ms) both interact with the tachycardia circuit and shorten the atrial electrogram intervals. The interesting termination suggests that the second extrastimulus retrogradely activated the atria via the "slow pathway" because of the significant prolongation of the stimulus to atrial electrogram interval and the subsequent antero-grade activation via the "fast pathway" as evidenced by the short PR interval. With this interpretation, the tachycardia terminated because of retrograde block in the "slow pathway."

AV block (as the PR or AV interval is relatively long), the premature ventricular stimuli could have terminated tachycardia by premature atrial depolarization, but the last QRS complex is problematic for the presence of atrial tachycardia or AVRT. For atrial tachycardia, if the QRS complex was produced by the last atrial depolarization, then why would first-degree AV block suddenly resolve? If the penultimate atrial depolarization was responsible for the QRS (with prolongation of the AV interval due to decremental conduction), then why wouldn't the last atrial depolarization also conduct, as the AV node would have had more time to recover (364 vs 352 ms)? For AVRT and retrograde conduction via an accessory pathway, it would be extremely unusual for the second premature ventricular contraction to cause such a dramatic delay in accessory pathway conduction, and even with this delay, because the AV node would be "engaged" at a shorter cycle length (364 ms) when compared to tachycardia (392 ms), why should AV node conduction suddenly improve? AVNRT with dual pathway physiology provides the best explanation for the unusual termination. In this case, the first ventricular stimulus activates the atria via the "fast pathway," and the second premature ventricular stimulus blocks in the "fast pathway" (because it was just depolarized by the first ventricular extrastimulus) and activates the atria via the "slow pathway" (explaining the dramatic prolongation in the VA interval). The wave of depolarization "turns around," and now the "fast pathway" is activated anterogradely and the resulting PR interval is short. It is obvious from this discussion that interpretation of electrograms can be complex and not always amenable to "tables and flowsheets." It is an important exercise that illustrates the principle of "explaining every beat."

From the aforementioned discussion, AVNRT is the most likely diagnosis, but all three supraventricular tachycardia mechanisms remain "in play," and continued evaluation and reinitiation of the tachycardia are required. Once tachycardia is reinitiated, ventricular overdrive pacing results in a V-A-V response, which "rules out" atrial tachycardia (Figure 4.11). Of the two possibilities left, AVNRT and AVRT using a septal accessory pathway comparing the VA conduction during supraventricular tachycardia and pacing can be useful. In this case, the VA conduction time during pacing at a rate slightly faster than the tachycardia cycle length leads to significant lengthening of the VA time. In general, if the tachycardia was using an accessory pathway, ventricular pacing should yield a relatively

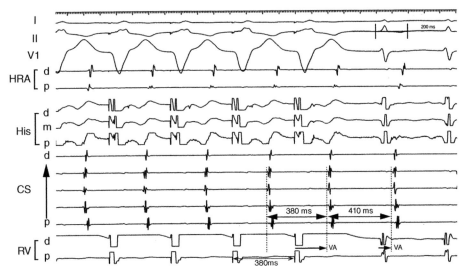

Figure 4.11 Response of the tachycardia to ventricular pacing. Once the tachycardia is entrained, cessation of pacing leads to a V-A-V response "ruling out" atrial tachycardia. Of the two remaining possibilities – AVRT using a septal accessory pathway and AVNRT, comparing the VA intervals between tachycardia and ventricular pacing can be extremely useful. In a tachycardia using a septal accessory pathway, the VA interval should be similar for both tachycardia and ventricular pacing. In this case, the VA interval is dramatically longer with ventricular pacing, making AVNRT a more likely diagnosis.

similar VA interval as during supraventricular tachycardia, although there can be differences (shorter if the ventricular pacing site is located close to the accessory pathway or longer if there is delay in intraventricular conduction), while in AVNRT, the VA is obligatorily longer than during ventricular pacing because the VA interval is a "pseudo interval," as there is simultaneous activation of the His bundle and the atrium, while in ventricular pacing, the VA interval is a "true" interval because of sequential activation of the His bundle and retrograde atrial activation (Figure 4.12). In this case, as shown in Figure 4.11, the VA interval is dramatically longer during ventricular pacing compared to tachycardia, making AVNRT the most likely diagnosis. Figure 4.13 shows ventricular pacing in another patient with a septal accessory pathway. In this case, notice that

the HA interval is actually longer than the stimulus to atrial electrogram interval during ventricular pacing. Several important points should be emphasized when using this form of analysis. Firstly, the pacing rate must be similar to the tachycardia rate (generally with a cycle length 20–30 ms faster), to minimize decrement in the retrograde pathway. Secondly, as pacing is occurring at a similar rate to tachycardia, entrainment of the atrium must be confirmed by an atrial rate that is equal to the pacing rate. Finally, evaluating the atrial electrogram intervals can help decide "what goes with what," as the last paced ventricular stimulus will yield the last atrial signal that occurs at the pacing interval. Another method for differentiating AVNRT and AVRT using a septal accessory pathway is shown in Figure 4.14. In this case, a His bundle premature beat is delivered when

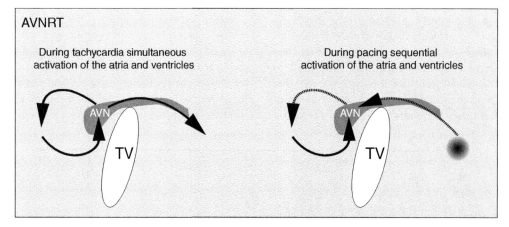

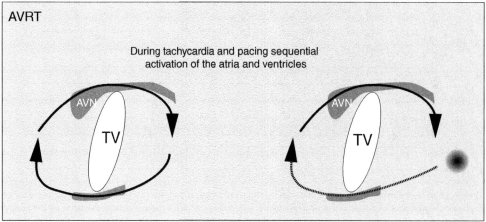

Figure 4.12 Schematic showing the reason for differences in retrograde conduction times between AVNRT and AVRT during tachycardia and ventricular pacing.

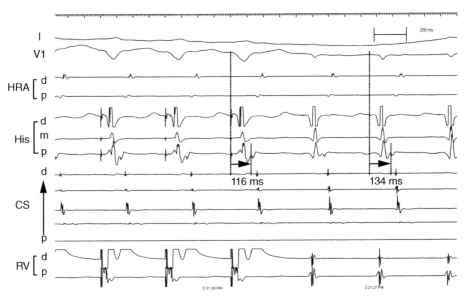

Figure 4.13 Morady maneuver in another patient with a septal accessory pathway. The patient is in supraventricular tachycardia at a cycle length of 430 ms. On cessation of ventricular pacing at 400 ms, a V-A-V response is noted. The ventricular stimulus to atrial electrogram interval (116 ms) is shorter than the HA interval (134 ms).

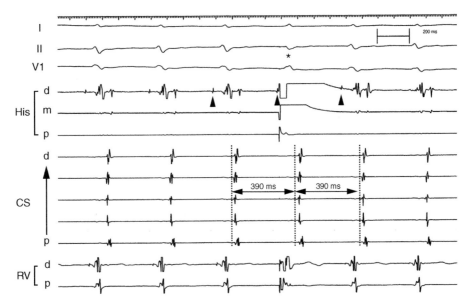

Figure 4.14 Pacing the His bundle during supraventricular tachycardia can also be useful. In this case, His bundle capture is confirmed by the slight change in the QRS complex that remains narrow (*), but the tachycardia is not reset, providing evidence that the distal is bundle is not participating in the circuit. The His bundle electrogram can be seen just before the pacing stimulus (arrowheads).

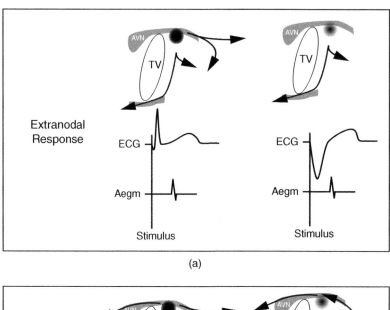

(a)

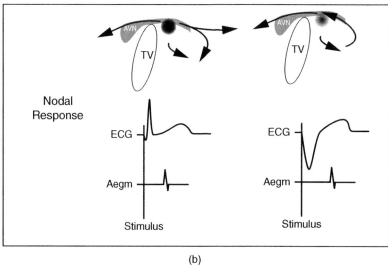

(b)

Figure 4.15 Schematic showing the use of His bundle pacing during sinus rhythm. On the left-sided drawings, a stronger stimulus strength leads to capture of the His bundle and adjacent ventricular myocardium. On the right-sided drawings, a decrease in the stimulus strength only captures ventricular myocardium. In the presence of an accessory pathway, an "extranodal" response will be observed where regardless of whether the His bundle is captured, the VA interval will remain relatively constant (a). In contrast, a "nodal" response is characterized by a shorter VA interval with His bundle capture, as the wave of activation has a "head start" when compared to ventricular depolarization only (b).

the His bundle has just depolarized. Distal ventricular capture is confirmed by the change in the QRS complex, but the tachycardia is not reset, suggesting that the lower portion of the His bundle (which would be necessary for AVRT using a septal accessory pathway) is not involved in the tachycardia circuit.

ParaHisian pacing during sinus rhythm can also be useful for identifying the presence of a septal accessory pathway (Figure 4.15). ParaHisian pacing takes advantage of the difference in conduction time that occurs when atrial activation occurs via an accessory pathway or the AV node when the His bundle is captured. In the setting of retrograde conduction via the AV node, capture of the His bundle should lead to shortening of the HA interval (as retrograde depolarization has a "head start"), often called a "nodal response." Conversely, if retrograde conduction is occurring via an accessory pathway, the conduction interval should be the same whether or not the His bundle is captured ("extranodal response"). ParaHisian pacing in our patient is shown in Figure 4.16. Although extremely useful, paraHisian pacing can sometimes be difficult because of problems capturing the electrically insulated His bundle. In addition, it is important to confirm that atrial capture is not present (Figure 4.16). Finally, it

is important to remember that ParaHisian pacing is useful for separating retrograde conduction due to septal accessory pathways from AV node conduction. In patients with free wall accessory pathways, a nodal response may be observed because activation via the AV node may be faster than an accessory pathway; that is, retrograde activation over the right bundle branch, His bundle, and AV node may be faster than retrograde activation via the accessory pathway due to relatively slow intraventricular activation (time from ventricular stimulus to the ventricular insertion point of the accessory pathway) and/or slow retrograde activation via an accessory pathway. Table 4.1 summarizes the paraHisian pacing technique and some of the exceptions to a "nodal response" and an "extranodal response."

Returning to our case, now that AVNRT has been confirmed, catheter ablation in the slow pathway is performed. An angiogram is performed to help delineate the septal anatomy (Figure 4.17). Although this technique is used in <5% of cases of patients with AVNRT, knowing the exact location of the coronary sinus can help differentiate a true septal position from a position actually within the coronary sinus if the clinician is uncertain. Regardless, orthogonal fluoroscopic views are required to ensure accurate catheter positioning.

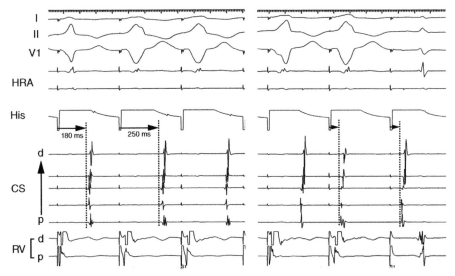

Figure 4.16 Electrograms from His bundle pacing. On the left panel, the narrower QRS complex (first QRS complex) is associated with a shorter stimulus to atrial time when compared to RV only capture (second and third QRS complexes). The stimulus to right ventricular electrogram is shorter during His bundle pacing due to more activation via the His Purkinje system. On the right panel, a problem associated with His bundle pacing is shown. In this case, atrial capture occurs on the second and third paced peats. The pacing stimulus to atrial electrogram interval is the same whether (second stimulus) or not (third stimulus) ventricular capture occurs.

Table 4.1 Technique for ParaHisian pacing.

- Electrograms should have atrial, His bundle, and ventricular components.
- Verify absence of RBBB. Although paraHisian pacing can be performed in the presence of RBBB, interpretation can be difficult.
- Pace at a rate slightly faster than the intrinsic rate (not during tachycardia).
- Verify ventriculoatrial conduction. If not present, the paraHisian pacing maneuver cannot be performed.
- Gradually decrease the pacing output and observe changes in the QRS morphology and in retrograde atrial activation.
- Ensure no atrial capture: stimulus to atrial EGM interval should be >50 ms.

• Nodal response	Stimulation to earliest atrial signal interval shorter with His bundle capture.
• Extranodal response	Stimulus to earliest atrial signal interval is the same regardless of whether the His bundle is captured.
• Exceptions:	***Extranodal response in the absence of an accessory pathway:***
	• Change in QRS morphology due to complete versus partial His bundle capture.
	Nodal response in the presence of an accessory pathway:
	• Nodal activation is faster than accessory pathway conduction (accessory pathway is located relatively far from the Hus bundle or retrograde AV node activation is very fast).
	• Accessory pathway conduction is faster with His bundle activation (early activation of the left bundle allows early activation of a left-sided accessory pathway).

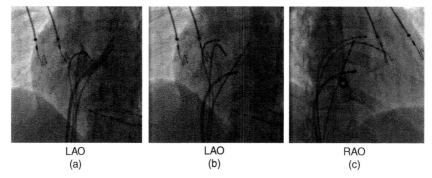

LAO   LAO   RAO
(a)   (b)   (c)

Figure 4.17 Coronary sinus angiography can to help define inferior septal anatomy. (a) The location and position of the coronary sinus in the left anterior oblique (LAO) view. (b) The catheter is located just outside the coronary sinus, but it is impossible to determine this from just a single image and requires corroboration from an orthogonal fluoroscopic view. The right anterior oblique (RAO) view confirms that the catheter is just between the coronary sinus and the tricuspid valve (c).

After ablation, the patient had no inducible arrhythmias and no evidence for dual pathway physiology with isoproterenol infusion. The patient has remained arrhythmia free for the last 2 years off medications.

KEY POINTS

- When the VA interval is >65 ms, then all three tachycardia mechanisms (AVNRT, AVRT, and atrial tachycardia) are possible.
- Several techniques may be required to "rule out" different possible arrhythmia mechanisms.
- In addition to evaluating the response after cessation of ventricular pacing, comparing electrograms between ventricular pacing and during supraventricular tachycardia can be an extremely fruitful source of information.
- ParaHisian pacing can be useful for identifying whether retrograde conduction is occurring over an accessory pathway.
- Defining the anatomy of the inferior right atrium near the coronary sinus and tricuspid valve can often be extremely useful.
- In complex cases, it is important to make sure that the diagnosis is clear and supported by firm electrophysiologic evidence before proceeding to ablation.

CHAPTER 5

Supraventricular tachycardia case 4

A 44-year-old woman has had a 10-year history of episodes of rapid heart rates that can sometimes last up to 8–9 hours. Currently, she has 7–10 episodes per year and had required emergency room evaluation and treatment for supraventricular tachycardia twice in the past year. Otherwise, her medical history is unremarkable, she takes no chronic medications, and her physical examination is normal. Her baseline ECG is shown in Figure 5.1.

It is reasonable to proceed with electrophysiology study and ablation if the patient understands the relative merits and risks of different strategies in the management of supraventricular tachycardia (Appendix, Table A5). In this patient, without other medical problems, daily medication would not be ideal for tachycardia episodes that occur once every 1–2 months. The use of medications only when episodes occur is reasonable, and although medications would likely lead to shorter episodes of tachycardia, oral medications would likely require 20–40 min before effective drug concentrations would develop.

At baseline, conduction intervals are normal with a PR interval of 153 ms, an AH interval of 84 ms, and an HV interval of 44 ms (Figure 5.2). The QRS duration is normal (100 ms) with no abnormalities. The astute reader will notice in Figure 5.2 that the fourth QRS complex is associated with a subtle change in the ventricular electrogram in the distal coronary sinus (earlier and lower amplitude) and the QRS complex itself (the S wave is not as deep).

With atrial pacing at a rate of 120 bpm (cycle length of 450 ms), there is 1:1 atrioventricular conduction, but every other QRS is now dramatically different and associated with a change in the AH and HV intervals (Figure 5.3). The second, third, and fourth atrial paced beats are associated with slight prolongation of the AH

interval from 84 to 105 ms, but more importantly, the HV interval of the second and fourth atrial paced beats is abnormally short (11 ms) and the QRS complex in V1 is now completely positive with loss of the terminal S wave. In addition, the low-amplitude ventricular signal recorded in the distal coronary sinus occurs earlier. Collectively, these findings are consistent with intermittent anterograde conduction over a left-sided accessory pathway located at the lateral portion of the mitral annulus. The ECG patterns associated with different types of accessory pathways will be covered in detail later, but for now, ventricular activation via left-sided accessory pathways is generally associated with prominent R waves in the right precordial leads (V1 and V2) because the left ventricle is behind the right ventricle and early activation of the left ventricle leads to a left to right and "back to front" activation of the portion of the ventricles activated via the accessory pathway. In Figure 5.4, the atrial pacing rate is increased to 150 bpm (cycle length of 400 ms), and the AH interval increases to 140 ms after the third paced beat, and there is no more evidence of accessory pathway conduction with any of the atrial paced beats. In both Figures 5.3 and 5.4, a right bundle potential can be observed on the proximal electrodes of the RV catheter.

With atrial premature beats, supraventricular tachycardia is induced (Figure 5.5). Close inspection of the electrograms suggests that the premature atrial stimulus results in prolongation of the AH interval with an additional low-frequency signal observed after the initial atrial signal in the distal His bundle electrograms. The etiology of this signal is unknown and could represent an atrial signal (suggesting local prolongation of atrial conduction) or a more proximal His bundle signal (suggesting intraHisian delay). Regardless, this delay initiates supraventricular tachycardia with a cycle length of 393 ms and an HA interval of 118 ms.

Understanding Intracardiac EGMs: A Patient Centered Guide, First Edition. Fred Kusumoto.
© 2015 John Wiley & Sons, Ltd. Published 2015 by John Wiley & Sons, Ltd.

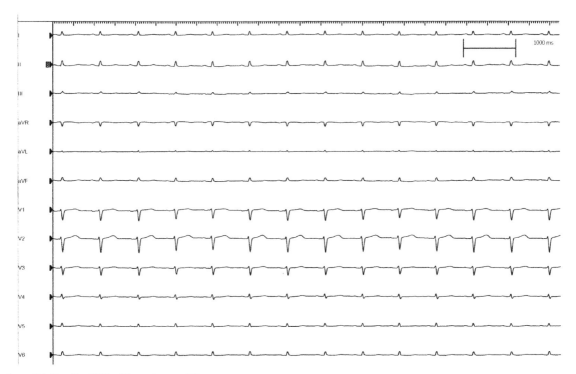

Figure 5.1 Baseline ECG with no abnormalities.

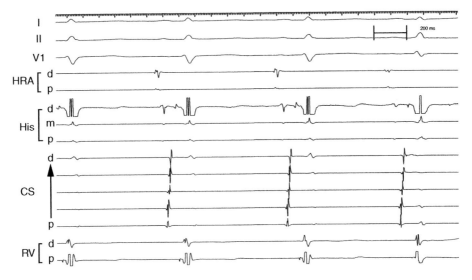

Figure 5.2 Baseline electrograms. The baseline cycle length is 770 ms. Atrioventricular conduction appears normal with a PR interval of 153 ms, an AH interval of 84 ms, and an HV interval of 44 ms. At first glance, the QRS appears normal with a QRS width of 101 ms.

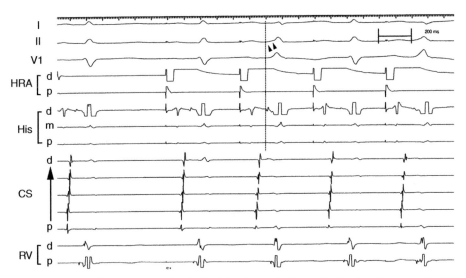

Figure 5.3 Atrial pacing at a rate of 450 ms is associated with 1:1 atrioventricular conduction, but changes in the QRS morphology are noted. With atrial pacing, as expected the AH interval increases, but in the QRS complexes associated with a monophasic R wave in V1, the onset of the QRS occurs simultaneously with His bundle depolarization. The onset of the QRS can often be difficult to identify particularly at faster sweep speeds, but in this case, subtle upward slurring can be observed in lead II (arrowheads).

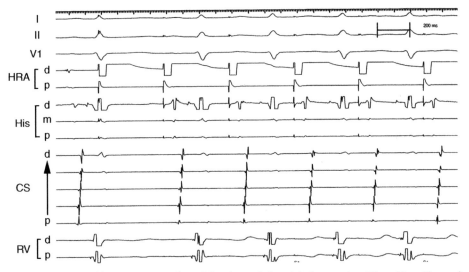

Figure 5.4 Atrial pacing continued from Figure 5.3. The atrial pacing cycle length is decreased to 400 ms. No evidence of anterograde activation via the accessory pathway is evident.

The tachycardia has an eccentric atrial activation pattern with initial atrial activation observed in the distal coronary sinus. The differential diagnosis in this situation would be AVRT using a left-sided accessory pathway (most likely), and as less likely possibilities, a left-sided atrial tachycardia associated with delayed atrioventricular conduction or AVNRT with a left-sided input (probably unlikely in the setting of such eccentric atrial activation) or with a bystander left-sided accessory pathway (Figure 5.6).

To differentiate among these possibilities for supraventricular tachycardia, it is reasonable to perform constant ventricular pacing at a rate just slower than the tachycardia cycle length to entrain

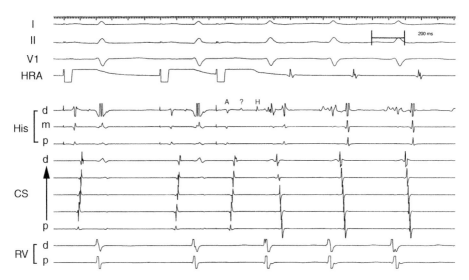

Figure 5.5 Initiation of tachycardia with premature atrial stimulation. After pacing at 600 ms, a premature atrial stimulus delivered at a coupling interval of 350 ms leads to a dramatic prolongation in atrioventricular conduction. Although the proximal atrial signal (A) and the His bundle electrogram (H) can be seen in the His bundle recording, the exact site of prolongation will depend on the definition of the intervening low-frequency signal (?): if defined as an atrial signal, there is local atrial delay in the AV node region, and if it is defined as a proximal His signal, then intraHissian delay is present. Regardless, the delay allows initiation of supraventricular tachycardia at a cycle length of 393 ms with an HA interval of 116 ms with the earliest atrial electrogram observed in the distal coronary sinus ("eccentric" activation).

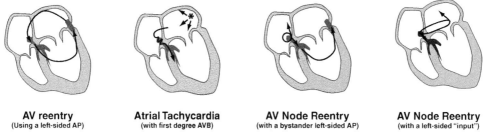

Figure 5.6 Schematic of the possible etiologies for a supraventricular tachycardia with an early signal in the left atrium and a short HA interval (and long AH interval). Of these possibilities, the most likely explanation is AVRT using a left-sided accessory pathway. The other options, while theoretically possible, are less likely.

the tachycardia and evaluate the subsequent response (Morady maneuver) or deliver scanning premature ventricular stimuli. In this case, with eccentric atrial activation making any of the possibilities with AVNRT as a basic mechanism highly unlikely the Morady maneuver can be useful for quickly ruling out atrial tachycardia. The advantage to scanning ventricular stimuli is that the electrophysiologist can specifically control the timing of the ventricular stimulus. Specifically, late coupled premature ventricular contractions can be delivered at a time when the His bundle is refractory or "committed" (Figure 5.7), so that there is no way the ventricular stimulus can travel retrogradely

to affect the AV node via the His bundle. In this case, a premature ventricular stimulus delivered 300 ms after the preceding QRS probably does not affect His bundle activation but does reset the tachycardia, as evidenced by the subsequent early atrial depolarization with the same activation sequence (Figure 5.8). Notice how difficult this maneuver can be sometimes. In this case, the electrophysiologist has to make a "best guess" that the signal after the ventricular stimulus represents an anterograde (or "committed") His electrogram. If true, finding "rules in" the diagnosis of AVRT using a left-sided accessory pathway. An earlier premature ventricular stimulus (coupling interval of 240 ms) leads

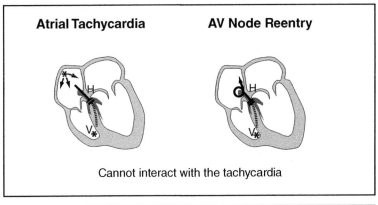

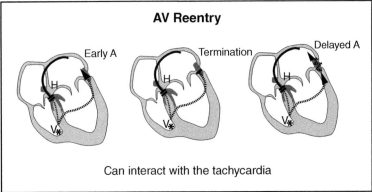

Figure 5.7 Schematic showing the usefulness of a premature ventricular stimulus during His bundle refractoriness. As the His bundle is "committed," unless there is also presence of an accessory pathway (an alternative path for retrograde ventriculoatrial conduction), the premature ventricular contraction will not interact with AVNRT or atrial tachycardia.

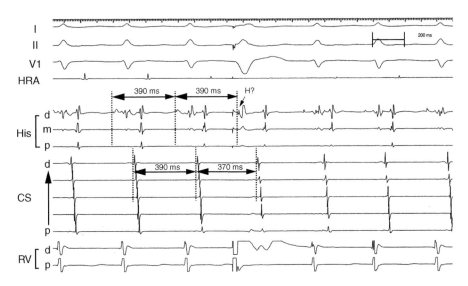

Figure 5.8 A premature ventricular stimulus at a coupling interval of 300 ms when the His bundle is refractory results in early activation of the atrium with the same pattern as baseline tachycardia. This finding "proves" the involvement of the left-sided accessory pathway as an integral part of the tachycardia, confirming the diagnosis of AVRT. One possible but *very* unlikely alternative explanation would be an atrial tachycardia located near or at the atrial insertion point of the accessory pathway.

to earlier activation of the atrium and termination of the tachycardia most likely due to anterograde block in the AV node (Figure 5.9). Unfortunately, this finding does not completely rule out atrial tachycardia because it is possible (although relatively unlikely) that the early atrial depolarization led to termination of the tachycardia. To completely rule out atrial tachycardia, the supraventricular tachycardia is reinduced and double ventricular stimuli are delivered (Figure 5.10). The first ventricular stimulus is delivered at a relatively long coupling interval to avoid interaction with the AV node but to facilitate ventricular activation and interaction with the accessory pathway. In this case, the tachycardia terminates because of retrograde activation into the AV node so that the AV node is refractory when it is engaged from above by the tachycardia wavefront. This finding of tachycardia "termination without an A" is evidence that the tachycardia is AV node dependent and "rules out" atrial tachycardia.

The method for evaluation with the Morady maneuver is shown in Figures 5.11 and 5.12. In Figure 5.11, ventricular pacing is delivered at a slightly shorter cycle length (370 ms) as compared to the tachycardia (393 ms). Atrial cycle lengths that are the same as the pacing interval confirm tachycardia entrainment, and on termination of pacing, a V-A-V response is noted,

"ruling out" atrial tachycardia (Chapter 2). Notice also that the first AH interval is longer than subsequent AH intervals. This common observation is due to either delayed conduction in the AV node because it is engaged sooner with pacing (atrial to atrial intervals of 370 ms) when compared to tachycardia (atrial to atrial intervals of 393 ms) or because of concealed retrograde activation into the AV node from the ventricular pacing stimuli. Regardless of the underlying mechanism, delay in the AV node results in more rapid AV conduction in the next beat of tachycardia. Despite these changes in AH intervals and changes in heart rate, the HA intervals remain constant or "hooked," suggesting that the H is associated with the following A. A constant HA interval despite tachycardia cycle length changes would not be observed in atrial tachycardia. It is also useful to examine the initial portion of the pacing train (Figure 5.12). Notice that ventricular pacing entrains atrial activation relatively early and before full ventricular capture. The ability to interact with the circuit early in the drive train suggests that the reentrant circuit is relatively large and makes AVRT using an accessory pathway the most likely diagnosis.

In addition to identifying a change in the tachycardia with the delivery of ventricular stimuli (either single or as a pacing "train"), changes in the behavior of the

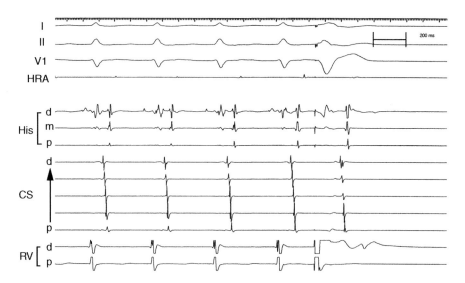

Figure 5.9 An earlier premature ventricular stimulus at a coupling interval of 240 ms results in early atrial depolarization and termination of the tachycardia. Although this would most likely be due to block in the AV node, it is possible (although unlikely) that the early atrial depolarization terminated an atrial tachycardia.

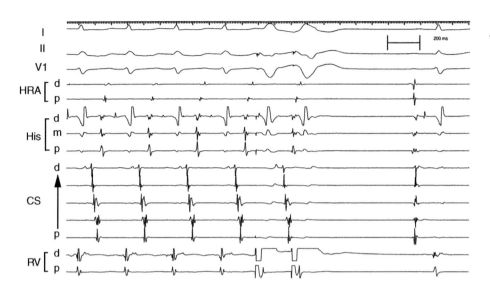

Figure 5.10 After tachycardia is reinitiated, two premature ventricular stimuli are delivered. The first ventricular extrastimulus delivered at a coupling interval of 230 ms is designed as a "conditioning" stimulus to shorten the retrograde refractory periods of the right bundle and His bundle and does not interact with the tachycardia. The second ventricular extrastimulus at a coupling interval of 230 ms leads to termination of the tachycardia without resetting the atrial electrogram. Termination is due to retrograde penetration into the AV node and AV node refractoriness when the anterograde wave of depolarization enters the AV node after atrial depolarization. This finding confirms AV node dependence of the tachycardia and "rules out" atrial tachycardia.

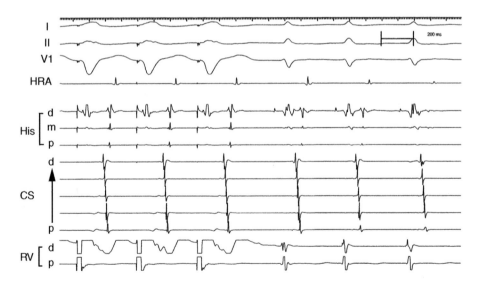

Figure 5.11 Pacing during tachycardia at a slightly faster cycle length entrains the tachycardia (shortening of the A-A intervals to the pacing cycle length), and on cessation of pacing, a V-A-V response is observed, thus "ruling out" atrial tachycardia that would have a V-A-A-V response (Figure 2.28). Notice also that the VA interval during pacing is similar to the HA interval during tachycardia, consistent with retrograde activation via an accessory pathway.

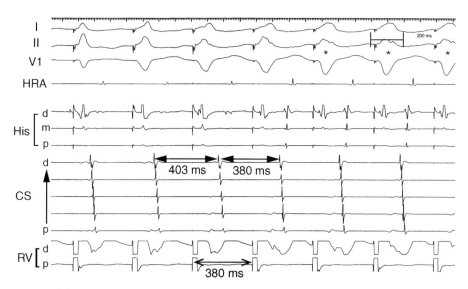

Figure 5.12 Inspection of the initial part of the pacing train can provide important clues to the arrhythmia mechanism. In this case, the tachycardia is reset before full ventricular capture (stable paced QRS complexes (*), a finding that suggests the tachycardia circuit is relatively large and uses ventricular tissue.

tachycardia during the development of bundle branch block can also be very useful. In the 1960s, Coumel described a decrease in the tachycardia cycle length with resolution of a bundle branch block suggesting the presence of AVRT using an ipsilateral accessory pathway (Figure 5.13). For example, in a patient with AVRT using a left-sided accessory pathway, resolution of left bundle branch block will be associated with shortening of the tachycardia circuit, as the left bundle is participating as a component of the reentrant circuit. In both AVNRT and atrial tachycardia, the left bundle would not be participating in the circuit, so resolution of left bundle branch block would not lead to a change in the cycle length. The electrograms illustrating "Coumels" sign during tachycardia are shown in Figure 5.14.

Although the diagnosis of AVRT using a left-sided accessory pathway has been confirmed in this patient, the clinician should acknowledge that a full electrophysiologic analysis has not been completed. At this point, anterograde properties of the AV node and the retrograde properties of the AV node and accessory pathway have not been assessed. It is always difficult to balance thoroughness and efficiency in the electrophysiology laboratory: more comprehensive evaluation reduces the likelihood of "missing something," but longer procedures may be associated with

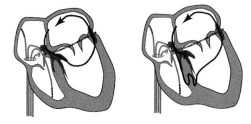

Normal His Purkinje conduction   Left bundle branch block

Figure 5.13 Schematic showing the mechanism of the Coumel's sign. Only in AVRT using an accessory pathway is the ipsilateral bundle an integral part of the tachycardia circuit. This means that if resolution of bundle branch block results in shortening of the tachycardia cycle length (an increase in heart rate) primarily mediated by shortening of the HA interval, the tachycardia must be using an accessory pathway located on the same side as the initial bundle branch block.

more complications due to sedation or vascular access problems. In this case, continuing gradual shortening of the atrial coupling interval will likely lead to repetitive episodes of tachycardia. Alternatively, the operator could start at very short atrial coupling intervals below the AERP and gradually increase the coupling interval until atrial capture occurs and evaluate whether AV node conduction follows. Generally, unless there is concern about atrioventricular conduction via the AV

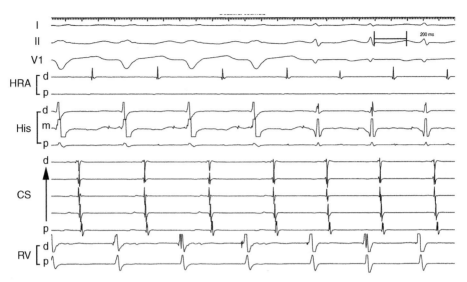

Figure 5.14 In this case, on resolution of left bundle branch block, the tachycardia cycle length shortens from 410 to 330 ms and the HA interval shortens from 235 to 135 ms. The AH interval increases slightly (175 ms during LBBB to 195 ms with normal ventricular depolarization) because more rapid atrial depolarization leads to some delay in the AV node.

node and His bundle, further definition of anterograde conduction properties of the AV node generally has a relatively low yield. In contrast, I believe that it is reasonable to at least generally assess the retrograde conduction properties of the accessory pathway and the AV node. Eccentric ventriculoatrial conduction during pacing is usually definitive proof that a nonseptal accessory pathway is present, although it does not prove that the accessory pathway is a necessary part of the clinical arrhythmia (it could be a "bystander"), and in *very* rare cases, retrograde activation via the AV node can be associated with eccentric activation of the coronary sinus. The response to ventricular pacing in our patient is shown in Figures 5.15 and 5.16; notice immediately the presence of eccentric atrial activation observed in the coronary sinus electrograms. The response to delivery of premature ventricular stimuli is shown in Figures 5.17–5.20. At a drive cycle length of 600 ms, a premature ventricular contraction at a coupling interval of 350 ms is associated with a VA conduction time of 150 ms with earliest atrial activation in the distal coronary sinus (Figure 5.17). When the coupling interval is shortened to 290 ms, notice the development of retrograde right bundle branch block, thus leading to a retrograde His bundle signal 135 ms after the ventricular stimulus (Figure 5.18). Notice that retrograde atrial activation in both the coronary

sinus and the His bundle region remains unaffected, which provides "proof" that retrograde conduction is independent of the His bundle. When the coupling interval is shortened to 280 ms, there is a dramatic change in the retrograde atrial activation pattern due to block in the accessory pathway, and now earliest atrial activation is in the proximal coronary sinus with a stimulus to earliest atrial electrogram interval of 324 ms, and the accessory pathway retrograde ERP is 280 ms (Figure 5.19). Further shortening of the coupling interval to 260 ms leads to loss of ventricular capture and a VERP of 260 ms (Figure 5.20). At this point, one could deliver double ventricular premature ventricular contractions to define the retrograde refractory period of the AV node, but again, the clinician must balance efficiency and thoroughness. Because the general characteristics of retrograde activation have been defined and there is no evidence of a second accessory pathway, it is reasonable for the electrophysiology study to move from the diagnostic to the therapeutic phase. The individual clinician will have to decide what is required for each study, and "the answer" will be different from practitioner to practitioner and from patient to patient.

One reason to perform catheter ablation in patients with accessory pathways is the small but measurable risk for sudden cardiac death in patients with accessory

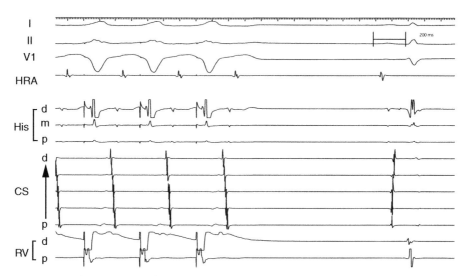

Figure 5.15 Constant ventricular pacing at a cycle length of 350 ms. Atrial activation is eccentric with first atrial depolarization in the distal coronary sinus.

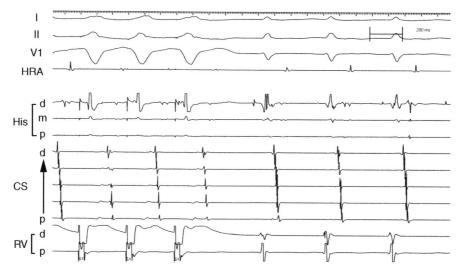

Figure 5.16 Continuation of ventricular pacing from Figure 5.15. Shortening the ventricular pacing cycle length (300 ms) reliably induces AVRT. The most likely explanation for this behavior is that at longer cycle lengths, concealed retrograde penetration into the AV node prevented anterograde activation of the AV node and initiation of AVRT. However, ventricular pacing at faster cycle lengths probably was associated with more proximal retrograde block in the His bundle–AV node axis so that anterograde AV node conduction could occur. This interpretation is supported by the alternating "long–short" atrioventricular intervals observed at the initial part of tachycardia.

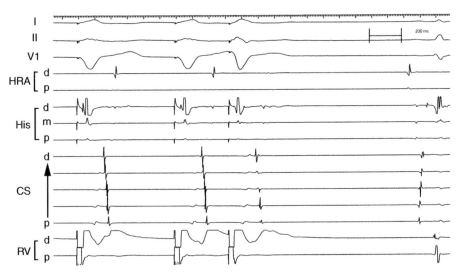

Figure 5.17 Ventricular premature stimulus at a coupling interval of 350 ms leads to a stimulus to atrial conduction time of 160 ms with earliest activation in the distal coronary sinus via the accessory pathway. Tachycardia does not start because the AV node is refractory (probably from concealed retrograde penetration into the AV node from the ventricular extrasimulus).

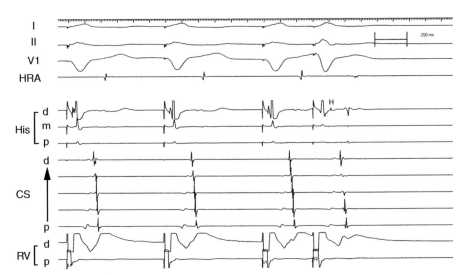

Figure 5.18 When the coupling interval is shortened to 290 ms, the stimulus to retrograde atrial activation remains the same at 160 ms, but in this case, a retrograde His recording (H) is observed with a stimulation to His interval of 105 ms. In this case, the retrograde His bundle signal is observed because of retrograde block in the right bundle. The unchanged stimulus to atrial activation interval proves that left-sided accessory pathway conduction is independent of conduction in the right bundle or His bundle. Tachycardia is not induced because of retrograde penetration (at least of the His bundle and likely the AV node).

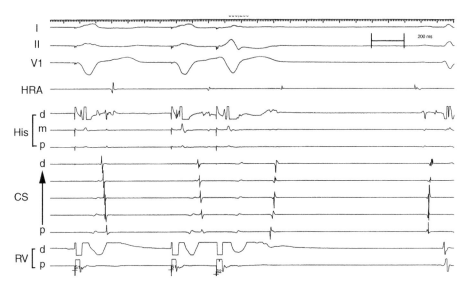

Figure 5.19 A coupling interval of 280 ms results in a dramatic change in the retrograde atrial activation pattern: earliest now in the proximal CS and with a stimulus to earliest atrial activation interval of 330 ms. This response is due to retrograde block of the accessory pathway and defines the retrograde APERP.

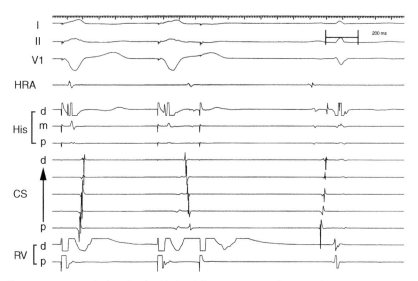

Figure 5.20 An earlier premature ventricular stimulus (260 ms) does not capture the ventricle thus defining the VERP.

pathways that can conduct anterogradely. This subject will be explored more fully in Chapter 7, but the very poor anterograde conduction properties of this accessory pathway suggests that this patient is at very low risk for sudden cardiac death. However, ablation is still a reasonable next step in this patient because of the symptoms associated with the supraventricular tachycardia.

There are several ways to map accessory pathways for ablation (Figure 5.21). Anterograde mapping is performed by identifying the earliest ventricular signal in the annular region during sinus rhythm or atrial pacing. Alternatively, retrograde mapping, identifying the earliest atrial signal, can be performed during ventricular pacing or during supraventricular tachycardia. The best and most efficient method for mapping will

Anterograde mapping

Retrograde mapping

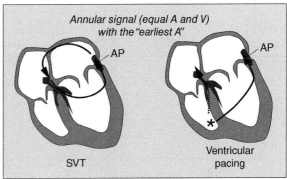

Figure 5.21 Schematic showing methods for ablation of accessory pathways. Anterograde mapping can by definition only be performed in accessory pathways with anterograde conduction. Mapping along the mitral and tricuspid annuli (equal atrial and ventricular electrogram amplitudes) and the earliest ventricular electrogram is identified. Retrograde mapping can be performed during supraventricular tachycardia or with ventricular pacing. Mapping during supraventricular tachycardia is advantageous because activation of the atria is solely through the accessory pathway, and concomitant depolarization via the AV node (dashed arrows) is not observed. However, with ablation of the accessory pathway during SVT, successful ablation will be associated with a dramatic change in heart rate.

vary from patient to patient. Anterograde mapping cannot be performed in patients who do not have manifest prexcitation and would be difficult in this patient with intermittent anterograde conduction. The effectiveness of retrograde mapping depends in the relative conduction properties of the accessory pathway and the AV node. With ventricular pacing, if the retrograde conduction properties of the AV node and the accessory pathway are similar, it may be difficult to map because of fusion between the two wavefronts. In supraventricular tachycardia, retrograde conduction is occurring solely through the accessory pathway, so fusion is not an issue, and the earliest atrial signal represents the atrial insertion point of the accessory pathway. The problem with this approach is the sudden rate change that occurs with ablation, which can sometimes lead to a shift in catheter position. In this patient, retrograde mapping during ventricular pacing is ideal because of the very different retrograde conduction properties of the accessory pathway and the AV node (fast conduction by the accessory pathway and slow conduction via the His AV node axis).

Although in the past a retrograde aortic approach was used for mapping and ablation of accessory pathways, this strategy has almost been completely supplanted by an atrial approach using transseptal puncture of the fossa ovalis to access the left atrium. Catheter stability is much easier to achieve with the left atrial approach, and older studies comparing the two techniques have shown the superiority of an atrial approach (both shorter procedure times and fewer complications). Catheter position using a catheter placed in the left atrium is shown in Figure 5.22.

Catheter ablation during ventricular pacing is shown in Figure 5.23. The earliest atrial signal during ventricular pacing is targeted. Generally, at the optimal site, the local ventriculoatrial conduction time will be short and the atrial and ventricular electrograms will be of similar amplitude (consistent with an annular position). Application of radiofrequency energy leads to

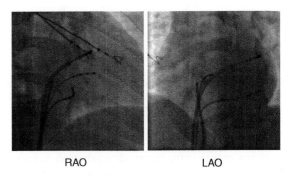

RAO　　　　　　　LAO

Figure 5.22 Fluoroscopic catheter positioning using a transseptal approach in the right anterior oblique (RAO) and left anterior oblique (LAO) projections.

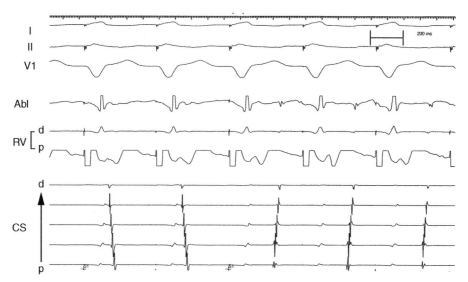

Figure 5.23 Ablation during ventricular pacing (cycle length of 450 ms). The catheter is moved along the annulus (equal atrial and ventricular electrogram amplitudes) until a site characterized by an early atrial signal is identified. Application of radiofrequency energy results in a change in the retrograde activation pattern due to block in the accessory pathway. The larger ventricular signal at this site suggests that the ablation catheter is located on the ventricular portion of the mitral annulus.

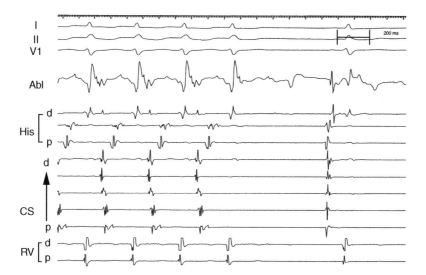

Figure 5.24 Another retrograde approach to ablation is identifying the earliest atrial signal during tachycardia. Although this strategy offers the advantage of eliminating fusion of retrograde activation via the AV node and the accessory pathway, sudden loss of accessory pathway conduction leads to termination of the tachycardia and a dramatic change in rate that can be associated with catheter instability.

an abrupt change in the retrograde conduction pattern during ablation. Figure 5.24 shows ablation during supraventricular tachycardia in another patient with a left-sided accessory pathway (in this case, earliest atrial activation in the coronary sinus is observed in the second to most distal electrode pair). The catheter is manipulated along the annulus to find the earliest atrial signal. Notice that the ablation catheter position is relatively ventricular (larger ventricular electrogram when compared to the atrial electrogram). Fortunately, in this case, when the tachycardia terminates with ablation, even with the dramatic rate change, the catheter remains fairly annular (equal atrial and ventricular electrogram amplitudes). One situation where retrograde mapping during supraventricular

tachycardia is arguably the best method for ablation is in the setting of a septal accessory pathway that is close to the His bundle. Figures 5.25 and 5.26 show the electrograms and fluoroscopic position of catheters in a patient undergoing ablation of a septal accessory pathway just above the His bundle. In supraventricular tachycardia, anterograde conduction via the AV node

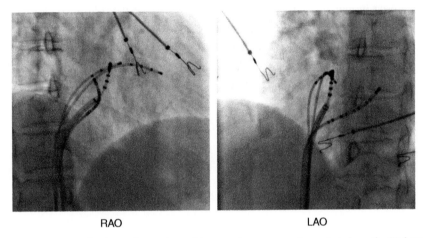

RAO   LAO

Figure 5.25 Fluoroscopic positions of catheters in a patient with a septal accessory pathway just above the His bundle.

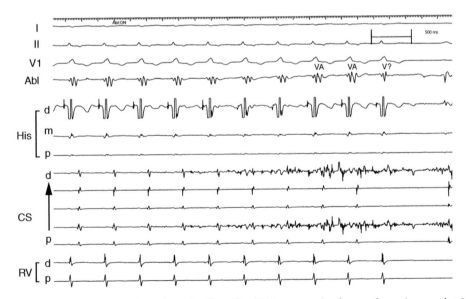

Figure 5.26 Ablation during supraventricular tachycardia allows the clinician to monitor for any change in normal atrioventricular conduction due to injury of the AV node. If any worrisome signs are observed, the ablation can be stopped quickly. With either anterograde mapping or retrograde mapping via ventricular pacing, normal atrioventricular conduction and accessory pathway conduction travel in the same direction, and identification of injury to the AV node may be delayed. An annular signal with equal ventricular (V) and atrial electrogram (A) amplitudes is identified. The tachycardia terminates with accessory pathway ablation (a ventricular signal without an accompanying atrial signal (?).

is completely separated from retrograde activation via the accessory pathway. Although catheter motion on termination can occur, this method allows the clinician to closely monitor normal AV node conduction and stop the ablation if any signs of AV nodal injury are observed such as prolongation of the AH interval or the development of transient atrioventricular block. Additional strategies for avoiding injury to the AV node for septal accessory pathways include mapping within the aortic cusps near the noncoronary and right coronary cusps, mapping the ventricular side of the tricuspid annulus by retroflexing the catheter underneath the tricuspid valve leaflets (because the His bundle may be separated from the ventricular insertion point of the accessory pathway by the fibrous annulus), or using cryoenergy (which often makes a smaller lesion than radiofrequency energy).

After ablation, pacing protocols are performed along with infusion of isoproterenol, and no evidence of recurrent accessory pathway conduction is observed. The patient has had no recurrent arrhythmias over a 2-year follow-up.

KEY POINTS

- Eccentric atrial activation during tachycardia usually "rules out" AVNRT, and the focus of the study is to differentiate AVRT from AT.

- Differentiating AT from AVRT focuses on confirming the participation of an accessory pathway as the retrograde limb during tachycardia (resetting or terminating the tachycardia when the AV node is refractory) or proving that the tachycardia is AV node dependent (spontaneous termination of the tachycardia with an atrial electrogram, termination of the tachycardia with a ventricular extrastimulus that does not reset the atrial signal) or that atrial activity is independent of the preceding ventricular electrogram (V-A-A-V response).

- Eccentric atrial activation during ventricular pacing generally confirms the presence of an accessory pathway and is the reason that many electrophysiologists perform ventricular pacing first during a diagnostic study.

CHAPTER 6

Supraventricular tachycardia case 5

A 64-year-old woman has had rapid heart rates since her 20s. Fifteen years ago, she underwent event recorder tracing, and supraventricular tachycardia was recorded (Figure 6.1). She has done well with conservative measures and has been able to control her arrhythmias with vagal maneuvers. Two years ago, she was started on atenolol with improvement in her symptoms. However, over the past year, the episodes of supraventricular tachycardias have become more frequent and more difficult to control despite atenolol.

Her physical examination is normal, and her baseline ECG shows no definitive evidence of preexcitation (Figure 6.2).

As mentioned in Chapter 2, drug refractory supraventricular tachycardia is an excellent reason to proceed to electrophysiologic testing. At electrophysiologic testing, catheters are placed in the standard positions: quadripolar catheters in the high right atrium, His position, and right ventricular apex and a decapolar catheter in the coronary sinus (Figure 1.3). Baseline conduction intervals are shown in Figure 6.3. The baseline cycle length is 830 ms (68 bpm), the QRS has a normal duration (90 ms) with no evidence of preexcitation, and the HV interval is 28 ms. Atrial pacing reveals an AVBCL of 350 ms without obvious changes in her QRS with atrioventricular block in the AV node (Figure 6.4).

Electrophysiologic response to atrial premature beats at a basic drive cycle length of 600 ms is shown in Figures 6.5–6.7. With atrial premature beats, a few "extra beats" are observed with earliest atrial activation on the distal coronary sinus (Figure 6.5). This could represent a clue to possible cause of the arrhythmia (perhaps a left-sided atrial tachycardia, a slowly conducting left-sided accessory pathway, or a left-sided input in the AV node) or simply be a nonspecific finding from interatrial reentry (often called "trash" in the

electrophysiology laboratory). Continued testing yields an AERP of 250 ms (Figure 6.6) and an AVNERP of 330 ms that requires the use of two premature atrial beats ("doubles") at coupling intervals of 340 and 330 ms (Figure 6.7).

Initial ventricular pacing at 600 ms reveals 1:1 ventriculoatrial conduction, and the astute reader will notice that there are subtle differences in the pattern of retrograde atrial activation between the first and subsequent ventricular paced beats (Figure 6.8). Although fusion from intrinsic sinus rhythm is always possible when this phenomenon is observed, this is unlikely in this case because of the change in activation sequence in the high right atrial electrograms. More likely, this represents two patterns of retrograde activation, either because of different "breakthrough points" from the AV node or because of the presence of a discrete accessory pathway. The response to progressively more premature ventricular stimuli (400, 380, 370, and 360 ms) is shown in Figures 6.9–6.12. Interestingly, this demonstrates the possibility of a third retrograde atrial activation pattern characterized by a long VA conduction time (stimulus to distal CS is 360 ms) that is similar to the extra beats identified during delivery of atrial extrastimuli (Figure 6.10). The sequence of premature ventricular stimuli demonstrates that the retrograde atrial activation pattern characterized by earliest atrial activation in the mid-coronary sinus (electrodes 5,6) has decremental conduction properties (Figures 6.9 and 6.11). At this point, we have possibilities rather than certainties. There are apparently three retrograde atrial activation patterns: earliest superiorly at the His catheter, earliest in the mid-coronary sinus, and earliest at the distal coronary sinus. It is likely that the first two responses simply represent different regions of initial retrograde atrial activation from the AV node (either superiorly or more inferiorly in the coronary sinus). The last response

Understanding Intracardiac EGMs: A Patient Centered Guide, First Edition. Fred Kusumoto.
© 2015 John Wiley & Sons, Ltd. Published 2015 by John Wiley & Sons, Ltd.

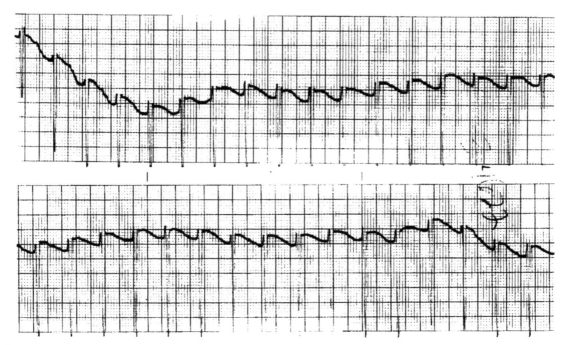

Figure 6.1 Event recorder tracing showing supraventricular tachycardia.

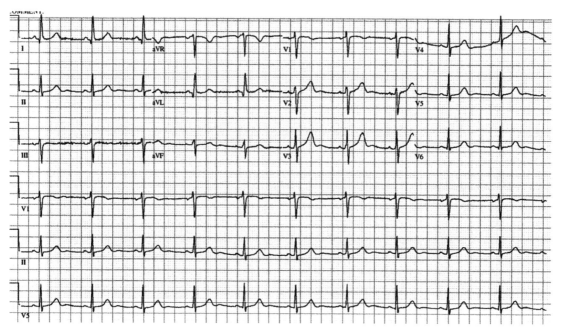

Figure 6.2 Baseline ECG is essentially normal although subtle QRS notching is noted in lead V3.

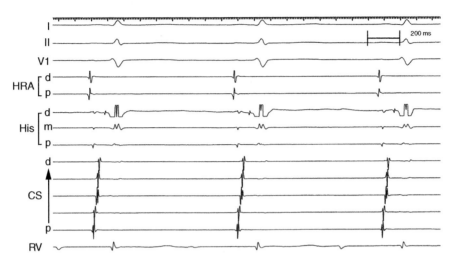

Figure 6.3 Baseline intervals. The basic cycle length is 881 ms (68 bpm), and the QRS duration is 90 ms with no evidence of preexcitation or other abnormalities. The HV interval is normal (28 ms).

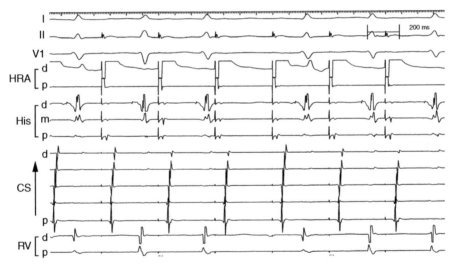

Figure 6.4 Atrial pacing at 350 ms leads to a Wenckebach response due to block within the AV node. Atrial pacing is not associated with any obvious large changes in the QRS complexes.

is more interesting, characterized by very eccentric retrograde atrial activation with similar "echo" beats noted from both atrial pacing and ventricular pacing maneuvers.

At this juncture in the electrophysiology study, it is critical to induce sustained tachycardia and an isoproterenol infusion is started. This leads to an increase in the basal heart rate to 90 bpm, and with atrial pacing at 400 ms, supraventricular tachycardia

is induced (Figure 6.13). The tachycardia cycle length is 370 ms with an HA interval of 271 ms with earliest atrial activation in the distal coronary sinus. Now that sustained supraventricular tachycardia is induced, the response to ventricular overdrive pacing or scanning premature ventricular stimulation can be performed. In this case, single scanning ventricular stimuli are delivered. A relatively late ventricular stimulus delivered at a time when the His bundle is refractory

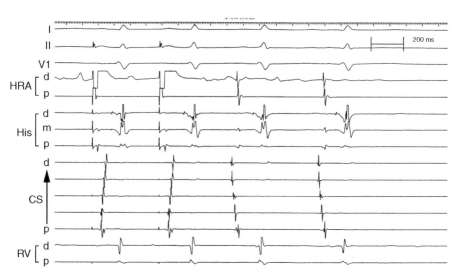

Figure 6.5 An atrial premature stimulus (420 ms) at a basic drive cycle length of 600 ms is associated with two additional beats characterized by a narrow QRS and earliest activation in the distal coronary sinus.

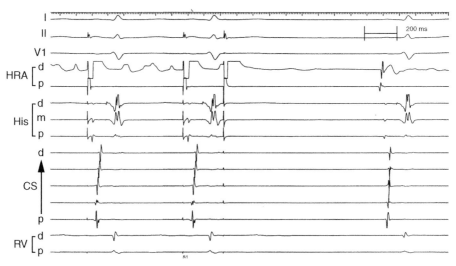

Figure 6.6 An atrial premature stimulus (250 ms) defines the atrial effective refractory period.

(R to stimulus interval of 350 ms) does not reset the tachycardia (Figure 6.14) – a finding that provides no information on tachycardia mechanism. However, an earlier ventricular stimulus (R to stimulus interval of 240 ms) terminates the tachycardia without resetting the atrial electrogram, thus providing strong evidence that the tachycardia is AV node dependent and ruling out a left atrial tachycardia (Figure 6.15). Supporting evidence ruling out a left atrial tachycardia is observed during spontaneous initiation of the supraventricular

tachycardia and is shown in Figure 6.16. In this case, a spontaneous premature atrial contraction from the right atrium (probably catheter-induced given the very early atrial activation observed in the distal high right atrial signal) initiates the tachycardia. Notice that the HA interval for both the first and second beats of tachycardia is the same despite changes in cycle length. This suggests that the HA intervals are "hooked" and thus related. Remember that in atrial tachycardia, the AH intervals are coupled and the HA intervals are

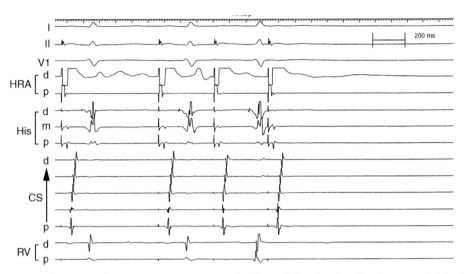

Figure 6.7 Double atrial premature beats (340 ms, 330 ms) are used to better define the AV node refractory period. In this case, the AV node effective refractory period (330 ms) is longer than the atrial effective refractory period obtained from Figure 6.7 because the first extrastimulus does interact with the AV node as evidenced by the prolongation of the AH interval when compared to the AH interval observed during the basic drive.

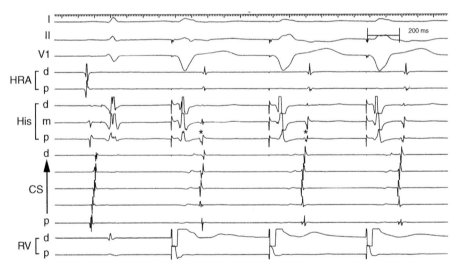

Figure 6.8 Initiation of ventricular pacing demonstrates subtle changes in retrograde atrial activation. The first ventricular paced beat leads to retrograde activation that is earliest in the proximal electrode of the His bundle (*) and the mid-portion of the coronary sinus, while the second ventricular paced beat has a longer VA interval and activation in the mid-portion of the coronary sinus precedes atrial activation in the His bundle. It is likely that these two atrial signals are from the ventricular paced beats because the interval between earliest atrial signals is the same as the ventricular paced rate, activation in the high right atrial electrodes is similar, and both are different from the sinus beat.

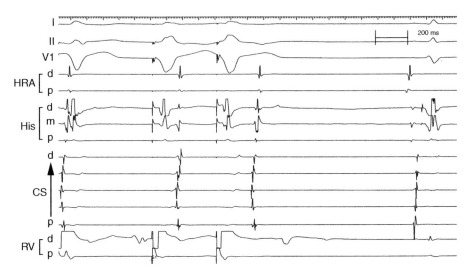

Figure 6.9 At a basic cycle length of 600 ms, a premature ventricular stimulus (400 ms) is associated with retrograde activation earliest in the coronary sinus and a stimulus to earliest atrial electrogram interval of 200 ms.

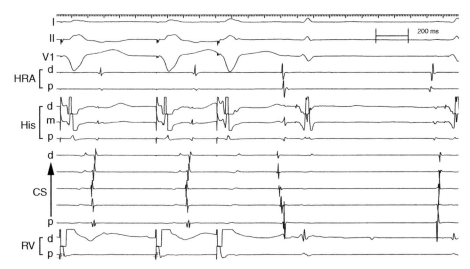

Figure 6.10 When compared to Figure 6.9, an earlier premature ventricular stimulus (380 ms) leads to an apparent change in the retrograde atrial activation pattern (earliest in the distal coronary sinus) and lengthening of the stimulus to atrial electrogram (380 ms) and an "echo" beat (the "extra" QRS complex).

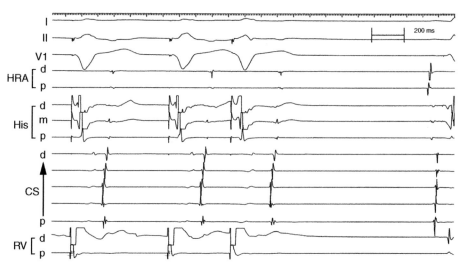

Figure 6.11 An earlier premature ventricular stimulus (370 ms) is associated with return of the atrial activation pattern observed in Figure 6.9 with lengthening of the stimulus to atrial electrogram interval (230 ms). Although this is likely due to decremental properties for this retrograde atrial activation pattern (suggesting that this may represent retrograde AV node conduction), intraventricular delay or delay in the right bundle or His bundle cannot be ruled out.

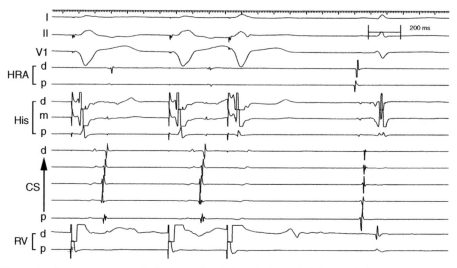

Figure 6.12 Shortening the premature ventricular interval to 360 ms leads to block in ventriculoatrial conduction, defining the baseline VAERP.

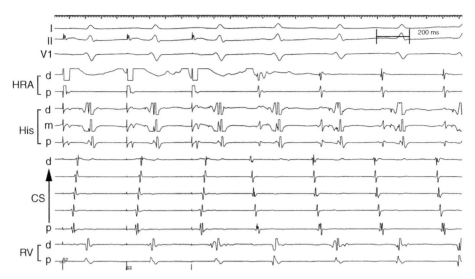

Figure 6.13 Atrial pacing induces a "long R-P" tachycardia associated with eccentric atrial activation with earliest atrial signal observed in the distal coronary sinus.

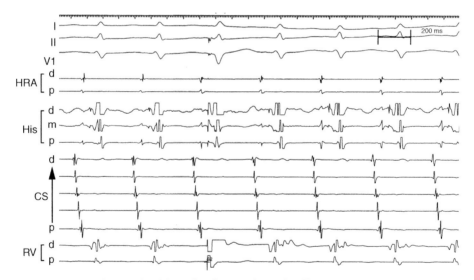

Figure 6.14 A premature ventricular stimulus delivered at the time the His bundle is "committed" does not reset the tachycardia. This response is not surprising given the QRS fusion, suggesting that a significant portion of the ventricles is being activated by the His Purkinje system.

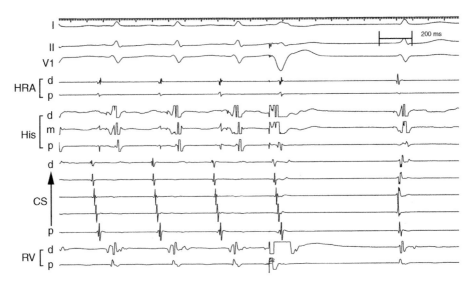

Figure 6.15 An earlier premature ventricular contraction is associated with more ventricular capture than the previous PVC (notice the QRS change), and importantly, this terminates the tachycardia without resetting the atrial electrogram. This important finding proves that the tachycardia is AV node dependent.

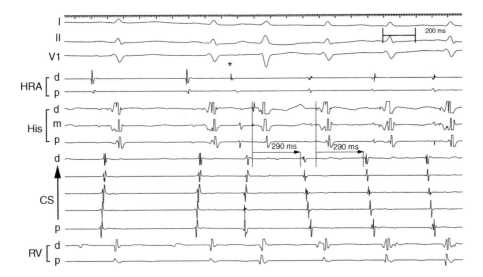

Figure 6.16 Spontaneous initiation of the tachycardia due to a premature atrial contraction (*) probably due to mechanical stimulation from the high right atrial catheter. In this case, the HA intervals during tachycardia are the same (290 ms), suggesting they are dependent on each other or "hooked." This is supporting evidence that an atrial tachycardia is not present and that some form of consistent retrograde conduction is a part of the tachycardia mechanism.

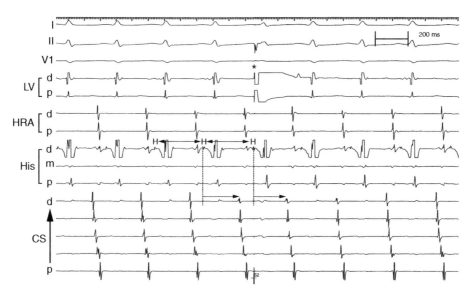

Figure 6.17 A left ventricular premature ventricular beat (*) delivered when the His bundle (H) is refractory leads to shortening of the VA interval with the same atrial activation pattern.

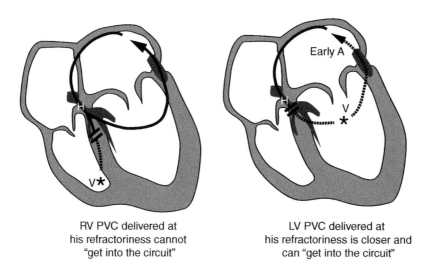

RV PVC delivered at
his refractoriness cannot
"get into the circuit"

LV PVC delivered at
his refractoriness is closer and
can "get into the circuit"

Figure 6.18 Schematic showing how a His refractory left ventricular premature ventricular stimulus is more likely to interact with a tachycardia using a left-sided accessory pathway.

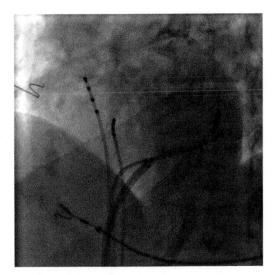

Figure 6.19 Left anterior oblique view with a steerable catheter advanced beyond the distal electrode of the coronary sinus.

accessory pathway (but not so slow that the left atrium is activated via the AV node) and AVNRT with a left-sided retrograde pathway. We will revisit this difficult issue in Chapter 9. However, a very useful maneuver for identifying the presence of a left-sided accessory pathway is the delivery of a His refractory left ventricular stimulus (Figure 6.17). Because a left ventricular stimulus will be closer to (or perhaps within) the reentrant circuit, it will more likely interact with a tachycardia that uses a left-sided accessory pathway (Figure 6.18). In this case, left atrial access is obtained and a catheter placed in the left ventricle. When a pacing stimulus is delivered (R-stimulus interval of 290 ms), the tachycardia is reset with the same retrograde activation pattern by 10 ms. This finding confirms the presence of AVRT using a slowly conducting left-sided accessory pathway.

Now that the mechanism of the tachycardia has been established, the focus of the study shifts to localizing the accessory pathway and successfully ablating it. As there has been no evidence of anterograde conduction, the accessory pathway must be mapped retrogradely. Unfortunately, because of competition between the AV node and the slowly conducting accessory pathway during ventricular pacing, the only effective way to map this slowly conducting left-sided accessory pathway is during tachycardia. As earliest atrial activation occurs in the distal coronary sinus, attempts are

independent (although they can be constant in a stable tachycardia with consistent AV conduction).

Although a tachycardia using a slowly conducting accessory pathway is "by odds" the most likely cause of this supraventricular tachycardia, two unlikely presentations of AVNRT have to at least be considered: an atypical AVNRT and a slowly conducting bystander

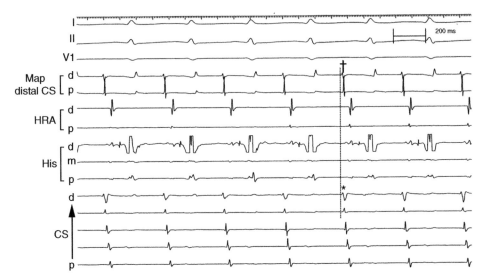

Figure 6.20 Electrograms recorded from the catheter positions noted in Figure 6.19. Notice that the more distal coronary sinus electrograms (†) are not substantially earlier than the electrograms recorded on the distal pair of electrodes of the decapolar catheter (*).

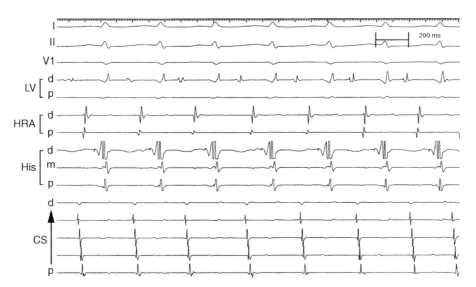

Figure 6.21 The endocardial surface of the mitral annulus is mapped, and the earliest atrial electrogram during tachycardia is measured at the lateral wall of the mitral annulus. The atrial electrogram is substantially earlier than the distal coronary sinus. Notice that the interval between ventricular and atrial signal remains relatively long when compared to the local conduction time usually recorded in accessory pathways, suggesting that this pathway has relatively slow conduction properties.

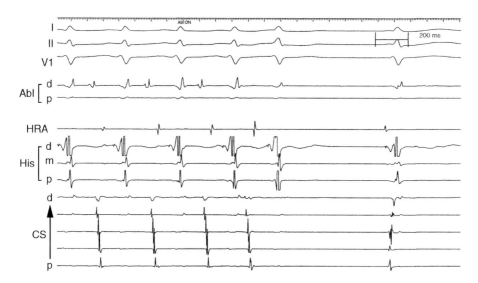

Figure 6.22 Application of radiofrequency energy leads to prompt termination of the tachycardia. However, notice that at termination, the atrial signal is early due to either a premature atrial contraction (spontaneous or catheter induced from the coronary sinus catheter) or transient improvement in accessory pathway conduction (destruction of a "more robust" slowly conducting branch of the accessory pathway, or facilitated conduction due to heating).

initially made to advance the coronary sinus catheter. However, because of a prominent Valve of Vieussens, the standard unidirectional deflecting catheter cannot be advanced farther, and a steerable mapping catheter is advanced more distally (Figure 6.19). Interestingly, the electrogram recorded in this case is not substantially different from the distal electrodes of the coronary sinus catheter (Figure 6.20), and it is elected to simply map the mitral annulus from the endocardial surface via transseptal access. The earliest atrial signal was observed at the true lateral mitral annulus (Figure 6.21), and delivery of radiofrequency energy led to termination of the tachycardia within several seconds (Figure 6.22). Radiofrequency energy delivery was continued, but it should be noted that the termination was "not clean." Notice that the tachycardia terminates with an early atrial that could be due to a premature atrial contraction or more rapid conduction in the accessory pathway. The apparent large ventricular electrogram on termination is due to simultaneous atrial depolarization from the sinus node (upright P wave in lead II) and a junctional escape beat. Fortunately, even after prolonged monitoring and higher doses of isoproterenol, no evidence of recurrent accessory pathway conduction was observed and the patient has remained arrhythmia free for 2 years.

KEY POINTS

- Although most accessory pathways exhibit relatively fast conduction properties, in some cases, accessory pathways can have slower conduction and in some cases decremental conduction.

- The diagnosis always focuses on differentiating among atrial tachycardia, AVNRT, and AVRT.

- Left-sided ventricular stimulation can be useful in confirming the diagnosis of AVRT in patients with left-sided accessory pathways.

- Ablation strategy depends on the electrophysiologic properties of the accessory pathway.

CHAPTER 7

Supraventricular tachycardia case 6: baseline preexcitation

A 17-year-old woman has known Wolff–Parkinson–White Syndrome. She underwent an attempted radiofrequency catheter ablation for a left inferior accessory pathway from a coronary sinus and retrograde aortic approach. Unfortunately, catheter ablation was not successful, and the patient has had continued palpitations associated with rapid narrow QRS tachycardia on 24-h ECG monitoring. Otherwise, she has no significant medical history, and her physical examination is normal.

Her baseline ECG is shown in Figure 7.1. This demonstrates obvious preexcitation with a short PR interval and delta waves. A number of excellent algorithms have been developed to help identify the location of an accessory pathway on the basis of the QRS morphology focusing on the initial portion of the QRS complex, as this reflects the portion of ventricular activation due solely to the accessory pathway (delta waves). From a practical standpoint, because the left ventricle is located leftward and more posteriorly relative to the right ventricle, left-sided accessory pathways are often associated with prominent R waves in leads V1 and V2 and an earlier precordial transition, while right-sided accessory pathways have a later precordial transition (see Figure 9.1 in Understanding Intracardiac EGMs and ECGs). Inferior accessory pathways are associated with negative delta waves in leads II, III, and aVF because depolarization via the accessory pathway leads to initial inferior to superior activation of the ventricles. Finally, right-sided accessory pathways are associated with more obvious delta waves. Remember that at baseline, ventricular depolarization represents a fusion of depolarization from the accessory pathway and the normal AV conduction system. As the

sinus node is located in the right atrium and the AV node and His bundle are septal structures, a left-sided accessory pathway is depolarized after the AV node, while a right-sided accessory pathway is depolarized before the AV node. A right-sided accessory pathway gets a "head start" as compared to the AV node, so more of the ventricles are activated via the accessory pathway. In contrast, left-sided accessory pathways are depolarized after AV node depolarization, and the amount of ventricular tissue activated via the accessory pathway may be very small and the delta wave is very subtle particularly in younger patients with more rapid AV node conduction. In this case, the QRS complexes are characterized by prominent R waves in V1 and V2, and the delta waves are negative in the inferior leads that localize this accessory pathway to the inferior and posterior portion of the left ventricle.

It is reasonable to consider a repeat electrophysiology study given the patient's symptoms. However, given the prior unsuccessful ablation attempt, it is important to consider what "can be different" this time to increase the likelihood of success. Firstly, although ablation of left inferior accessory pathways can be performed using a retrograde aortic approach, a transseptal approach is often simpler and provides more stable catheter placement. The second issue is coronary sinus anatomy. Some patients with left inferior accessory pathways may have venous anomalies, including unusual venous branches or diverticulum that can make ablation particularly challenging.

The patient is brought to the electrophysiology laboratory, and her baseline electrograms are shown in Figure 7.2. The QRS complex is very wide (160 ms), the PR interval is extremely short, the QRS complex appears to be continuous with the P wave (no isoelectric segment), and an obvious His bundle

Understanding Intracardiac EGMs: A Patient Centered Guide, First Edition. Fred Kusumoto.
© 2015 John Wiley & Sons, Ltd. Published 2015 by John Wiley & Sons, Ltd.

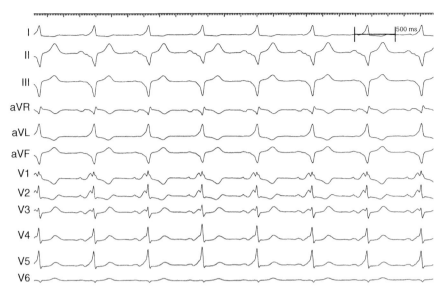

Figure 7.1 Baseline ECG. The QRS is wide and bizarre with prominent R waves in the right precordial leads (V1 and V2) and an initial negative deflection in the inferior leads. These findings suggest a left-sided inferior accessory pathway.

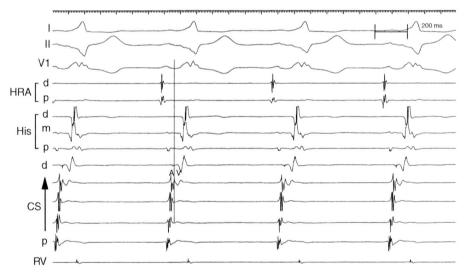

Figure 7.2 Baseline electrograms show no obvious His bundle deflection. An early ventricular signal (V) is observed in the second-to-most-distal electrode pair in the coronary sinus. It can often be difficult to distinguish atrial signals (A) form ventricular signals, but generally in the coronary sinus, the atrial signal has higher frequency ("is sharper") than the ventricular signal.

electrogram cannot be observed. Close inspection of the electrograms suggests that the tip of the coronary sinus catheter may be in a ventricular branch (relatively large ventricular signal and a very small atrial signal) and that the far-field ventricular signal (suggested because of the broad low-amplitude and low-frequency characteristics) in the second-to-most

distal coronary signal is extremely early. This finding of early ventricular activation provides an important clue that this electrode pair may be very close to the ventricular insertion point of the accessory pathway. Atrial pacing helps define the electrophysiologic properties of the accessory pathway (Figures 7.3 and 7.4). As increasing the atrial pacing rate slows AV

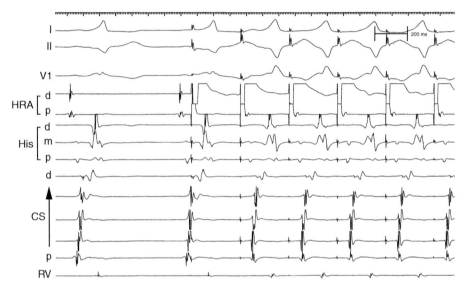

Figure 7.3 Atrial pacing at a cycle length of 300 ms results in a broader, "more bizarre" QRS complex because a larger portion of the ventricles is depolarized by the accessory pathway rather than the AV node.

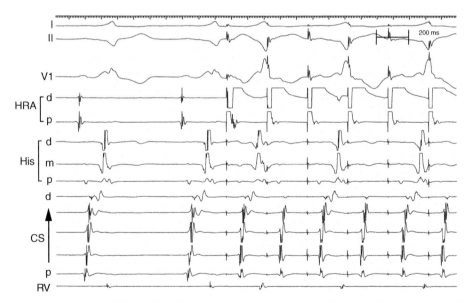

Figure 7.4 At a pacing cycle length of 250 ms, 2:1 atrioventricular block is noted due to block in both the accessory pathway and the AV node.

conduction without generally changing conduction via the accessory pathway, the QRS complex becomes more "bizarre," as more of the ventricles are depolarized via the accessory pathway relative to ventricular activation from the His Purkinje system (Figure 7.3). At an atrial pacing rate of 250 ms, 2:1 atrioventricular conduction develops due to block in both the accessory pathway and the AV node (Figure 7.4). The behavior in response to more rapid pacing will depend on the relative refractory properties of the accessory pathway and the AV node and whether retrograde penetration is present. For example, in this case, the AV node may not conduct because of an intrinsically long ERP or because accessory pathway conduction from the prior atrial paced beat was associated with retrograde activation into the AV node as shown in Figure 7.5 (this phenomenon is called concealed penetration). Because ventricular depolarization in the presence of an accessory pathway is due to both the accessory pathway and the AV node, pacing from a site closer to the accessory pathway will lead to more ventricular tissue depolarized by the accessory pathway as compared to the AV node and a wider and more bizarre QRS complex (Figure 7.6).

After atrial pacing at a constant rate is performed, the anterograde electrophyiologic properties of the accessory pathway can be further evaluated by the use of atrial extrastimuli (Figures 7.7 and 7.8). At a basic cycle length of 600 ms, a premature atrial contraction with a coupling interval at 260 ms is associated with ventricular depolarization via the accessory pathway, and at a coupling interval of 250 ms, there is block in the accessory pathway. The baseline effective refractory period for the accessory pathway is 250 ms. Careful inspection of the His electrograms shows a high-frequency His signal during pacing at the drive cycle length that is not observed with the premature stimuli.

The anterograde conduction properties of the accessory pathway have important clinical ramifications. Patients with accessory pathways that can be associated with rapid ventricular activation due to a short refractory period of the accessory pathway may be at risk for sudden cardiac death. The absolute risk for sudden death is controversial, and data from the Mayo Clinic and other large registries have estimated a risk of 0.09–0.60%, while a more recent analysis from Milan found a much higher risk, up to 2% in children. Regardless of the absolute risk, the data consistently show that patients with accessory pathways with very rapid anterograde conduction are more likely to have sudden cardiac death. An accessory pathway ERP <250 ms or a shortest R–R interval of 250 ms during atrial fibrillation has been historically used as cut-offs for defining patients at risk for sudden cardiac

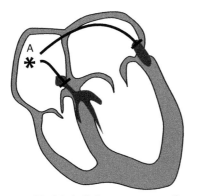

Block in both the accessory pathway and the AV node because of intrinsic electrophysiologic properties

(a)

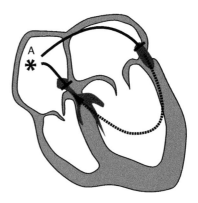

Block in both the accessory pathway and the AV node because of concealed retrograde penetration from the preceding ventricular depolarization

(b)

Figure 7.5 Schematic showing two possible explanations for the development of 2:1 atrioventricular block: intrinsic electrophysiologic properties of both the AV node and accessory pathway (a) or concealed penetration into the AV node from prior depolarization of the accessory pathway represented by the dashed arrow (b).

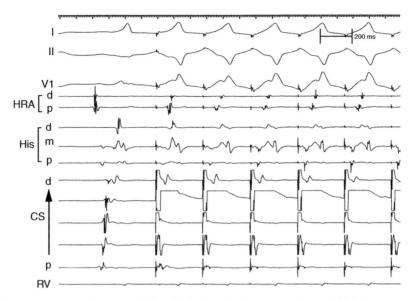

Figure 7.6 Pacing from the coronary sinus at a cycle length of 280 ms leads to a very abnormal QRS due to more ventricular depolarization via the left-sided accessory pathway.

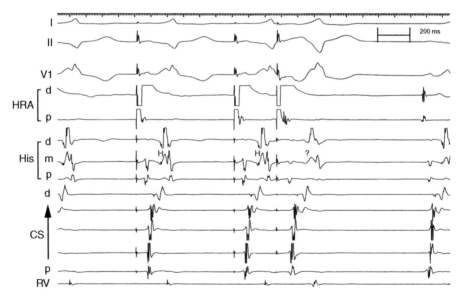

Figure 7.7 At a basic pacing cycle length of 600 ms, a premature atrial stimulus at a coupling interval of 260 ms is associated with ventricular activation via the accessory pathway. Notice that a His deflection (H) can be observed with pacing at the basic drive cycle length but not with the premature atrial stimulus (?) because of either block or delay in the AV node.

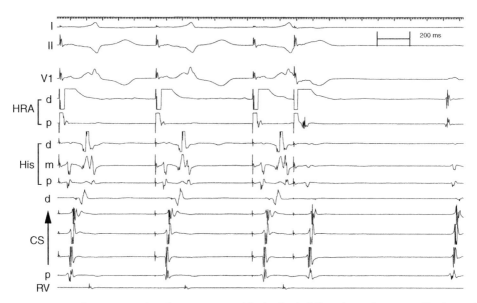

Figure 7.8 In continuation of Figure 7.7, when the premature atrial stimulus is delivered at a shorter coupling interval (250 ms), accessory pathway conduction is blocked, thus defining the ERP of the accessory pathway (250 ms). As atrial depolarization is not associated with depolarization via the AV node and a narrow QRS complex, the likely explanation for the findings in Figure 7.7 is block in the AV node rather than delay.

death, although it should be acknowledged that the great majority of patients, even those with accessory pathways with rapid conduction properties, will not have sudden cardiac death because the absolute rate is low regardless of the estimate used.

Once the anterograde properties of the accessory pathway and the AV node are defined, ventricular pacing is used to evaluate retrograde conduction properties. In a patient with an accessory pathway, retrograde conduction usually can occur via the His bundle and AV node or the accessory pathway, although a very small percentage of accessory pathways can only conduct anterogradely. With ventricular pacing at a cycle length of 400 ms, 1:1 ventriculoatrial conduction is observed, and although earliest atrial activation is difficult to define (it appears to be earliest in the proximal coronary sinus region or the His bundle region), the atrial electrogram precedes retrograde His depolarization (Figure 7.9). With more rapid ventricular pacing, the retrograde atrial activation sequence changes with earliest atrial activation in the second-to-most distal electrode pair in the coronary sinus that clearly precedes atrial depolarization in the His bundle (Figure 7.10).

With the onset of pacing, there is prolongation of the ventriculoatrial interval that "settles down" to 2:1 conduction. The two patterns of retrograde atrial activation suggest two ways for atrial activation to occur: either via the His bundle and the AV node or via an accessory pathway. Delivery of premature ventricular beats defines the ventricular ERP but does not define the retrograde refractory period for the accessory pathway (Figures 7.11 and 7.12).

At this point, there are several options. Isoproterenol can be started to induce supraventricular tachycardia and to provide additional information on the electrophysiologic properties of the accessory pathway. If the patient was asymptomatic and the goal of electrophysiologic testing is to define risk for sudden cardiac death, this would be the next step. However, in a patient with obvious preexcitation and documented supraventricular tachycardia, an alternative strategy is to map and ablate the accessory pathway and after ablation evaluate whether tachycardia is present and use isoproterenol then if required. The latter strategy has the advantage of performing the ablation without relative tachycardia and perhaps catheter instability due

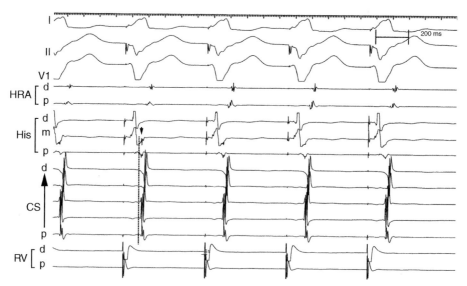

Figure 7.9 With ventricular pacing at a cycle length of 400 ms, 1:1 ventriculoatrial conduction is observed ("for every V there is an A), and atrial activation appears to occur simultaneously in the coronary sinus and the His bundle region (dashed vertical line) and precede His bundle depolarization (arrow).

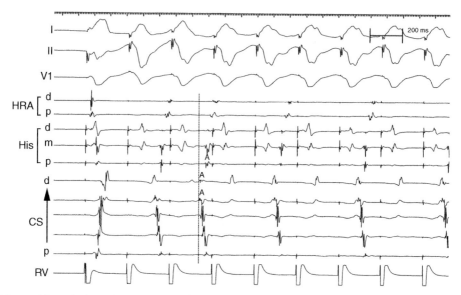

Figure 7.10 More rapid ventricular pacing (280 ms) results in 2:1 retrograde ventriculoatrial conduction, and atrial signals (A) in the coronary sinus clearly precede those recorded in the His bundle region.

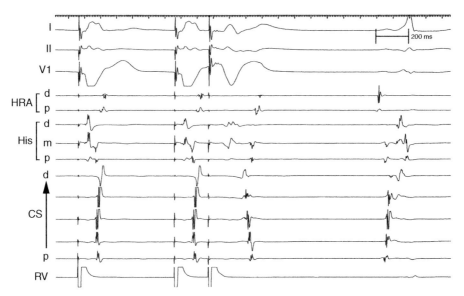

Figure 7.11 Ventricular pacing at a drive cycle length of 400 ms is followed by a premature ventricular stimulus at a coupling interval of 210 ms. During the drive cycle, retrograde depolarization appears to be occurring in the AV node, but with the premature ventricular stimulation, there is retrograde block in the AV node and conduction solely up the accessory pathway characterized by a change in the atrial activation pattern with late atrial activation of the His bundle region.

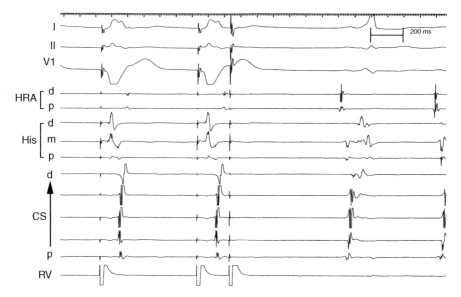

Figure 7.12 Continuation of Figure 7.11. The coupling interval is shortened to 200 ms and results in loss of ventricular capture, defining the VERP.

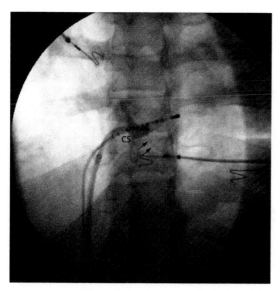

Figure 7.13 Angiogram of the coronary sinus (CS) showing normal anatomy and a small posterolateral vein (arrows).

to residual isoproterenol and shortening the procedure time but has the disadvantage of not fully defining the accessory pathway's electrophysiologic properties and identifying the exact mechanisms of sustained arrhythmias.

In this case, direct mapping of the accessory pathway is chosen, and as a first step, an angiogram of the coronary sinus is performed to identify any unusual venous anatomy. Angiography demonstrates no abnormal venous anatomy (Figure 7.13). Transseptal puncture is performed to obtain left atrial access and the mitral annulus is mapped. Mitral annular position is identified by atrial and ventricular electrograms with equal amplitude and consistent electrogram recordings suggesting stable catheter position. In Figure 7.14, the catheter position is unstable and moves from a more atrial position in the first beat, annular signals for the second and third beats, and a ventricular location for the fourth beat. Although it is reasonable to use a short or fused "local" atrioventricular conduction time as a first estimate for a possible accessory pathway location, as shown in Figure 7.15, it is important to identify a site where the ventricular signal is earlier than any ventricular signal (an early "global" signal). Compare Figures 7.14 and 7.16. In Figure 7.16, the electrograms are stable, have a short "local" atrioventricular interval (the two signals are continuous), and the ventricular signal precedes the earliest ventricular signal identified on the coronary sinus electrograms. The onset of the QRS complex should also be used, but in this case, the onset of the QRS is difficult to identify because of

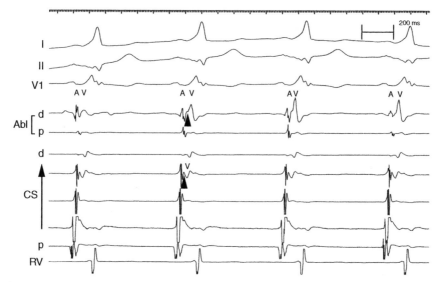

Figure 7.14 Ablation catheter placed along the mitral annulus. The changes in relative amplitudes of the atrial and ventricular signals suggest that while the catheter is located near the mitral annulus it has an unstable position. Notice that although the "local" atrioventricular time appears excellent (the atrial and ventricular signals are almost fused), the ventricular signal (V) on the ablation catheter is significantly later than the earliest ventricular signal recorded by the decapolar coronary sinus catheter (arrowheads).

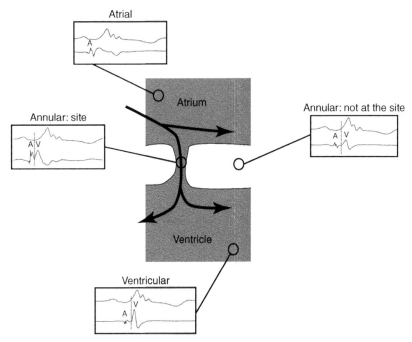

Figure 7.15 Schematic of anterograde mapping the location of the accessory pathway during sinus rhythm. The catheter tip is moved to different sites. Annular sites can be identified by comparing the relative sizes of the atrial (A) and ventricular (V) electrograms. If the catheter tip is at the annulus, the atrial and ventricular electrograms will have similar amplitudes. Atrial locations will have larger atrial signals, and ventricular sites will have larger ventricular signals. Once on the annulus, the site of the accessory pathway can be identified by locating the site with the earliest ventricular signal relative to the onset of the QRS complex. (Adapted from Kusumoto 2009.)

fusion with the P wave. In Figure 7.17, application of radiofrequency energy leads to a progressive change in the QRS complex with final normalization.

After the ablation, as shown in Figure 7.18, although the QRS complex has changed dramatically from baseline and an isoelectric portion of the PR interval can now be observed, the HV interval remains short. However, atrial pacing demonstrates prolongation of the AH interval, and the His bundle signal always precedes the QRS complex. This response is characteristic of a fasciculoventricular accessory pathway that leads to relatively early ventricular activation in the His bundle region (See Figure 9.29 in Understanding Intracardiac EGMs and ECG for further explanation). This type of accessory pathway can cause an abnormal QRS due to partial depolarization of the ventricles via the accessory pathway but is not associated with arrhythmias. Even after

ablation, ventricular pacing is associated with eccentric atrial activation in the coronary sinus (Figure 7.19). However, unlike baseline ventricular pacing, the atrial electrogram recorded from the His bundle precedes the earliest coronary sinus atrial depolarization, emphasizing the importance of evaluating both the timing and pattern of atrial activation. In this case, retrograde AV nodal conduction is associated with an "eccentric" atrial activation pattern in the coronary sinus. This is likely due to the positioning of the coronary sinus catheter with the more proximal electrodes actually outside the body of the coronary sinus and stresses the importance of making sure catheters are stably positioned. The patient is observed and isoproterenol is infused, but no tachycardia or evidence for recurrent accessory pathway conduction is observed. After 5-year follow-up, the patient remains asymptomatic.

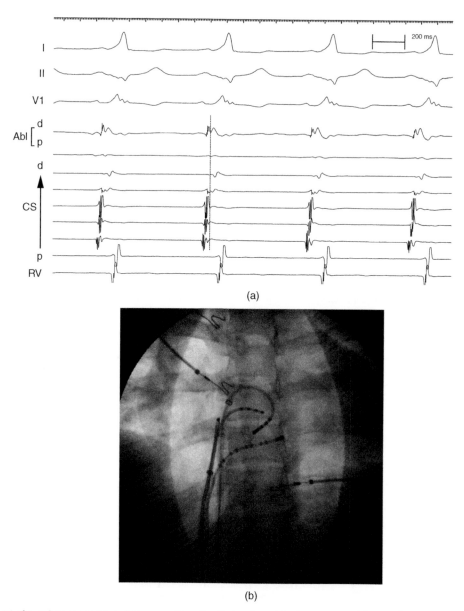

(a)

(b)

Figure 7.16 (a) The catheter is positioned at a promising site. Notice the stable electrograms with an early ventricular electrogram relative to the earliest ventricular signal recorded in the coronary sinus. (b) Corresponding fluoroscopic position of the catheters in Figure 7.16a.

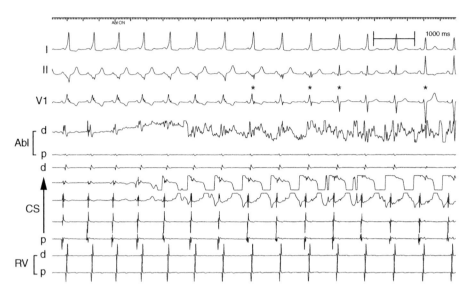

Figure 7.17 Application of radiofrequency energy leads to progressive change in the QRS complex (*) until normalization and development of an isoelectric PR interval.

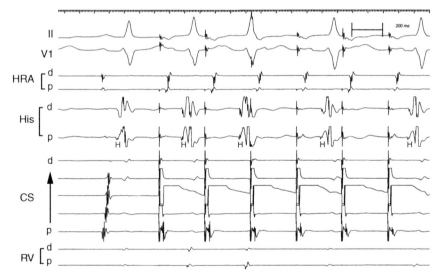

Figure 7.18 After ablation, the HV interval remains short but atrial pacing demonstrates no change in the QRS morphology with AH prolongation and the His bundle electrogram (H) always precedes the QRS complex. This finding is consistent with a fasciculoventricular fiber.

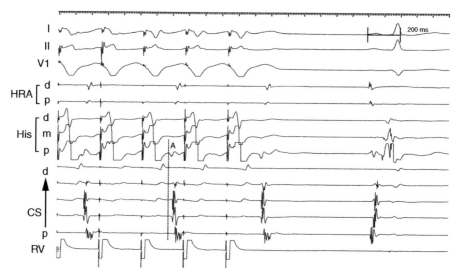

Figure 7.19 Ventricular pacing after ablation reveals earliest activation in the coronary sinus electrograms in the mid-portion. However, atrial activation of the coronary sinus occurs after the initial atrial signal is recorded in the His bundle region. In this case, relatively "eccentric" coronary sinus activation is produced by retrograde AV nodal depolarization. This finding is probably due to the proximal position of the coronary sinus catheter (Figure 7.16b) with the proximal electrodes actually outside the coronary sinus.

KEY POINTS

- The morphology of the QRS complex will provide clues to the location of an accessory pathway that can conduct anterogradely.

- Because the QRS morphology represents fusion between activation via the AV node and the accessory pathway, maneuvers that delay AV nodal activation (more rapid atrial pacing, adenosine) will lead to more ventricular depolarization via the accessory pathway and a wider more bizarre appearing QRS complex.

- Accessory pathways with rapid conduction and short refractoriness can lead to more rapid ventricular depolarization and increase the risk for sudden cardiac death.

- Fasciculoventricular accessory pathways can cause abnormal appearing QRS complexes but can be identified because His bundle depolarization precedes the QRS complex.

CHAPTER 8

Supraventricular tachycardia case 7: baseline preexcitation

A 39-year-old nurse with a long-standing arrhythmia history of a Mahaim accessory pathway tachycardia comes to you for evaluation. He began having episodes of rapid heart rates in his teens associated with palpitations and light-headedness. Eleven years ago, after an episode of atrial fibrillation, the patient underwent electrophysiology study and attempted ablation and was told he had a Mahaim-type accessory pathway that was located near his AV node and that successful ablation would likely lead to requirement of permanent pacing. He has done reasonably well on atenolol 25 mg daily but does continue to have some breakthrough arrhythmias and does note fatigue with atenolol. Otherwise, the patient has no significant medical problems, and his physical examination is normal. His ECG is shown in Figure 8.1.

Inspection of his ECG demonstrates obvious preexcitation with a relatively normal transition and negative delta wave in V1. The normal transition suggests that the location of the accessory pathway is septal and perhaps right inferior along the tricuspid valve annulus.

A few words about Mahaim-type accessory pathways are important in this case. Generally, accessory pathways have rapid conduction properties similar to atrial or ventricular tissue. However, some accessory pathways display slow conduction and anterograde only conduction and are collectively called Mahaim accessory pathways in honor of Ivan Mahaim who carefully evaluated the connections arising from the Bundle of His in the late 1930s. There is an interesting history on the nomenclature of accessory pathways. Kent originally described nodal appearing tissue in the trisuspid annulus and thought these represented the pathway of normal atrioventricular conduction.

Although the work of Tawara conclusively showed that normal activation occurs via the AV node and His bundle, the term "Kent bundle" has been used to describe accessory pathways with rapid conduction properties found in the Wolff–Parkinson–White Syndrome. Actually, Kent probably described specialized accessory pathways that had AV nodal histologic properties. For many years, these slowly conducting accessory pathways were thought to branch off the AV node and insert into ventricular fibers or distal portions of the fascicles and were anatomically referred to as nodoventricular or nodofascicular fibers, respectively. However, important work by Tchou and colleagues showed that these specialized pathways with slow conduction properties were actually most commonly observed along the tricuspid valve with insertion into the fascicles and are best described as atriofascicular fibers. In this work, they showed that these pathways exhibited only slow anterograde conduction. This should raise the first question about the patient's diagnosis of a "Mahaim" fiber, as most of these patients do not have a delta wave at the beginning of the QRS complex because the accessory pathway has slow conduction properties. Careful inspection of ECGs in patients with proven Mahaim fibers suggests that the ECG manifestation may be sharp components in the middle or at the end of the QRS complex, which is not surprising given the slow conduction characteristics of these unique accessory pathways. As ECG localization of accessory pathway depends on evaluation of the delta waves, accessory pathways with slow conduction properties may be particularly difficult to localize accurately.

Given the patient's continued symptoms, it is reasonable to have the patient undergo repeat electrophysiologic testing, although it is important to have

Understanding Intracardiac EGMs: A Patient Centered Guide, First Edition. Fred Kusumoto.
© 2015 John Wiley & Sons, Ltd. Published 2015 by John Wiley & Sons, Ltd.

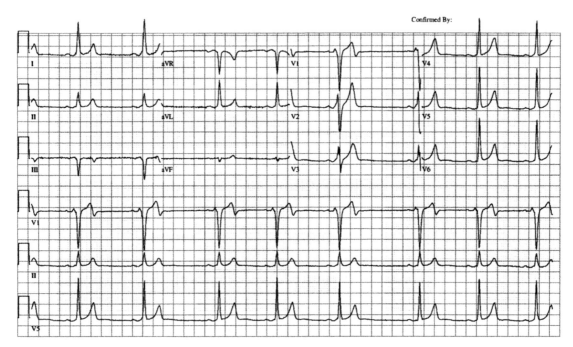

Figure 8.1 Baseline ECG. A delta wave is present and negative in lead III. Transition is normal, which places the accessory pathway on the septum.

a frank preprocedure discussion about the risk of pacemaker and a decision on strategy if an accessory pathway with a higher likelihood of being complicated by AV block is identified. In this case, it is decided that electrophysiologic testing and ablation will be performed unless the risk is "too high." Although the instructions given by patients often are vague, it is always important to have these discussions before electrophysiology study and ablation.

Baseline electrograms are shown in Figure 8.2. When placing catheters for a patient who may have a fascicular insertion for an accessory pathway, it is often very helpful to have electrodes that record a right bundle branch potential. In our laboratory, as shown in this case, the right ventricular quadripolar catheter is placed septally to allow for RB potential recording. In this case, the HV interval is short and the His bundle depolarization precedes right bundle depolarization. A premature ventricular contraction leads to apparent retrograde activation via the AV node with first atrial depolarization possibly in the His bundle region (very low frequency signal can be seen) with first definitive atrial electrogram recorded in the proximal coronary sinus.

Atrial pacing is performed first at 500 ms (Figure 8.3). In this case, the His bundle is "driven into" the QRS because of progressive AV nodal delay. In the second paced beat, it appears that the His-right bundle potential relationship is maintained, suggesting that even with greater preexcitation the right bundle is being depolarized by the His bundle, making a fascicular ventricular insertion point less likely. Also notice that the accessory pathway has fairly slow conduction properties because the QRS complex has a right-sided pathway morphology (left bundle branch block morphology in V1 suggesting that the right ventricle is depolarized before the left ventricle), and yet pacing from the right atrium yields a fairly long interval between the stimulus and the onset of ventricular depolarization. Continued atrial pacing leads to the development of right bundle branch block defining the AP blocked cycle length (Figure 8.4). It is interesting to note that once block in the accessory pathway develops, it persists, suggesting that retrograde penetration into the ventricular insertion point is present (similar to the sustained bundle branch block observed in the Ashman's phenomenon as discussed in Understanding ECGs and EGMs).

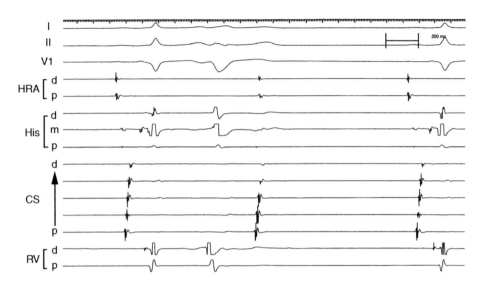

Figure 8.2 Baseline electrograms show obvious preexcitation with a short HV interval. The second QRS represents a premature ventricular contraction and retrograde conduction with earliest atrial electrogram in the His bundle catheter.

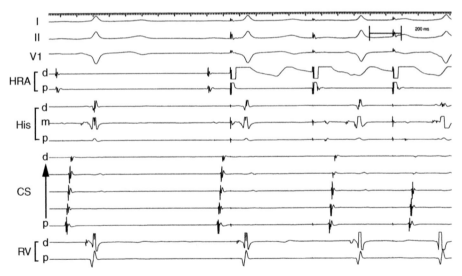

Figure 8.3 Atrial pacing at a cycle length of 500 ms leads to a dramatic change in the QRS complex with LBBB morphology. In addition, there is an increase in the AH interval and the HV internal becomes more negative.

The electrophysiologic response to premature atrial extrastimuli is shown in Figures 8.5 and 8.6. In Figure 8.5, two atrial extrastimuli are delivered at coupling intervals of 450 and 490 ms. Notice that premature atrial stimuli are associated with more preexcitation due to prolongation of AV node conduction. In Figure 8.6, a more closely coupled second premature atrial stimulus

(480 ms) results in block in the accessory pathway and conduction to the AV node with right bundle branch block.

Ventricular pacing at a cycle length of 600 ms shows no evidence of retrograde accessory pathway conduction (Figure 8.7). As there is no apparent ventriculoatrial conduction via the accessory pathway or the AV node,

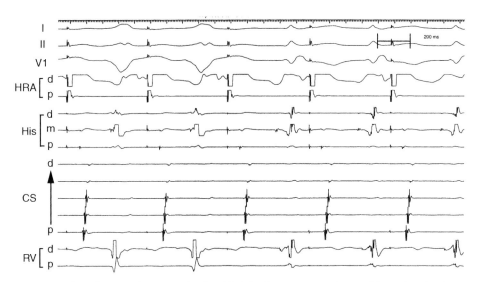

Figure 8.4 With continued atrial pacing, the patient develops block in the accessory pathway with continued atrioventricular conduction with right bundle branch block. It is interesting that the putative RB potential is still present without a change in timing, suggesting that it may not be a right bundle potential or more likely the patient has block in a more distal portion of the right bundle.

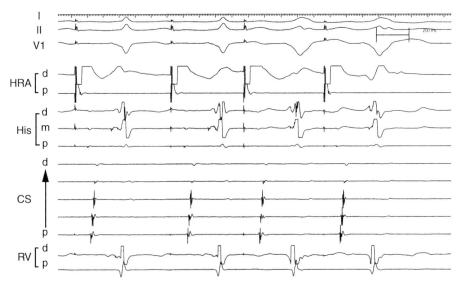

Figure 8.5 Premature atrial stimuli at coupling intervals of 450 and 490 ms. The premature atrial depolarization leads to a more abnormal QRS complex, as a larger portion of the ventricles is being activated via the accessory pathway.

further shortening of the ventricular pacing cycle length or the use of ventricular premature ventricular stimulation protocols would not provide any additional information.

At this point, the electrophysiologist can choose to simply map and ablate as in Case 7 or continue to try to induce tachycardia. There are no fast and hard rules for making this decision. However, attempts at initiation of tachycardia are elected in this case because of the unusual conduction properties of the accessory pathway and for an extremely important clinical issue. In sustained tachycardia, activation of the accessory

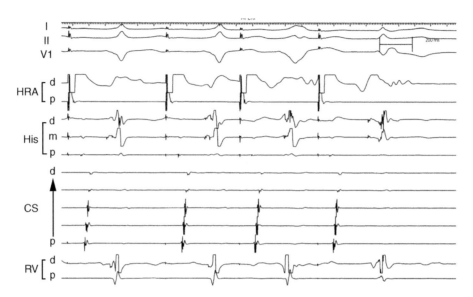

Figure 8.6 Premature atrial stimulus protocol continued from Figure 8.5. The second atrial extrastimulus is given slightly earlier (480 ms), and this leads to a sudden change in the QRS complex (RBBB morphology) and the appearance of a His bundle deflection. This change occurred because of block in the accessory pathway.

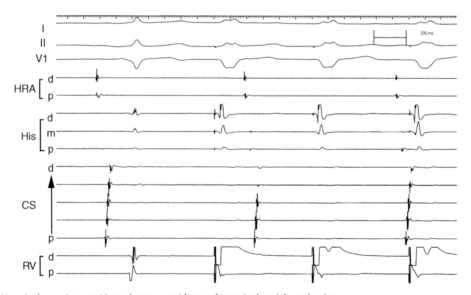

Figure 8.7 Ventricular pacing at 600 ms shows no evidence of ventriculoatrial conduction.

pathway will likely be maximally separated from AV node conduction and facilitates mapping of both structures – an issue important in this patient in whom the accessory pathway has been previously localized near the AV node. Double atrial stimuli initiate a wide complex tachycardia with an approximate cycle length of 380 ms and cycle length variability (Figure 8.8). In wide complex tachycardia, the electrophysiologist must distinguish between four basic possibilities: atrial tachycardia with aberrant conduction (bundle branch block or activation via the accessory pathway), AVNRT with aberrant conduction, ventricular tachycardia, and

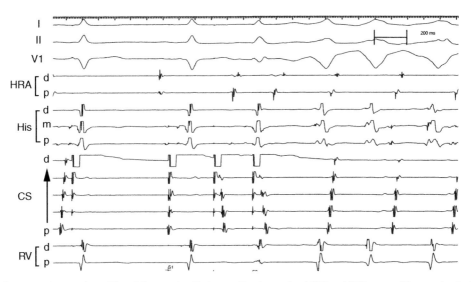

Figure 8.8 Coronary sinus pacing with atrial extrastimuli. At coupling intervals of 280 and 250 ms, a wide complex tachycardia is initiated with a cycle length of 380 ms with a 1:1 ventriculoatrial relationship with a ventriculoatrial concduction time of 167 ms and an atrioventricular conduction time of 217 ms.

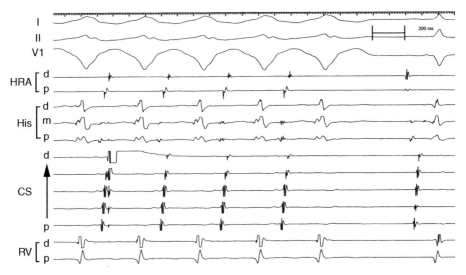

Figure 8.9 The tachycardia terminates with a ventricular signal, thus ruling out ventricular tachycardia. Earliest atrial activation appears to be in the His bundle region, suggesting that the tachycardia is dependent on retrograde AV nodal conduction.

AVRT (either orthodromic reciprocating tachycardia with aberrant conduction or antidromic tachycardia).

Inspection of the surface ECG demonstrates a QRS complex with a left bundle branch block morphology and normal frontal axis (positive QRS complexes in I and II). Initial evaluation of the electrograms reveals a 1:1 relationship between ventricular and atrial activity.

Atrial activation appears to be first in the His bundle recordings. The wide complex tachycardia spontaneously terminates on a ventricular signal without preceding changes in the VA conduction. This implies that the tachycardia is dependent on ventriculoatrial conduction, thus ruling out ventricular tachycardia (Figure 8.9).

To help evaluate a patient with a right-sided accessory pathway, particularly a patient with a Mahaim pathway, it is extremely useful to place a multielectrode catheter on the tricuspid annulus (Figure 8.10). The electrograms from this catheter position during an atrial premature stimulation protocol are shown in Figures 8.11–8.13. In Figure 8.11, a premature atrial stimulus from the high right atrium (the proximal electrodes of the ten-pole catheter on the tricuspid annulus) is delivered, and the first interesting finding is the early ventricular activation recorded in the distal electrodes of the tricuspid annulus catheter. Evaluation of the premature atrial contraction

shows more preexcitation due to delay in the AV node and apparent delay in the His electrogram but that there is also accompanying delay in ventricular activation via the accessory pathway. In Figure 8.12, a more closely coupled premature atrial contraction leads to even more delay in the accessory pathway. Finally, in Figure 8.13, the premature atrial contraction blocks in the accessory pathway, and no ventricular activation is present (due to prior block in the AV node). It is interesting to speculate when AV node block occurred. The local electrograms recorded at the His bundle region show a similar relationship for a coupling interval of 290 and 260 ms,

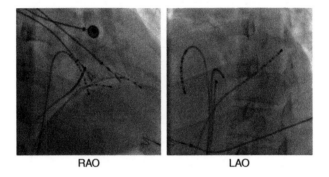

RAO   LAO

Figure 8.10 Fluorscopic images showing a decapolar catheter placed along the tricuspid annulus.

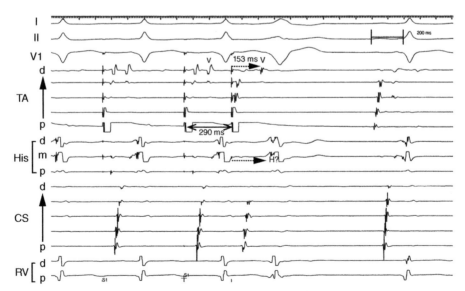

Figure 8.11 Atrial extrastimulus protocol. An atrial premature stimulus delivered at a coupling interval of 290 ms appears to be associated with AV node delay and slowed conduction in the inferolateral tricuspid annulus (dashed arrows). The putative ventricular signal (V) recorded in the distal electrodes of the tricuspid annulus (TA) has a delayed conduction time, and the His bundle electrogram (H?) is obscured by ventricular activation.

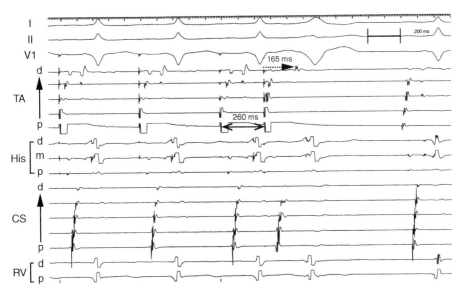

Figure 8.12 Atrial extrastimulus protocol continued from Figure 8.11. An atrial premature stimulus is delivered at a shorter coupling interval (260 ms), and delay in the stimulus to putative ventricular signal increases to 165 ms.

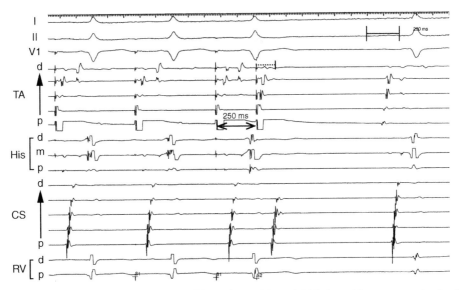

Figure 8.13 Atrial premature stimulus protocol continued from Figures 8.11 and 8.12. An atrial premature stimulus delivered at a coupling interval of 250 ms results in atrioventricular block due to block both in the accessory pathway and in the AV node. Loss of the second electrogram in the distal electrodes provides evidence that this signal was due to local ventricular activity. The APERP is 250 ms, so that although this accessory pathway has slow conduction properties, it has a relatively short refractory period. At this point, it is unclear when block in the AV node actually occurred, although it is suspicious that the local electrogram recorded in the His bundle catheter is similar for both a coupling interval of 300 and 260 ms, suggesting the possibility that block in the AV node had already occurred and the high-frequency multicomponent signals actually represent retrograde His bundle depolarization.

which suggests that the multicomponent high frequency signals suggestive of a His bundle recording could be due to retrograde activation from the accessory pathway.

With the initiation of wide complex tachycardia (Figure 8.14), the diagnostic strategy is similar to supraventricular tachycardia, but instead of delivering a ventricular stimulus when the His bundle is refractory, an atrial depolarization is delivered when the atrial tissue near the AV node has already depolarized. An example of this strategy is shown in Figures 8.15 and 8.16. In this case, an atrial stimulus delivered after atrial depolarization in the His bundle catheter leads to early ventricular activation with the same QRS morphology as tachycardia, providing strong evidence that the accessory pathway is participating in the tachycardia as the anterograde limb of the tachycardia circuit. An even earlier premature stimulus terminates the tachycardia by early His depolarization and retrograde termination in the AV node (Figure 8.16).

Mahaim accessory pathways are generally divided into atriofascicular and atrioventricular pathways, and atrioventricular pathways are divided arbitrarily into long and short accessory pathways. In this case, since most of the delay is at the annulus, it appears that the patient has a short atrioventricular accessory pathway with slow conduction properties.

Catheter ablation for most Mahaim pathways requires initiating wide complex tachycardia and searching for pathway potentials. In this case, as preexcitation is present, anterograde mapping in sinus rhythm can be performed identifying the earliest ventricular signal (Figure 8.17). The fluoroscopic position of the ablation catheter is shown in Figure 8.18. Application of radiofrequency energy at this site leads to an abrupt change in the QRS morphology after 7 s, suggesting elimination of the accessory pathway (Figure 8.19). In some cases, ablation of the ventricular insertion site is required. Generally, this is more difficult because of the branching nature of the distal insertion point of the accessory pathways, but in some cases, this is the only option available.

After ablation, the patient had no evidence of recurrent accessory pathway conduction and no evidence of tachycardia. He has now been arrhythmia free off medications for the last 2 years.

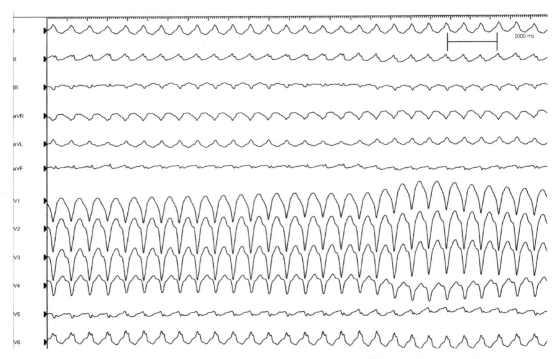

Figure 8.14 12-lead ECG from sustained wide complex tachycardia showing a left bundle branch block morphology.

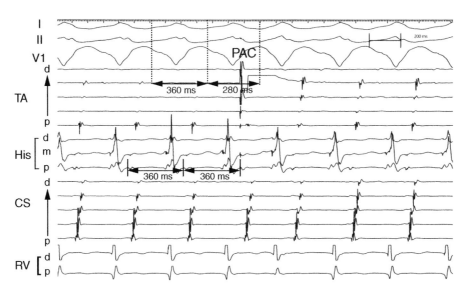

Figure 8.15 An atrial premature stimulus at a coupling interval 300 ms (when the His bundle near the atrium has already depolarized) preexcites the ventricle with the same QRS morphology.

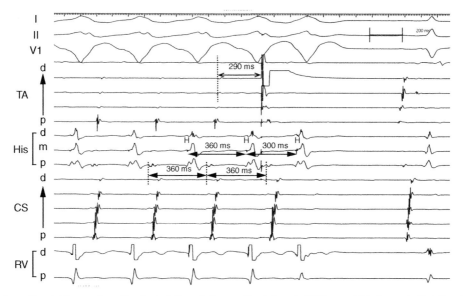

Figure 8.16 An earlier atrial premature stimulus is delivered at a coupling interval of 290 ms, which does not affect the atrial electrogram timing in the His bundle recording (the atrial electrogram is "committed," and the atrial to atrial electrogram interval remains 360 ms), preexcites the ventricle and the His bundle (300 ms), and terminates the tachycardia.

Another accessory pathway with slow conducting properties leads to a supraventricular tachycardia called permanent junctional reciprocating tachycardia (PJRT). This tachycardia was first identified by Gallaverdin and Veil in 1937 and more completely evaluated by Coumel in 1967, who first coined the term PJRT to describe an incessant (hence "permanent") tachycardia that appeared to arise from the septal region ("junctional") and involve reentry between the atria and the ventricles ("reciprocating"). Although these accessory pathways exhibit slow and decremental conduction similarly to the Mahaim fibers described in our patient,

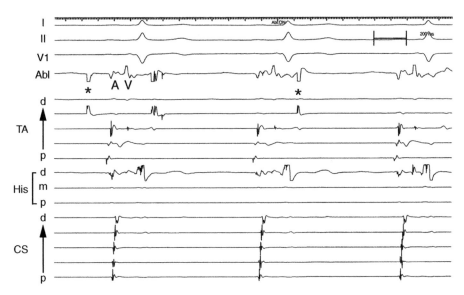

Figure 8.17 Electrograms obtained from the catheter positions in Figure 8.18. Notice the coincident artifact (*) on the distal electrode of the ablation catheter and electrode pair 3,4 of the tricuspid annulus, confirming that these electrodes are in the same location. The ventricular signal is relatively early.

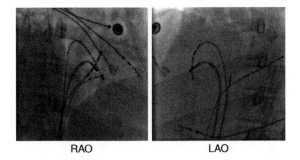

RAO   LAO

Figure 8.18 Fluoroscopy showing the ablation catheter in the inferolateral wall of the tricuspid annulus in the RAO and LAO projections.

clinically, they activate solely in the retrograde manner. Interesting studies in patients with PJRT in whom AV nodal ablation has been purposely or inadvertently been performed has suggested that these fibers can conduct anterogradely but very slowly and appear to have slow conduction properties because they are thin and serpiginous. Patients with PJRT often present at a younger age, and 20–50% will initially come to medical attention because of heart failure due to tachycardia-induced cardiomyopathy.

Figure 8.20 shows the telemetry strips from a young patient with PJRT with the characteristic findings.

The patient has an incessant tachycardia and is given adenosine, which terminates the tachycardia by blocking retrograde conduction. Retrograde termination can be identified by the absence of the deeply negative deflection that is coincident with the T wave. As this signal is not present on the immediate subsequent beats, the clinician can infer conclusively that the deflection was due to atrial depolarization. However, almost immediately after the effects of adenosine "wear off" tachycardia begins again. Because the reentrant circuit has two "slow limbs," the AV node and the slowly conducting accessory pathway, there is a large excitable gap that is the reason that these arrhythmias are incessant. As shown in the 12-lead from another patient with PJRT, slow retrograde conduction leads to a P wave in the terminal portion of the T wave, which is most often evident in the lateral leads (Figure 8.21).

Fortunately, ablation is extremely effective for the treatment of these patients. Generally, the earliest retrograde atrial electrogram is targeted. Although the accessory pathways can be located anywhere on the valvular annuli, most are located in the inferior septal portion of the heart near the coronary sinus os. Ablation in the coronary sinus requires special attention to reduce the risk of perforation and injury to the coronary arteries. When radiofrequency energy is used,

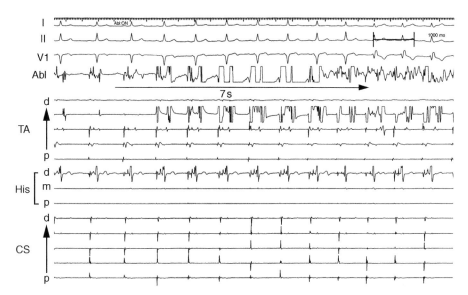

Figure 8.19 After 7 s of radiofrequency energy application, the QRS complex abruptly changes to a right bundle branch block (RBBB) morphology suggestive of successful elimination of the accessory pathway.

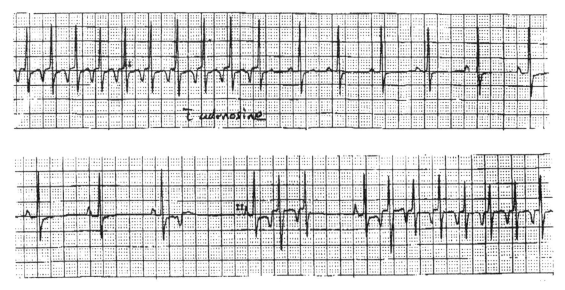

Figure 8.20 Rhythm strip from a young boy with incessant tachycardia and a severe cardiomyopathy (LVEF 10%). Infusion with adenosine led to transient termination of the tachycardia. Comparison of sinus beats and tachycardia can be extremely useful for identifying atrial depolarization.

low power should be used (20–30 W) for relatively short periods with careful monitoring of the impedance during ablation. Alternatively, cryoablation has been described as a method that can be used to ablate safely within the coronary sinus. A site just within the coronary sinus os is found in the patient described in Figure 8.20. Application of radiofrequency energy leads to prompt termination of the tachycardia (Figure 8.22).

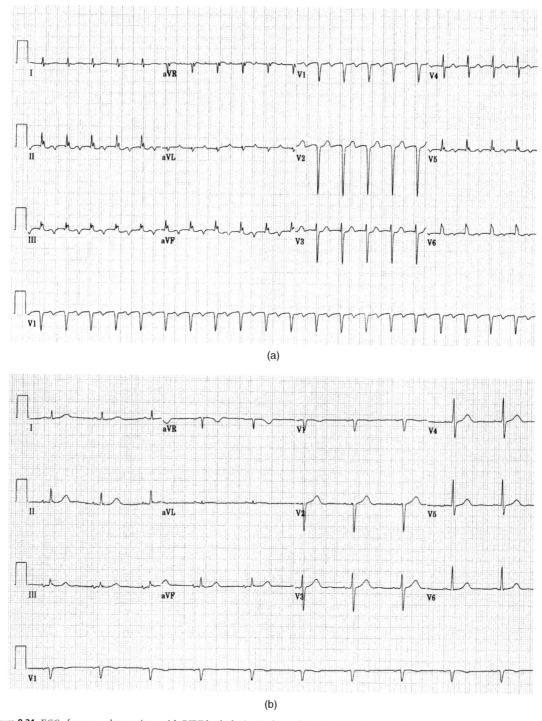

(a)

(b)

Figure 8.21 ECGs from another patient with PJRT both during tachycardia (a) and during normal sinus rhythm (b). Comparison of the ECGs helps to identify the characteristic inverted P waves in the inferolateral leads during tachycardia.

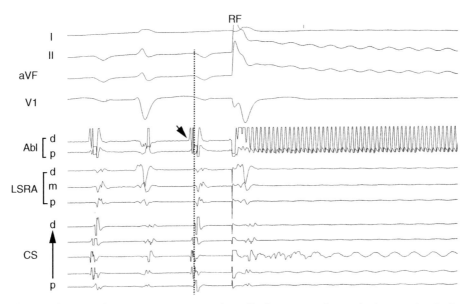

Figure 8.22 Ablation in the patient from Figure 8.20. During tachycardia, the coronary sinus region is mapped and a site with earliest atrial depolarization is identified. Radiofrequency energy application results in prompt termination of the tachycardia. (Adapted from Kusumoto 2009.)

The patient did not have any spontaneous or inducible arrhythmias after the procedure. The patient's ejection fraction, which was 10% at the time of procedure, became normal by 4-month follow-up.

KEY POINTS

- Accessory pathways can exhibit slow conduction properties.
- The most commonly encountered slowly conducting accessory pathways are Mahaim fibers that is a phrase used to collectively describe atriofascicular and atrioventricular pathways with slow conduction properties and anterograde only conduction.
- Mahaim accessory pathways generally present with a wide complex tachycardia due to anterograde conduction via the accessory pathway and retrograde activation via the AV node.

- Involvement of the accessory pathway in the wide complex tachycardia can be confirmed by delivering an atrial extrastimulus when the atrial region around the His bundle region is "committed," which results in early activation of the ventricles with the same QRS morphology.
- Ablation is generally performed by identifying discrete electrograms often called "Mahaim" potentials along the path of the Mahaim fiber.
- Another type of slowly conducting accessory pathway is involved in PJRT. This accessory pathway conducts slowly but clinically only in the retrograde direction and causes an incessant supraventricular tachycardia that can be associated with tachycardia-induced cardiomyopathy.

CHAPTER 9

Supraventricular tachycardia case 8

A 31-year-old emergency room nurse has a 1-year history of rapid heart rates and palpitations following exercise. When she exercises aggressively, her heart rate will reach 170 bpm and then suddenly increase to a rate >200 bpm with the development of chest pressure and light-headedness. After several minutes, her heart rate will return to 100–120 beats per minute. An event monitor is shown in Figure 9.1. She underwent prior electrophysiology study and had no inducible arrhythmias but an occasional single AV node "echo" and underwent an empiric slow pathway modification. Unfortunately, she has had continued episodes of symptomatic rapid heart rate that have worsened in frequency and duration. Her ECG is shown in Figure 9.2.

The patient's event recorder tracings clearly show sudden onset of a rapid narrow complex tachycardia. Several small single-center studies have described the effectiveness of empiric slow pathway modification in patients with documented supraventricular tachycardia who are not inducible for sustained tachycardia at electrophysiology study. The cohorts all included patients who had no underlying cardiac disease and evaluated the effects of an empiric slow pathway modification. In most but not all studies, ablation was performed only in those patients with evidence for dual pathway physiology. Over short- and longer-term follow-up, the patients generally did well with >90–95% free of supraventricular tachycardia. This strategy is in part successful because AVNRT will be the most common cause of regular SVT in almost all populations of nonelderly adults. If this approach is taken, great care on the relative advantages and disadvantages of the empiric ablation is necessary. The electrophysiologist must always remember that supraventricular tachycardia is not life-threatening, that recurrent arrhythmia is not a "bad" outcome, and that a repeat ablation is far better than permanent pacemaker implantation in a young patient, particularly when the diagnosis has not been completely established.

However, given her continuing symptoms, it is reasonable to have the patient undergo repeat electrophysiologic testing. Baseline conduction intervals are shown in Figure 9.3. The baseline cycle length is 1016 ms, and the patient has normal AV conduction with a PR interval of 174 ms, an AH interval of 114 ms, and an HV interval of 39 ms. As the patient is undergoing a repeat electrophysiology study and was noninducible at her prior study (perhaps making atrial tachycardia a more likely possibility), a decopolar catheter is placed along the lateral wall of the tricuspid annulus (position similar to that shown in Figure 8.10).

Baseline atrial pacing shows an AV blocked cycle length of 350 ms with block in the AV node. Atrial premature stimulation protocols reveal normal decrement in the AV node without AH "jumps" and an AVN effective refractory period of 390 ms. Baseline ventricular pacing reveals a VA blocked cycle length of 450 ms with concentric septal activation. At a basic pacing cycle length of 600 ms, the ventriculoatrial refractory period was 450 ms with no evidence of decrement of the septal retrograde atrial activation.

Clearly in this patient, sustained arrhythmia is required, and the patient is started on isoproterenol. Atrial overdrive pacing from the coronary initiates supraventricular tachycardia with a cycle length of 350 ms with earliest atrial activation in the distal coronary sinus (Figure 9.4). Not surprisingly, the tachycardia cycle length does not change with the development of right bundle branch block (Figure 9.5). A Morady maneuver is performed and this leads to

Understanding Intracardiac EGMs: A Patient Centered Guide, First Edition. Fred Kusumoto.
© 2015 John Wiley & Sons, Ltd. Published 2015 by John Wiley & Sons, Ltd.

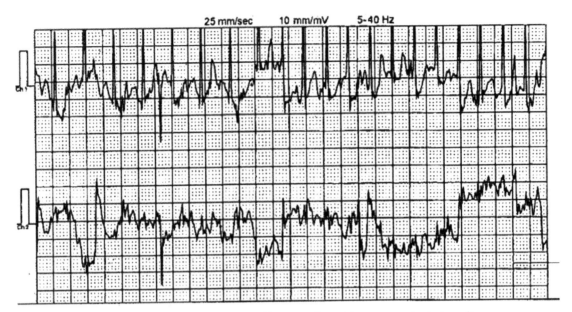

Figure 9.1 Event recorder tracings at peak exercise show sudden onset of a rapid narrow complex tachycardia.

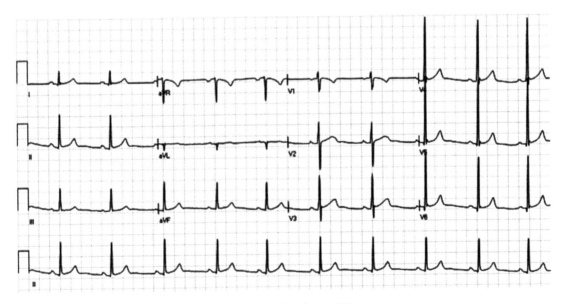

Figure 9.2 Baseline ECG shows no evidence of preexcitation or other abnormalities.

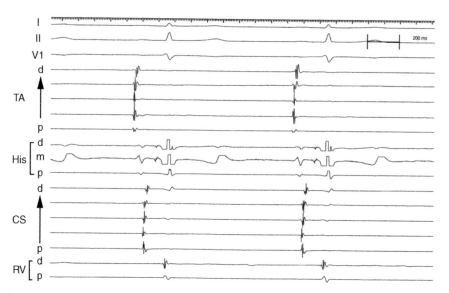

Figure 9.3 Baseline electrograms are normal.

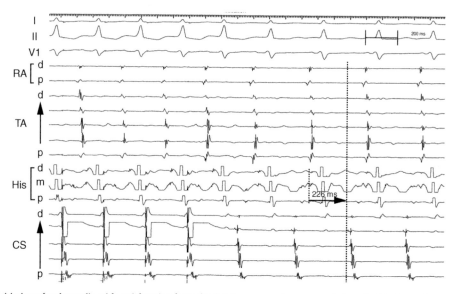

Figure 9.4 Initiation of tachycardia with atrial pacing from the distal coronary sinus at a cycle length of 260 ms. The supraventricular tachycardia has a cycle length of 350 ms, and the HA interval is 226 ms with earliest atrial activation observed in the distal coronary sinus either at the distal electrodes or at the second-most-distal electrode pair.

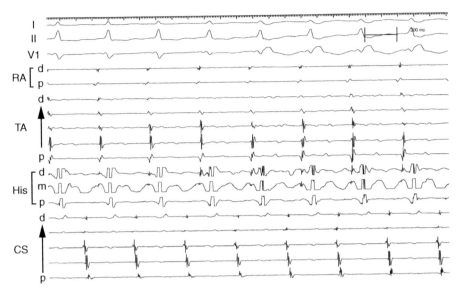

Figure 9.5 The tachycardia unaffected by the development of RBBB.

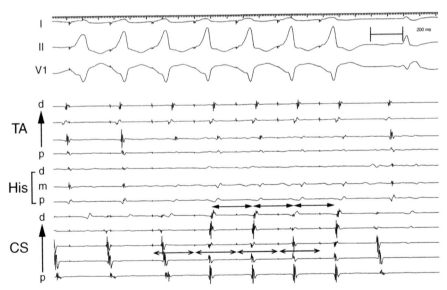

Figure 9.6 Morady maneuver during tachycardia. Tachycardia cycle length is 340 ms, and ventricular pacing is performed at a cycle length of 260 ms. Atrial capture is identified by the shortening of the atrial electrogram cycle length to the paced cycle length and a change in the retrograde atrial activation pattern. On cessation of pacing, there is a V-A-A-V response and then termination of the tachycardia.

a "V-A-A-V" response and a change in the coronary sinus electrogram, thus suggesting a diagnosis of atrial tachycardia (Figure 9.6). Tachycardia is now essentially incessant, and a spontaneous initiation of tachycardia is shown in Figure 9.7. Tachycardia simply appears to start with the first atrial activation pattern matching subsequent atrial activation during tachycardia, suggesting that automaticity and atrial tachycardia are the likely cause. Adenosine is given and demonstrates continuation of the tachycardia despite AV block, thus

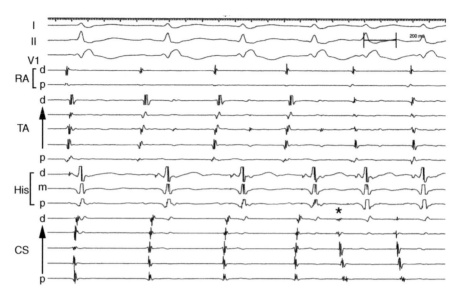

Figure 9.7 Spontaneous initiation of the tachycardia. There is a slight decrease in the sinus node cycle length, and the tachycardia simply appears "to start" with the first atrial electrogram (*) similarly to subsequent atrial electrograms.

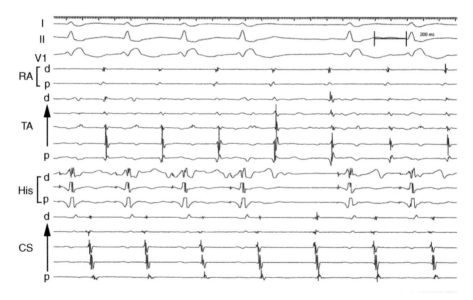

Figure 9.8 The tachycardia continues despite the development of AV block; a finding that definitively "rules out" AVRT using a slowly conducting left-sided accessory pathway.

conclusively ruling out a slowly conducting accessory pathway (Figure 9.8). However, later the tachycardia appears to terminate with the development of AV block and terminates with an atrial signal (Figure 9.9). As we learned in Chapter 2, spontaneous termination of a supraventricular tachycardia on an atrial

electrogram suggests AV node dependence and generally rules out an atrial tachycardia. In this case, this finding could also represent spontaneous termination of atrial tachycardia at the same time that AV block develops – perhaps statistically unlikely but certainly theoretically possible.

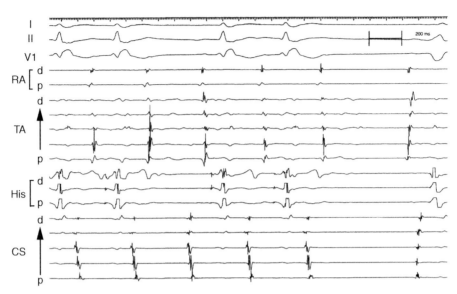

Figure 9.9 Termination of the tachycardia with an atrial electrogram although at a time when AV block might be expected due to prior Wenckebach behavior of AV conduction. Although still consistent with the diagnosis of atrial tachycardia, it would mean that the tachycardia terminated coincidentally at a time when AV block was expected.

Generally, eccentric activation of the coronary sinus rules out AVNRT. However, a small percentage of patients with AVNRT will display eccentric activation. Making a definitive diagnosis is critical because the distinction between the two possibilities will potentially have a large impact on ablation strategy. In this case, although we have conclusively "ruled out" an accessory pathway and have important evidence favoring atrial tachycardia (Morady maneuver with a V-A-A-V response, eccentric atrial activation, and initiation that appears to start with tachycardia), the unusual termination of the tachycardia with an atrial signal in the setting of AV block, while still "explainable," is rather unexpected.

There are several methods to help make this distinction if the diagnosis is still unclear. Atrial pacing maneuvers are shown in Figures 9.10–9.12. In Figures 9.10 and 9.11, notice that capture of the entire right atrium and the proximal coronary sinus electrograms does not affect the arrhythmia. Only when there is capture of the distal coronary sinus does the tachycardia terminate. The importance of the tissue depolarization recorded on the distal coronary sinus electrogram is confirmed with coronary sinus pacing (Figure 9.12). Sudden termination of tachycardia with

only slight advancement of atrial depolarization begins to tip the balance toward a reentrant tachycardia such as AVNRT. Both of these responses would be unusual for an automatic atrial tachycardia. More compelling evidence for AV node dependence of the tachycardia can be observed with careful inspection of the response to ventricular pacing. Ventricular pacing would reproducibly interact with the tachycardia by causing an increase in the tachycardia cycle length (Figure 9.13). This response would not occur in atrial tachycardia in response to ventricular pacing (unless there was a random atrial tachycardia rate change) and provides important evidence that the patient has AVNRT and the earliest atrial activation in the distal coronary sinus represents a left-sided input into the AV node.

How then to reconcile the V-A-A-V response observed in response to ventricular pacing? Ventricular pacing was associated with rapid retrograde activation via a "fast pathway." Importantly, activation of the "fast pathway" did not appear to affect the tachycardia (Figures 9.10 and 9.11). However, the AV node is a complex structure and may have more than two "inputs." In this case, the best explanation is a reentrant circuit that involves a left-sided AV nodal input that is separate from the electrograms recorded in the

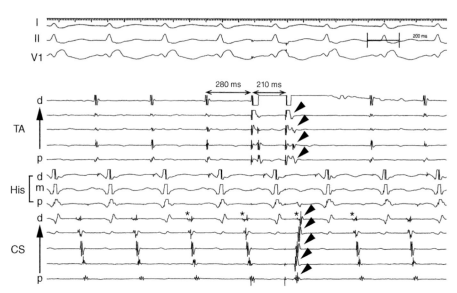

Figure 9.10 Double atrial stimuli from the right atrium at coupling intervals of 280 and 210 ms. Notice that the right atrium and almost all of thecoronary sinus electrograms can be captured by the extrastimuli (arrowheads) without affecting the tachycardia (*).

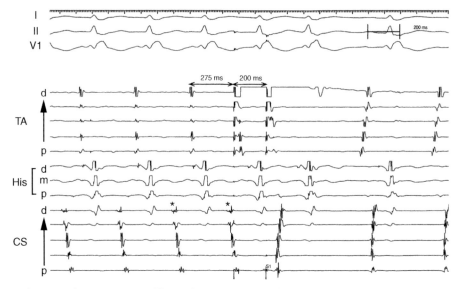

Figure 9.11 Continuation of Figure 9.10. Double atrial extrastimuli at slightly shorter coupling intervals (270 and 200 ms) are delivered. Only when the initial component of the distal coronary sinus electrogram (*) is captured does termination occur.

coronary sinus with a "slow left atrial input" either on the endocardial surface of the inferior left atrium or on the roof of the coronary sinus (Figure 9.14). This circuit would have decremental properties (which would offer an explanation for Figure 9.13), have V-A-A-V response because it is essentially an "atrial tachycardia," and

would not require the involvement of the proximal coronary sinus. Unusual arrhythmias are more likely to be identified after a prior failed ablation either because they were complex to begin with or because the prior ablation altered the electrophysiologic properties of critical tissues.

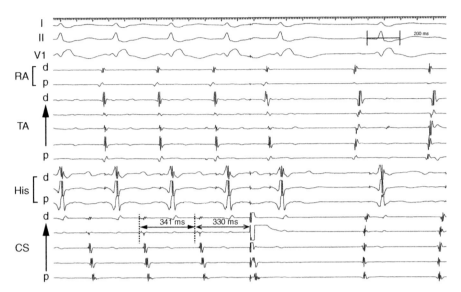

Figure 9.12 The importance of the distal coronary sinus for maintaining tachycardia is confirmed. In this case, a "late A" delivered at the coronary sinus just 10 ms before expected atrial depolarization terminates the tachycardia.

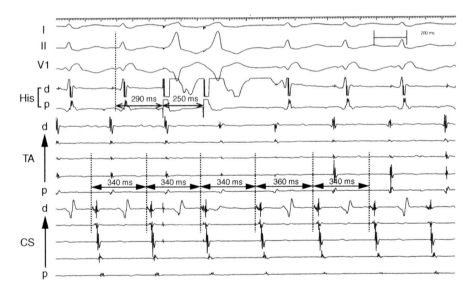

Figure 9.13 Scanning ventricular stimuli are delivered during tachycardia. When double extrastimuli are delivered at coupling intervals of 290 and 250 ms reproducibly elicited prolongation in the tachycardia cycle length measured at the distal coronary sinus. This finding is characteristic of AVNRT and would not be found in atrial tachycardia.

There are several approaches to ablation in this setting. One option would be to map the earliest atrial signal during tachycardia while others ablate in the typical slow pathway region. In my experience, relatively early sites just within the endocardial surface of the left atrium can often be found. In addition, early areas can also be found in portions of the coronary sinus, suggesting that the eccentric coronary sinus activation

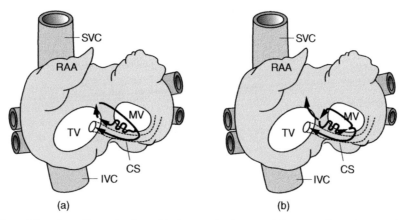

Figure 9.14 Several possible tachycardia mechanisms. (a) Slow conduction travels from septally in the same direction as coronary sinus activation; (b) slow conduction travels laterally and travels in the opposite direction of the electrograms recorded in the coronary sinus.

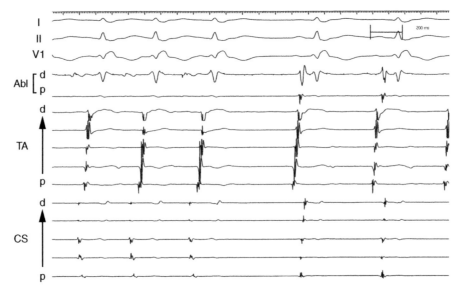

Figure 9.15 A catheter is placed on the roof of the coronary sinus, and an early atrial electrogram is recorded, which suggests that retrograde atrial activation travels from the septum to the lateral wall (Figure 9.14(b)). After placement of the catheter at this site, tachycardia could not be reinduced. Radiofrequency energy was applied, and the patient was noninducible despite aggressive pacing protocols.

may be due to local block in portions of the coronary sinus. In this case, a site just within the coronary sinus was found with early activation during supraventricular tachycardia (Figure 9.15). With a catheter positioned here, the tachycardia terminated and could no longer be induced. Radiofrequency energy was applied, and the patient had no inducible arrhythmias after the ablation.

She has been arrhythmia free for the last several years. Given her excellent clinical response, in retrospect, the findings suggest that slow retrograde activation proceeded from the septum laterally and the apparent early depolarization of the distal coronary sinus was due to complex patterns of depolarization within the coronary sinus. It is possible that the prior slow pathway ablation contributed to this unusual finding and also worsened her arrhythmia.

KEY POINTS

- The arrhythmia mechanism in some cases may be unclear, and it is important to make a diagnosis before proceeding to designing a therapy plan.

- It is important to keep several maneuvers in mind to determine the tachycardia mechanism and understand what maneuvers completely "rule out" a tachycardia mechanism; for example, continuation of tachycardia during AV block conclusively rules out involvement of an AV accessory pathway in a reentrant circuit, while others provide "strong evidence" with some very unusual exceptions.

- Prior ablations may contribute in producing unusual presentations and electrogram patterns due to the production of regions of block (this issue is more obvious in Chapters 15–18).

CHAPTER 10

Supraventricular tachycardia case 9

A 53-year-old businessman had a first episode of a rapid heart rate 4 years ago. Three years ago, he had another episode of tachycardia and at electrophysiology study was found to have dual AV node physiology and underwent slow pathway modification. Unfortunately, he has had continued episodes of rapid heart rate and is referred for evaluation. He is otherwise healthy, and his physical examination is normal. Baseline ECG and a recording during tachycardia are shown in Figures 10.1 and 10.2.

The baseline ECG shows mild ST segment changes but otherwise shows no significant abnormalities. The event recorder tracing suggests the presence of discrete P waves in lead V1 that are positive and separated by an isoelectric period.

A few words about rapid atrial tachycardias and nomenclature are important in this case. Used generally, the term atrial tachycardia refers to any arrhythmia that is confined to atrial tissue (Figure 1.2) and would include atrial fibrillation, atrial flutter, focal atrial tachycardia, and multifocal atrial fibrillation. Of these, focal atrial tachycardia and atrial flutter would yield rapid but regular atrial rates. Atrial flutter is generally used to describe an atrial arrhythmia caused by reentry. Atrial flutters are often subdivided into macroreentry and microreentry depending on the size of the circuit. Focal atrial tachycardias appear to arise as a point source and are often due to abnormal automaticity. Obviously, it can sometimes be difficult to differentiate between a focal tachycardia source and a very small reentrant circuit (Chapter 11). The distinction is often important for determining the ablation strategy. In patients with atrial flutter, the reentrant circuit must be defined with specific attention to defining a critical

isthmus that can be targeted for ablation. Conversely, in atrial tachycardia, the ablation strategy is to find "the source" of abnormal activity, although as mentioned earlier, small reentrant circuits may be approached therapeutically as a point source. In practical terms, for atrial flutter ablation, regions of critical conduction are identified (using entrainment mapping as described in later chapters), and for atrial tachycardia ablation, the site of earliest atrial activation is sought. Remember, in atrial flutter, as there is continuous electrical activity, there is "no early and no late" electrograms.

The ECG can provide some clues on whether the patient has atrial flutter or atrial tachycardia. In macroreentrant atrial flutter, continuous atrial activity can be observed and careful inspection of all leads simultaneously will reveal that there is no discrete isoelectric period. Because atrial tachycardias are due to abnormal automaticity, there will be periods when atrial depolarization is not occurring, so discrete isoelectric periods separating the P waves will be observed. Unfortunately, often, the distinction can be difficult for several reasons. Firstly, atrial activity can often be obscured by the QRS complex and T waves. Secondly, often all 12 leads are not available for analysis from ambulatory ECG monitors, and while discrete P waves can be observed in one lead (often V1), other leads that might show continuous activity are not present. Thirdly, even if all 12 leads are available for analysis, slow conduction through an isthmus may be associated with such a small amount of atrial depolarization that a deflection away from baseline will not be observed. A common correlate to this phenomenon is supraventricular tachycardia due to AVRT or AVNRT where depolarization of the AV node usually cannot be observed clinically with current electrophysiologic recording equipment and must be

Understanding Intracardiac EGMs: A Patient Centered Guide, First Edition. Fred Kusumoto.
© 2015 John Wiley & Sons, Ltd. Published 2015 by John Wiley & Sons, Ltd.

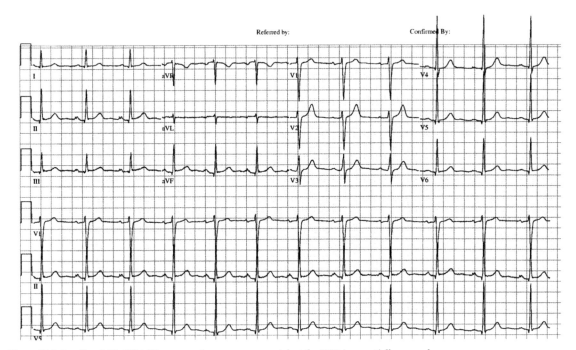

Figure 10.1 Baseline ECG. Mild ST segment changes are present, but the ECG is essentially normal.

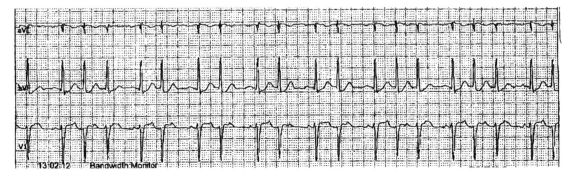

Figure 10.2 Irregular tachycardia recorded during ambulatory ECG monitoring. Discrete P waves appear in lead V1 that are positive and appear to be separated by an isoelectric period.

inferred. Fourthly, atrial flutter due to microreentry will have a similar ECG pattern as atrial tachycardia from an automatic source.

Returning to our case, during tachycardia, the patient appears to have discrete P waves in all three leads – negative in aVL, positive in lead II, and biphasic (initially flat or negative and then positive) in lead V1 suggestive of an atrial tachycardia due to abnormal automaticity. The baseline electrograms are normal.

Atrial pacing protocols are also normal with an AVBCL of 280 ms and an AVNERP of 236 ms. Ventricular pacing reveals no evidence of accessory pathway conduction and normal retrograde VA conduction properties. Double atrial extrastimuli induce unsustained atrial tachycardia.

As sustained tachycardia will again be important in this situation, the patient is started on isoproterenol. Atrial overdrive pacing induces a supraventricular tachycardia with a cycle length of 280 ms with variable AV conduction (Figure 10.3). The 12-lead ECG is shown in Figure 10.4. Notice that it is often difficult to discern the specific shape of the P wave, so it is often helpful to increase the gain of the ECG leads (Figure 10.5). Inspection of the ECG does suggest that the P waves are separated by a true isoelectric period and importantly confirms that this arrhythmia is similar to his clinical arrhythmia with generally similar morphology: upright P wave in lead II and a biphasic P wave in lead V1.

In order to provide more electrogram coverage of the right atrium, a decapolar catheter is placed along

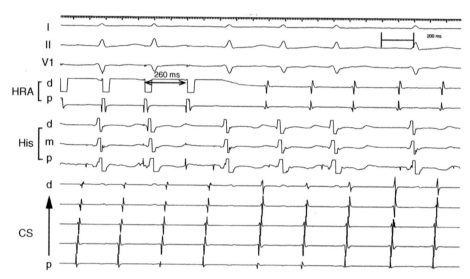

Figure 10.3 Rapid pacing from the right atrium at a cycle length of 260 ms induces an atrial tachycardia with a cycle length of 280 ms.

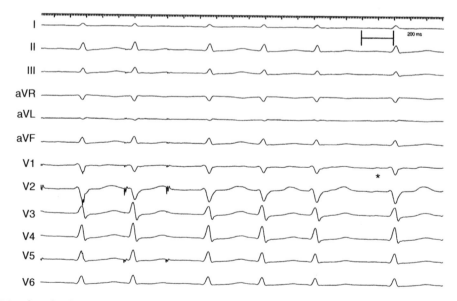

Figure 10.4 ECG of atrial tachycardia at "normal" gains. Specific P wave morphology and the earliest P wave deflection are difficult to assess even after AV block (*).

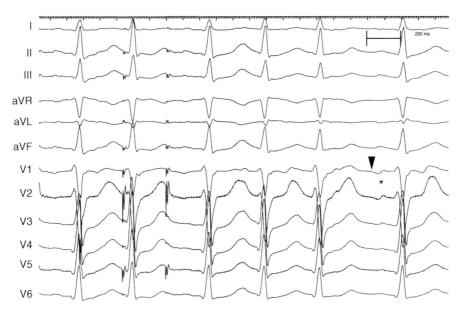

Figure 10.5 Gaining up the ECG allows the P wave morphology to be assessed (*) and identification of the earliest P wave deflection (arrowhead).

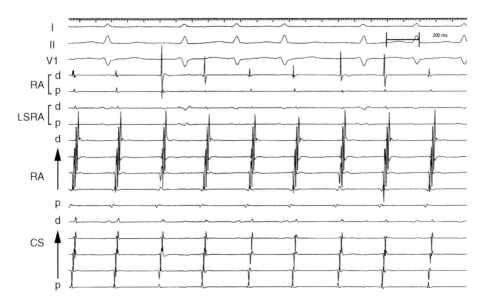

Figure 10.6 Addition of a right atrial catheter on the roof of the right atrium demonstrates a relatively early signal at the superior septum.

the roof of the right atrium with the distal electrode laterally on the free wall and the proximal electrode septally. Initial inspection of the electrograms "rules out" both an accessory-pathway-mediated tachycardia because the tachycardia continues even in the presence of AV block and AVNRT because atrial activation is "high to low" with initial atrial depolarization in the high right atrium (Figure 10.6). Now that it has been determined that the patient has an atrial tachycardia (using the more general definition), the focus of the study switches to determining whether the patient has a large reentrant circuit or a point source as the cause of his tachycardia.

Initial inspection of the electrograms shows that the left and right atria are activated almost simultaneously and that in the right atrium and on the surface ECG the P waves appear to be separated by an isoelectric period. Both findings suggest an automatic site but can be misleading. In particular, patients with left-sided atrial flutters will often have discrete flutter waves that are separated by isoelectric periods on the surface ECG (Chapters 10.15–10.18). The septal region of the

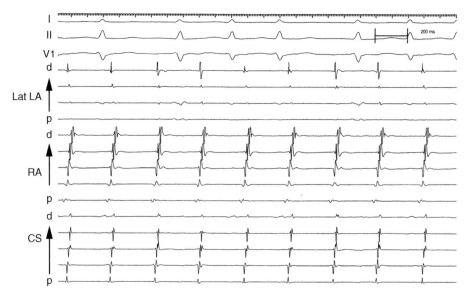

Figure 10.7 A decapolar catheter placed in the lateral wall of the left atrium demonstrates late activation of this region.

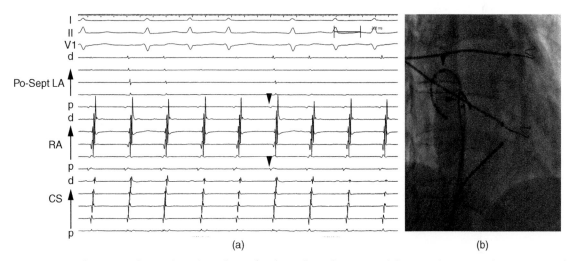

(a)   (b)

Figure 10.8 (a) Electrograms from a decapolar catheter placed septally in the posterior left atrium demonstrate late activation of this region. The earliest atrial signals are recorded in the superior electrodes of the left atrial and right atrial multielectrode catheters (arrowheads), which localizes the likely focus to the superior portion of the interatrial septum. (b) Fluoroscopic position of the catheters with the electrograms recorded on (a).

right atrium is the earliest initial electrogram on first evaluation, but it is critical to evaluate more posterior regions of the left atrium. Although the tachycardia may ultimately be localized to the right atrium, it is prudent to map the left atrium before proceeding with ablation.

Left atrial access is obtained and a multielectrode catheter is placed at the lateral wall and all of the recorded electrograms are late (Figure 10.7). This finding is not surprising as the coronary sinus is being activated in proximal to distal manner. Importantly, a multielectrode catheter placed on the posterior left atrial septum near the pulmonary vein ostia demonstrates that this area is also late (Figure 10.8). Taken together, all of the electrograms appear to occur simultaneously and make a focal source for tachycardia far more likely. The mapping strategy can now focus on identifying the earliest electrogram relative to the P wave. Early and stable intracardiac electrograms are observed on the superior portion of the left atrial side of the septum (Figures 10.9 and 10.10). Delivery of radiofrequency energy at this site leads to prompt termination of the

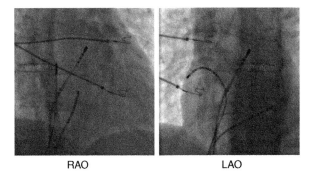

RAO   LAO

Figure 10.9 Mapping/ablation catheter placed in the superior portion of the left atrial side of the septum. RAO, right anterior oblique; LAO, left anterior oblique.

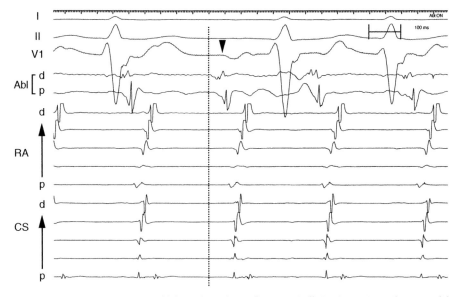

Figure 10.10 Electrograms from the superior septal left atrial site shown fluoroscopically in Figure 10.10. The onset of the electrogram precedes the earliest identifiable portion of the P wave (arrowhead) by 39 ms.

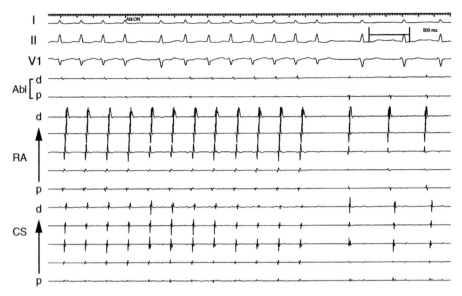

Figure 10.11 Radiofrequency energy application leads to cessation of tachycardia in 2.5 s.

atrial tachycardia in <3 s (Figure 10.11). During ablation in this region, it is important to avoid injury to the AV node, and continuous careful monitoring of the PR interval during ablation is required.

Automatic atrial tachycardias occur in characteristic anatomic locations. As a general rule of thumb, atrial tachycardias often arise at the confluence of anatomic structures. For example, in the right atria, automatic tachycardias are often located most commonly at the Crista terminalis (the anatomic site where the sinus venosus and the primitive right atium meet) and less frequently at the tricuspid annulus or the orifices of the superior vena cava, inferior vena cava, or coronary sinus. In the left atrium, the most common tachycardia sites are at the mitral annulus and from the pulmonary veins. Of course, there are many exceptions, and automatic atrial tachycardias from the atrial appendages, the posterior left atrium, and the septal region (as in our patient) have been described.

- Focal atrial tachycardias arise most commonly from specific sites: in the left atrium from the pulmonary veins and posterior left atrium but also less commonly from the septal region, the mitral annulus, and the left atrial appendage, while in the right atrium most commonly from the crista terminalis and less commonly the vena cavae, the coronary sinus, and the tricuspid annulus.

- In the setting of normal atrial tissue, in a focal atrial tachycardia, most of the atria will be depolarized in a relatively short period, often within 100–120 ms (consider the width of a P wave).

- Once focal atrial tachycardia has been identified as the mechanism of arrhythmia, sustained tachycardia facilitates the ablation and the earliest atrial electrogram is sought.

- Because the P wave represents global atrial depolarization, the atrial electrogram of the tachycardia source should occur earlier than the P wave and precede all recorded intracardiac electrograms.

KEY POINTS

- Regular atrial tachycardias can be due to reentry (atrial flutter) or automaticy (most accurately a focal atrial tachycardia but also commonly called atrial tachycardia).

CHAPTER 11

Supraventricular tachycardia cases 10 and 11

A 64-year-old woman has episodes of palpitations that began 10 years ago but now have become very frequent. She has been given beta-blockers with no change in her symptoms. Her physical examination is normal, other than irregular heartbeats, and her ECG is shown in Figure 11.1.

Her ECG shows bursts of atrial tachycardia. Inspection of the P wave provides some insight into the possible location of the tachycardia site. The P waves are positive in aVR, which suggests a left atrial site that is likely inferior given the very negative P waves identified in the inferior leads. At this point, the clinician can choose between more aggressive medical therapy or an invasive approach with electrophysiology study and ablation. A comprehensive discussion of the nuances of antiarrhythmic medications is far beyond the scope of this discussion. Generally, all medications can be thought of as "poisons with desirable side effects" and particularly for antiarrhythmic medications: "stronger poisons equals more efficacy but more risk" (Figure 11.2). The specific grouping and positions of the drugs in the figure are offered only as an opinion, and obviously, many experts will differ on the details and relative positions of specific drugs.

In this case, after discussion, the patient opts for an invasive approach and is taken to the electrophysiology laboratory. Because the patient clearly has an atrial tachycardia on initial noninvasive testing, the main strategy for the electrophysiology study is identification of the mechanism and anatomic location of the atrial tachycardia. Two decapolar catheters are positioned in the coronary sinus and the lateral wall of the right atrium, respectively, and are kept in the same position throughout the study. Initially, a quadripolar catheter is placed in the His bundle position.

Initial electrograms associated with a burst of atrial tachycardia are shown in Figure 11.3. As expected, baseline conduction is normal with an AH interval of 56 ms and an HV interval of 33 ms. Initiation of tachycardia is very suggestive of automaticity with the atrial electrograms from the first beat of tachycardia similar to subsequent beats. The tachycardia is regular with a cycle length of 253 ms, and initial evaluation of depolarization demonstrates near simultaneous depolarization of the lateral wall of the right atrium, the coronary sinus, and the septal atrial tissue near the AV node and His bundle. Coronary sinus activation is from proximal to distal, and of all the atrial electrograms present, the proximal coronary sinus appears the earliest. Because the P wave in V1 is almost entirely positive, a site from the posterior left atrium is the most likely site for tachycardia.

Left atrial access is obtained, and the roving multielectrode catheter is placed in the left atrium. Initially, the catheter is placed in the lateral wall of the left atrium (I believe it is prudent to first go to regions where you "don't think the focus is" and confirm your earlier clinical suspicion), and not surprisingly, given the proximal-to-distal coronary sinus activation pattern, this area is "late" (Figure 11.4). The catheter is moved to the posterior LA and the electrograms from this region are earlier than those from the lateral wall of the left atrium, but not the proximal CS (Figure 11.5 and 11.6). Finally, the circular mapping catheter is placed in the right inferior pulmonary vein, and importantly, activation appears to be "going into" the vein rather than "going out" (Figure 11.7). A site on the posterior wall just outside the inferior border of the right inferior

Understanding Intracardiac EGMs: A Patient Centered Guide, First Edition. Fred Kusumoto.
© 2015 John Wiley & Sons, Ltd. Published 2015 by John Wiley & Sons, Ltd.

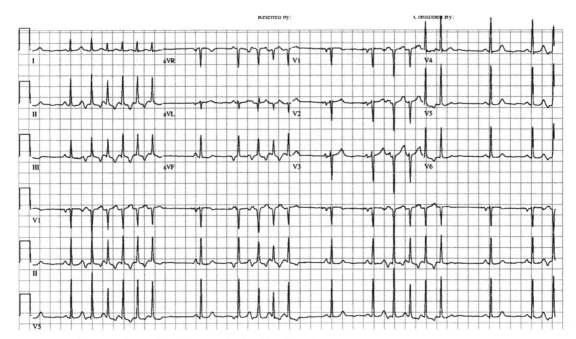

Figure 11.1 Baseline ECG shows salvos of nonsustained atrial tachycardia.

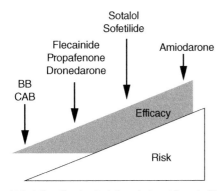

Figure 11.2 "Classification" of the relative risk and efficacy of commonly used antiarrhythmic medications. Generally, efficacy and risk go "hand in hand," and more effective drugs generally have more risks or side effects.

pulmonary vein is associated with a very early electrogram (Figures 11.8 and 11.9). Ablation at this site leads to prompt resolution of her salvos of atrial tachycardia (Figure 11.10). The patient had no recurrence during the procedure and had done well without symptoms or atrial tachycardias for the past 3 years.

In a second case, a 33-year-old woman with episodes of rapid heart rate has undergone prior ablation for a crista terminalis tachycardia and has continued episodes of tachycardia confirmed by event recorder tracings. She has had continued arrhythmias and has been referred for electrophysiology study and ablation.

When she arrives at the electrophysiology laboratory, she has incessant tachycardia (Figure 11.11). Initial electrograms from the patient during tachycardia are shown in Figure 11.12. At high gains, a broad low-frequency signal is identified on the high right atrial catheter placed at the superior vena cava and right atrial junction that is significantly earlier than the other electrograms. Because atrial depolarization is "high-low" and from "posterior to anterior," it is clear that the patient has an atrial tachycardia rather than AVNRT or AVRT, and attention can be focused on mapping the atrial tachycardia. Similarly to the first case, atrial activation is almost simultaneous, making a point source for her tachycardia the most likely possibility.

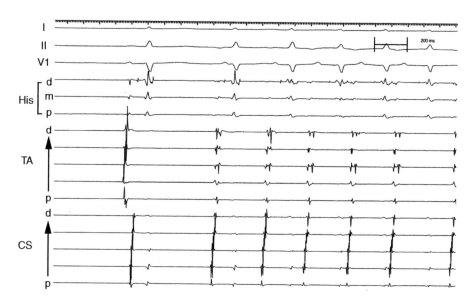

Figure 11.3 Baseline electrograms showing sinus rhythm and a salvo of atrial tachycardia. Earliest atrial electrogram is observed in the proximal coronary sinus. During tachycardia, the recorded electrograms occur simultaneously, favoring the diagnosis of an automatic atrial tachycardia. Because the coronary sinus is activated in a proximal-to-distal fashion, the tachycardia site is not in the lateral wall of the left atrium.

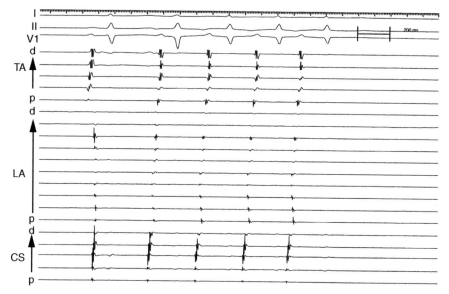

Figure 11.4 A multielectrode catheter placed on the lateral wall shows that this region of the atria is "late."

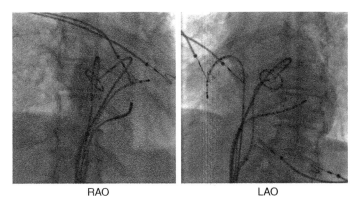

RAO   LAO

Figure 11.5 Fluoroscopy showing a circular mapping catheter placed on the inferior posterior wall in the right anterior oblique (RAO) and left anterior oblique (LAO) projections.

Again, it is important to obtain left atrial access, and in this case, a 64-electrode "basket" catheter is placed in the right superior pulmonary vein (Figure 11.13). Analysis of these electrograms demonstrates extremely early atrial activation emanating from deep within the right superior pulmonary vein (Figure 11.14). From the fluoroscopic images, it can be seen that the right superior pulmonary vein travels just behind the superior vena cava and that the early low-frequency signal recorded at the superior vena cava–right atrial junction represents the "far-field" recording of electrical activity from the right superior pulmonary vein.

Ablation within the pulmonary vein may lead to development of scar tissue and pulmonary vein stenosis; therefore, in this case, ablation was performed in the left atrium just outside the right superior pulmonary vein with termination of her tachycardia when the vein was isolated. Reevaluation of the right superior pulmonary vein with the basket catheter confirmed that the atrial tachycardia continued but the venous depolarization could not propagate to the left atrium because of the lesion set around the pulmonary vein. Interestingly, although the basket catheter recording suggests a point source for the tachycardia with no areas

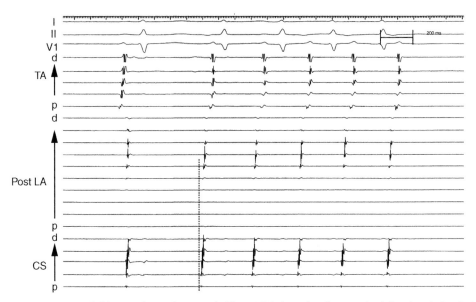

Figure 11.6 Electrograms recorded from catheter placement in Figure 11.5 show that the posterior left atrium is depolarized earlier as compared to the lateral wall but still does not "beat" the proximal coronary sinus.

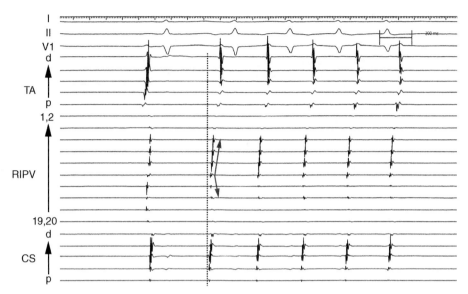

Figure 11.7 When the circular mapping catheter is placed in the right inferior pulmonary vein itself, the signals are even later, suggesting that the tachycardia site is "outside" the right inferior pulmonary vein and traveling into the veins.

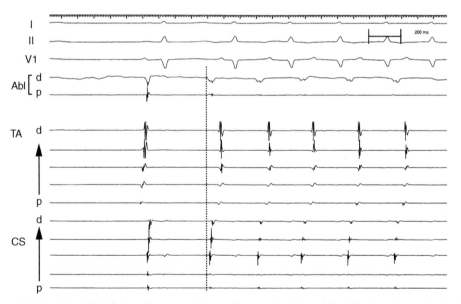

Figure 11.8 A site below the right inferior pulmonary vein near the posterior floor of the left atrium is associated with an early electrogram.

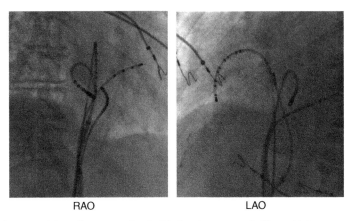

RAO   LAO

Figure 11.9 Fluoroscopic location of the catheters associated with the electrograms in Figure 11.8.

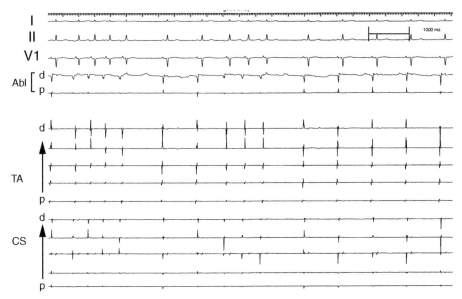

Figure 11.10 Radio-frequency energy at this site results in prompt cessation of the tachycardia.

of continuous activity that would be consistent with reentry, three extrastimuli within the pulmonary vein led to termination of the tachycardia (Figure 11.15). This finding certainly does not prove the mechanism but does suggest the possibility of reentry. The patient had been arrhythmia-free for the past 6 years.

These two cases are presented together to show the different approaches to atrial tachycardias that are located near the pulmonary vein region. In the first case, the tachycardia focus was located outside the pulmonary vein and a direct ablation approach could be performed. In the second case, the tachycardia focus emanated from deep within the pulmonary vein; therefore, the approach was to ablate within the left atrium just beyond the pulmonary vein os with a goal to isolate the pulmonary vein. Once the mechanism of tachycardia is identified, a therapeutic strategy can be individually tailored on the basis of the circumstances.

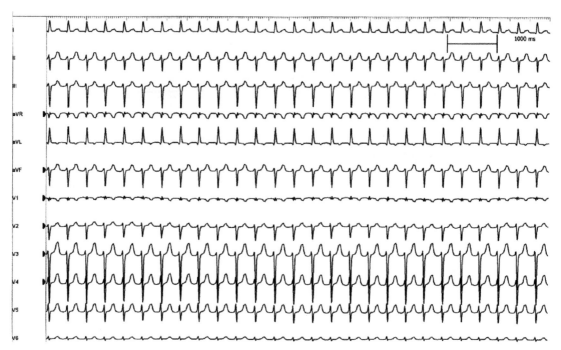

Figure 11.11 ECG showing incessant atrial tachycardia on arrival at the electrophysiology laboratory.

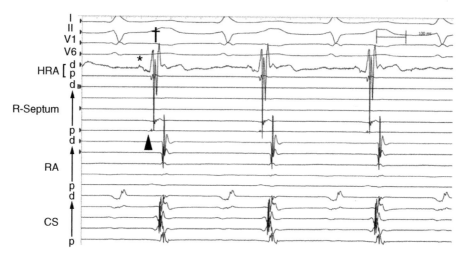

Figure 11.12 Initial electrograms during tachycardia. The earliest atrial electrogram was recorded at the superior vena cava–right atrial junction (high right atrium (HRA)). Notice that there are two components of the electrogram: a low-frequency early signal (*) and a later high-frequency signal (†). Low-frequency signals should always arouse suspicion of a "far-field" source of the electrogram – the electrograms are produced by an adjacent structure rather than from where the catheter is placed. Additionally, notice the relatively early electrogram recorded from the more proximal region of the coronary sinus relative to the right atrium.

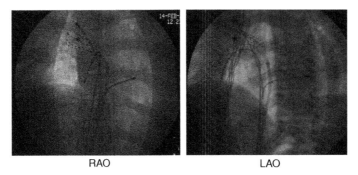

RAO   LAO

Figure 11.13 Fluoroscopy with a 64-electrode basket placed in the right superior pulmonary vein in the right anterior oblique (RAO) and left anterior oblique (LAO) projections.

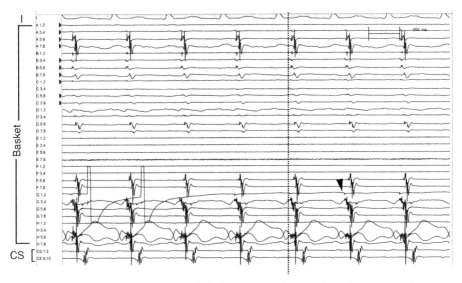

Figure 11.14 Electrograms recorded from the 64-electrode basket catheter placed in the right superior pulmonary vein shown in Figure 11.13. Earliest atrial signals are recorded in the third and the fourth electrode of the G and H splines that are shown by an asterisk in Figure 11.13 in the RAO and LAO projections.

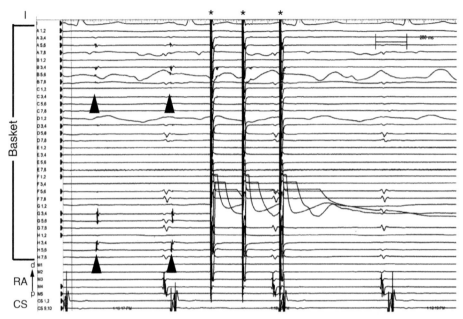

Figure 11.15 Termination of the tachycardia within the pulmonary vein with three extrastimuli delivered from within the pulmonary vein.

KEY POINTS

- In some cases, the diagnosis of an automatic focal atrial tachycardia can be established before electrophysiologic testing; however, it is important to analyze the available electrograms to make sure they are consistent with the diagnosis.

- Careful evaluation of the electrograms during mapping is often facilitated by a systematic approach using multielectrode catheters.

- The ablation strategy may differ on the basis of the location of a focal atrial tachycardia (direct ablation vs. isolation).

CHAPTER 12

Supraventricular tachycardia case 12

A 57-year-old retired police officer comes to your office complaining of rapid heart rate and tiredness for the past week. He had a similar episode 6 months ago when he was found with atrial flutter and required cardioversion. His physical examination reveals a rapid regular heart rate but is otherwise unremarkable without evidence for valvular abnormalities, left ventricular dysfunction, or heart failure. His ECG is shown in Figure 12.1.

The patient is with an arrhythmia characterized by organized rapid atrial activity. For our discussion, we have used a more generalized definition of atrial tachycardia as any arrhythmia that arises solely from atrial tissue. Electrophysiologists will use the term atrial flutter to describe an atrial arrhythmia due to a reentrant mechanism. In 1911, using the newly developed scientific tool, the ECG, Jolly and Ritchie were the first to describe the sawtooth atrial activity associated with atrial flutter and to distinguish between atrial flutter and fibrillation. Importantly, during the same era, using a canine model, Lewis noted that atrial flutter was associated with continuous atrial activity around the inferior and superior vena cavae.

Later on, during the 1980s and 1990s, investigators from multiple laboratories described the "typical" atrial flutter circuit that traveled around the right atrium, bounded anteriorly by the tricuspid valve (Figure 12.2). In typical atrial flutter, the critical isthmus that facilitates the development of a stable reentrant circuit is defined anteriorly by the tricuspid valve and posteriorly by the inferior vena cava. The usual reentrant circuit travels from lateral to medial in this isthmus and then activates the septum and left atrium in an inferior-to-superior direction. The wave of depolarization travels medial to lateral along the roof of the right atrium and then

down the lateral right atrial wall. When "looking" into the right atrium "through" the tricuspid valve, the wave of depolarization travels counterclockwise around the tricuspid valve, and the typical atrial flutter is often also called "counterclockwise atrial flutter" or cavotricuspid isthmus (often called the CTI) dependent atrial flutter.

From a clinical standpoint, atrial flutter generally occurs with atrial fibrillation and the decision on ablation of atrial flutter must always take the management of atrial fibrillation into account. For example, in the patient with both atrial fibrillation and atrial flutter, an isolated atrial flutter ablation will do very little for the patient's future outcome. However, in some cases, patients may have only paroxysmal atrial fibrillation that is minimally symptomatic, and it is only the development of sustained atrial flutter that leads to symptoms. In the latter case, it may be reasonable to perform an atrial flutter ablation. Another reasonable clinical situation to perform ablation of atrial flutter is for the patient with both atrial fibrillation and atrial flutter where an antiarrhythmic drug effectively treats the atrial fibrillation but persistent episodes of atrial flutter remain (Appendix, Table A7).

In addition to the discussion of clinical goals, the electrophysiologist must also carefully assess and discuss the risk of the procedure with the patient. Generally, the risk for an ablation performed solely in the right atrium is less than that for an ablation in the left atrium. Not only does access to the left atrium via transseptal puncture add a small but measurable risk, procedures in the left atrium that require extended mapping are associated with increased risk of stroke and other embolic events and bleeding (because intraprocedural anticoagulation is required). Table A5 in the Appendix compares the risks for ablation of supraventricular

Understanding Intracardiac EGMs: A Patient Centered Guide, First Edition. Fred Kusumoto.
© 2015 John Wiley & Sons, Ltd. Published 2015 by John Wiley & Sons, Ltd.

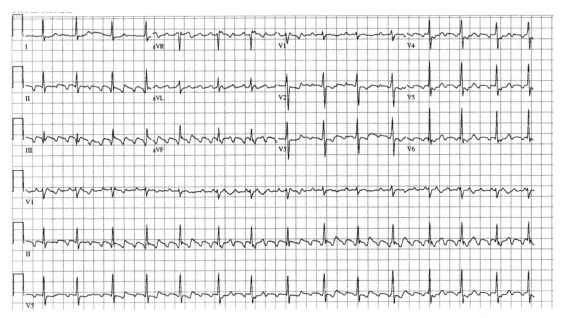

Figure 12.1 Baseline ECG is suggestive of typical atrial flutter with negative flutter waves in the inferior leads and no true isoelectric period for atrial depolarization.

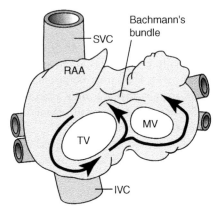

Figure 12.2 Schematic showing the atrial flutter circuit in typical "counterclockwise" atrial flutter. TV, tricuspid valve; MV, mitral valve; SVC, superior vena cava; IVC, inferior vena cava. (Kusumoto 1999. Reproduced with permission of Harris Barton Press.)

tachycardia, atrial flutter, and left-sided ablation of atrial tachyarrhythmias (both left-sided atrial flutter and atrial fibrillation).

Examination of the ECG from our patient reveals predominantly negative flutter waves in the inferior leads that are consistent with typical counterclockwise atrial flutter using the cavotricuspid isthmus. Atrial

flutter is the likely mechanism because there is no true isoelectric period that can be identified on the ECG. Even the "flatter" part of the flutter waves has a very gradual downward course. Remember, in atrial flutter, a portion of the atrium is always being depolarized, and if a macroreentrant circuit is present, relatively continuous atrial depolarization will be observed. In this patient with recurrent typical atrial flutter without atrial fibrillation, electrophysiology study and catheter ablation are a reasonable approach. For electrophysiology studies for the typical atrial flutter, we generally use two or three venous access sites. Two for the coronary sinus and the ablation/mapping catheter, and if a third catheter is used, it is placed along the lateral wall of the right atrium (Figure 12.3). Techniques among different operators vary significantly. For example, some will place a catheter in the cavotricuspid isthmus itself to evaluate the activation within this area.

Regardless of the catheter set used, once the catheters are placed, the first step is to identify the general pattern of atrial activation (Figure 12.4). In our patient, atrial depolarization travels from superior to inferior along the lateral wall of the right atrium (from proximal to distal electrodes), followed by activation of the cavotricuspid isthmus, which is followed by activation of the

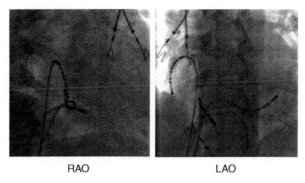

RAO   LAO

Figure 12.3 Initial fluoroscopic position of catheters in the right anterior oblique (RAO) and left anterior oblique (LAO) orientations. CS, coronary sinus; RA, right atrium; CTI, cavotricuspid isthmus.

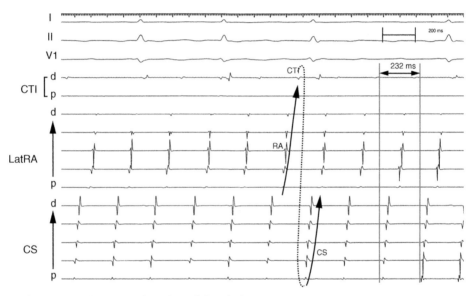

Figure 12.4 Initial electrogams showing a tachycardia cycle length of 232 ms with almost the entire tachycardia cycle length "covered" by catheters placed in the right atrium (RA), the cavotricuspid isthmus (CTI), and the coronary sinus (CS).

coronary sinus from the proximal electrodes to the distal electrodes. This activation pattern is consistent with the typical atrial flutter. Notice the electrogram equivalents of a macroreentrant flutter circuit: electrograms can be recorded through almost the entire cycle length of the tachycardia and the sequential activation of the right and left atria.

Once the general atrial activation sequence has been identified, the next step is to perform entrainment mapping by evaluating the tachycardia response to pacing (Figure 12.5). In entrainment mapping for atrial flutter, different sites of the atria are paced at a slightly shorter cycle length as compared to the

tachycardia (10–20 ms less) to minimize the likelihood of arrhythmia termination or cause slower conduction during one of the components of the tachycardia circuit. Once the circuit is entrained (as evidenced by a shortening of the tachycardia cycle length to the paced cycle length), pacing is stopped and the electrograms are evaluated. Entrainment mapping is arguably the most important concept for understanding the mechanism and ablation of atrial flutter and has two basic parts.

The first part of entrainment mapping is to determine how pacing affects the pattern of atrial activation. Generally, the closer a pacing site is to the exit site from a critical isthmus, the more similar the paced atrial

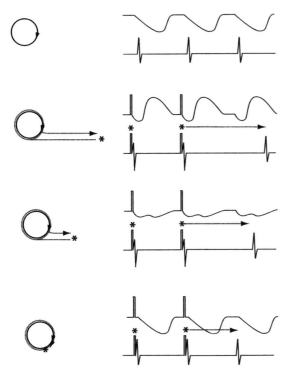

Figure 12.5 Conceptual schematic of entrainment mapping. When pacing from a site far from the circuit, the pattern of atrial depolarization changes leading to a change in the flutter morphology and a change in the electrograms. In addition, when pacing is stopped, the return cycle length is longer because the wave of depolarization has to travel to the reentrant circuit, interact with the circuit, and then return. As pacing is performed at a site closer to the reentrant circuit, the paced flutter wave looks more like spontaneous atrial flutter, there is a corresponding increase in the match between electrograms during pacing when compared to the electrograms during tachycardia, and on cessation of pacing, the timing is less. When pacing is performed from within the critical isthmus, the pattern of atrial depolarization is the same for both pacing and tachycardia and the return cycle length matches the tachycardia cycle length. This combination of findings is called concealed entrainment. (Kusumoto 2009. Reproduced with permission of Wiley.)

activation pattern (evaluated from the surface ECG and the intracardiac electrograms) will be to the spontaneous flutter waves. Figure 12.6 shows the effect of pacing from the high right atrium. Oftentimes, in atrial flutter, it is difficult to assess the surface ECG because of the relatively small atrial flutter waves; however, notice that activation in the right atrium is different during pacing when compared to atrial flutter and that, although the pattern of activation of the coronary sinus

is the same as that for pacing and atrial flutter, the timing from the stimulus to the coronary sinus electrograms differs between pacing and atrial flutter. Figure 12.7 shows the effect of pacing from the coronary sinus os (the proximal coronary sinus electrodes). In this case, the activation of the atria is the same during pacing and tachycardia as measured by the electrogram timing.

The second part of entrainment mapping is to evaluate the return cycle length on cessation of pacing. The farther the pacing site is from the critical isthmus, the longer is the return cycle length. In Figures 12.6 and 12.7, the return cycle length after cessation of pacing is much shorter from the coronary sinus as compared to the high right atrium that provides additional evidence that the coronary sinus is located very near the tachycardia circuit.

The findings from entrainment mapping confirm the presence of a cavotricuspid isthmus–dependent atrial flutter. In this case, the two barriers required for an isthmus of slow conduction are very well defined: the tricuspid annulus and the anterior wall of the inferior vena cava. A series of radiofrequency lesions are placed from the tricuspid valve to the inferior vena cava (Figure 12.8). Several important points are worth emphasizing during atrial flutter ablation. First, it is important to acknowledge the shortcomings of fluoroscopy. Most importantly, the LAO projection is often not in the same plane as the tricuspid valve, and catheter orientation may change as the catheter is moved from distal positions to proximal positions. In addition, fluoroscopy obviously cannot provide direct visualization of structures and often the operator must infer the position of the Eustachian ridge by the behavior of the catheter tip. Despite these issues, fluoroscopy can be extremely helpful, particularly if biplane fluoroscopy is available. By switching between the RAO and the LAO projection during ablation, the RAO projection provides important information on the position of the ablation catheter in relation to the tricuspid valve and the inferior vena cava, while the LAO projection allows the clinician to provide some guidance that he is following a "linear" path and is not inadvertently ablating more septally or more laterally. In the LAO projection, I will generally perform the ablation at the 6:00 position (with the tricuspid annulus positions arranged like a clock with 6:00 directly inferior, 12:00 directly superior, and septal is 2:00 to 5:00), although other operators will ablate more septally (e.g.,

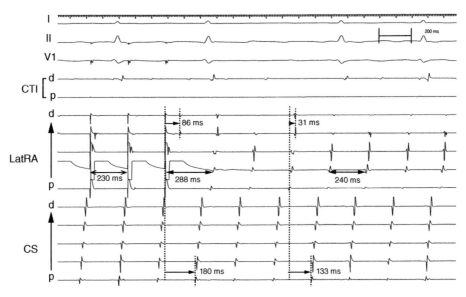

Figure 12.6 Entrainment mapping. Pacing from the high right atrium at a cycle length of 230 ms (the tachycardia cycle length has increased slightly from baseline to 240 ms). Notice that the stimulus to right atrial electrogram has shortened dramatically during pacing when compared to the electrogram-to-electrogram interval in atrial flutter. In addition, although the pattern of atrial activation within the coronary sinus is the same during pacing and atrial flutter (suggesting that the general direction of activation in both cases is the same), the stimulus to the electrogram interval during pacing is longer than the electrogram-to-electrogram interval during atrial flutter. In atrial flutter, it can often be difficult to identify the subtle changes in the flutter waves; however, the use of intracardiac electrograms provides a valuable surrogate for assessing the difference in atrial activation between pacing and atrial flutter. The return cycle length is longer than the tachycardia cycle length (288 ms vs. 240 ms), providing evidence that the pacing site is located at a distance from the tachycardia circuit.

5:30 or 5:00) or more laterally (6:30 or 7:00). The specific position of where the cavotricuspid isthmus ablation is performed is not that important as long as the operator tries to achieve a consistent "line." Oftentimes, as the ablation is being performed, pouches and ridges in the cavotricuspid isthmus will be encountered, which will tend to push the ablation catheter more septally or more laterally making achieving a line of block particularly challenging. It is important to understand that the Eustachian ridge is at the anterior portion of the inferior vena cava and often there are deep pouches within the cavotricuspid isthmus that must be negotiated to achieve a block. During ablation, it is important to monitor for any change in atrioventricular conduction to identify possible damage to the AV node. The clinician must pay close attention to any decrease in the ventricular response rate or development of a slow regular QRS rhythm and rate that could be due to complete heart block. During ablation, the tachycardia terminates (Figure 12.9).

Although tachycardia termination during ablation provides comfort and does suggest the ablation strategy is correct (some jokingly call this "thermal mapping"), it does not indicate in itself a successful ablation. In atrial flutter, the goal of ablation is to cause a line of conduction block across a critical isthmus: in this case, the cavotricuspid isthmus. In order to increase the likelihood of a successful ablation, it is important to confirm the presence of a line of block across the cavotricuspid isthmus. Assessing the presence of cavotricuspid isthmus block requires pacing from both sides of the line of block. Returning to our patient, in Figure 12.10, pacing is performed from the low lateral right atrium at a cycle length of 250 ms and atrial depolarization is first identified in the lateral right atrium followed by depolarization of the coronary sinus. The interval between the pacing stimulus and the proximal coronary sinus is 69 ms. Although the conduction pattern of the atrium is consistent with cavotricuspid isthmus block, the relatively short conduction time

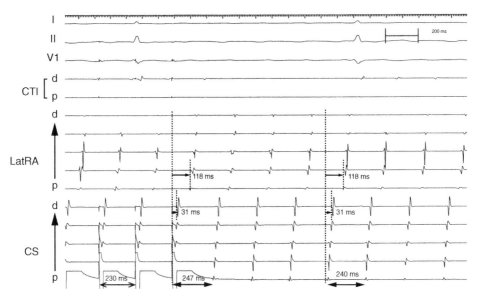

Figure 12.7 Entrainment mapping continued from Figure 12.6. In this case, pacing is performed from the coronary sinus and the stimulus to electrogram intervals match the electrogram-to-electrogram intervals whether measured at the right atrium or the coronary sinus. This provides strong evidence that, although the surface flutter waves cannot be observed, atrial activation is very similar for pacing when compared to spontaneous tachycardia. In addition, notice that the return cycle length after cessation of pacing almost matches the tachycardia cycle length. These two pieces of evidence suggest that the coronary sinus is very close to the reentrant circuit and provides strong evidence favoring a cavotricuspid isthmus–dependent atrial flutter.

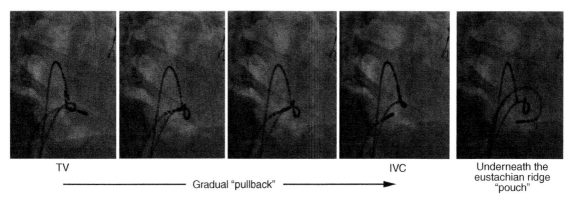

TV   IVC   Underneath the
                                                                                                                        eustachian ridge
─────────────────── Gradual "pullback" ──────────────▶   "pouch"

Figure 12.8 Ablation at the cavotricuspid isthmus in the RAO projection. On the left is a simple pullback of the catheter with downward force placed on the catheter from the tricuspid valve to the inferior vena cava. Oftentimes, patients will have deep pouches that are covered by a prominent Eustachian ridge.

from the stimulus to the proximal coronary sinus suggests that cavotricuspid isthmus conduction block has not been achieved. This suspicion becomes evident when pacing at a cycle length of 200 ms induces atrial flutter (Figure 12.11). The ECG of the induced atrial flutter is shown in Figure 12.12 in comparison to the original baseline atrial flutter. Notice that the flutter wave morphology is very different between the two atrial flutters. However, entrainment mapping confirms that this atrial flutter is also dependent on the cavotricuspid isthmus. When doing additional ablation in the cavotricuspid isthmus region, it is prudent to try and "stay in the original line" and identify the areas of tissue that remain viable. Higher frequencies ("sharper

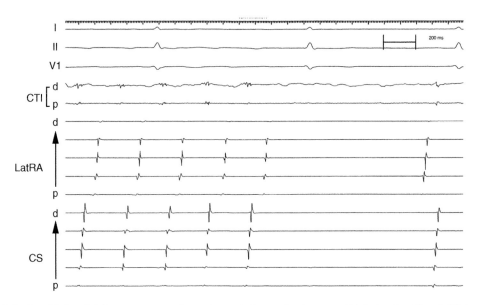

Figure 12.9 During ablation, it is important to monitor atrioventricular conduction to avoid injuring the AV node/His bundle axis. If the ablation is performed during atrial flutter (and you have correctly defined the tachycardia circuit!), the tachycardia will often terminate.

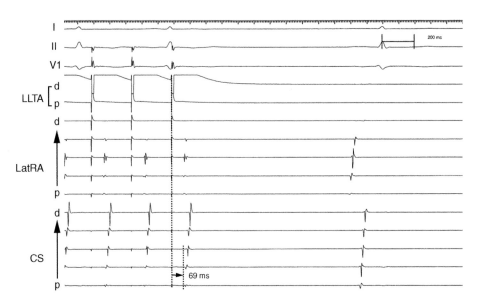

Figure 12.10 Pacing from the low lateral tricuspid annulus (LLTA) at a cycle length of 250 ms leads to an atrial activation pattern consistent with cavotricuspid isthmus block: Lateral right atrium (Lat RA) depolarization preceding coronary sinus depolarization. However, the stimulus to proximal coronary sinus electrogram is relatively short (69 ms), suggesting that cavotricuspid isthmus conduction is still present.

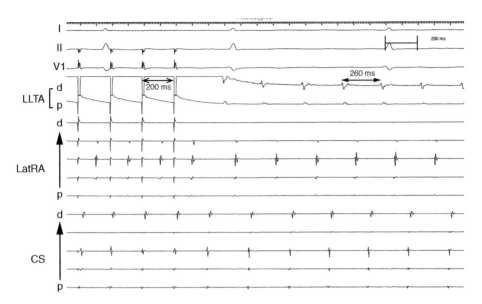

Figure 12.11 Pacing from the low lateral right atrium at a cycle length of 200 ms initiates atrial flutter with a tachycardia cycle length of 260 ms (30 ms longer than the initial atrial flutter) with sequential right atrial and left atrial depolarization consistent with a macroreentrant atrial flutter.

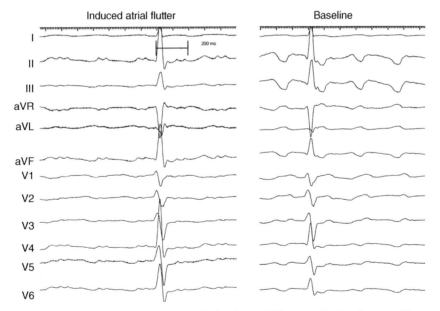

Figure 12.12 ECG of the induced atrial flutter as compared to the baseline atrial flutter. Notice that there are differences in the flutter wave morphology.

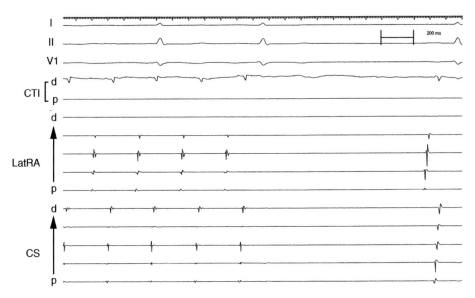

Figure 12.13 Viable tissue in the ablation line is identified by electrogram amplitude, and ablation on the right atrial side of the Eustachian ridge leads to termination of atrial flutter.

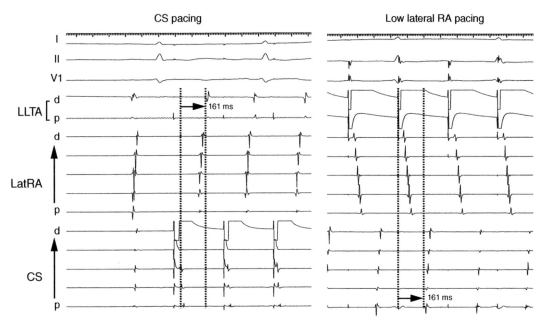

Figure 12.14 After additional ablation in the cavotricuspid isthmus, bidirectional block is confirmed by pacing from either side of the cavotricuspid isthmus line and recording a significant delay that is relatively constant regardless of the pacing cycle length or the direction that the pacing wavefront is traveling.

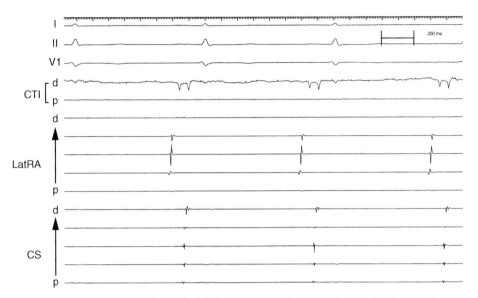

Figure 12.15 Another sign of cavotricuspid isthmus block is the presence of split potentials along the line of block.

or spikier") and larger amplitudes are characteristics of viable tissue. Areas within the cavotricuspid isthmus that are commonly missed are the right atrial side of the Eustachian ridge, deep pouches within the cavotricuspid isthmus (remember that ablation must be performed on both the anterior and posterior "sides" of a pouch, and apically near the tricuspid valve). Ablation at a site on the right atrial side of the Eustachian ridge terminates the tachycardia (Figure 12.13).

After this ablation, atrial pacing from the low lateral right atrium and the coronary sinus is associated with a dramatic increase in the conduction time across the cavotricuspid isthmus (Figure 12.14), and importantly, the conduction time remains constant at different paced rates and in both directions whether pacing from the lateral right atrium or the left atrium. Differential pacing is another method for evaluating whether an effective line of block is present. Pacing is performed at two sites on the same side of block and the interval to a fixed point is compared. In the presence of cavotricuspid isthmus block, pacing from a site closer to the line of block should yield a longer conduction time. In addition to pacing maneuvers, evaluation of the electrograms along the line of block can also be useful. If block is present, split potentials should be recorded (Figure 12.15). Double potentials signify that the area recorded by the electrode pair is being activated by two wavefronts.

After the ablation, the patient has done well without any symptomatic arrhythmias. Ambulatory ECG monitoring reveals short bursts of atrial fibrillation of 6–10 beats. In this case, episodes of atrial fibrillation likely facilitated development of sustained atrial flutter. Identification of atrial fibrillation may be clinically important particularly in patients for whom anticoagulation may be appropriate.

KEY POINTS

- Macroreentrant atrial flutter can be associated with continuous atrial activity on surface ECG; however, in some cases, a relatively isoelectric period between flutter waves will be observed.

- Macroreentrant atrial flutter often is associated with electrogram recordings that span a large portion of the tachycardia circuit.

- Once atrial flutter is identified, the goal of ablation is to produce a line of block across a critical isthmus.

- The most common form of atrial flutter uses the isthmus formed by the inferior vena cava and the tricuspid valve.

- After ablation, it is important to confirm that a line of conduction block has been produced.

CHAPTER 13

Supraventricular tachycardia case 13

A 43-year-old woman underwent an open atrial septal defect repair for an ostium secundum defect in 1991. Five months ago, she developed rapid heart rate with shortness of breath and severe fatigue. She was found to have a rapid narrow complex rhythm that resolved after 4 days of hospitalization. Since then, she had intermittent symptomatic arrhythmias that have become increasingly frequent and now constant for the past 2 months.

Her current medications include metoprolol 37.5 mg twice daily and diltiazem 180 mg daily for rate control, and she has been anticoagulated with warfarin. In her physical examination, only a rapid irregular heart rate was noted. Her ECG is shown in Figure 13.1. Transthoracic echocardiography shows no evidence of an interatrial shunt, mild left atrial enlargement, normal left ventricular function, and no significant valvular abnormalities.

Her ECG shows rapid regular atrial activity and an irregular but rapid ventricular response. Atrial activity is most prominent in lead V1 and appears biphasic, but is predominantly positive. In the inferior leads, the flutter waves are less prominent and are minimally negative in lead III and flatter with multiple components in leads II and aVF. The flutter waves are positive in I and aVL and negative in lead aVR. As mentioned in the previous chapter, inspection of the flutter wave morphology can be useful for identifying whether the atrial flutter depends on the cavotricuspid isthmus. However, in the setting of prior atrial surgery or prior ablations, flutter wave morphology becomes a less reliable tool for identifying the underlying type of atrial flutter.

Given her symptoms, the patient is referred for electrophysiology study and her preoperative laboratory analysis is normal (including a pregnancy test), but her INR is only 1.5.

Her subtherapeutic INR necessitates a preprocedural transesophageal echocardiography that demonstrates no left atrial thrombus and confirms normal left and right ventricular function and the absence of any significant valvular abnormalities or interatrial shunt. Interestingly, evaluation of her septum suggests relatively normal anatomy and an atrial patch cannot be identified.

When approaching an electrophysiology study and likely ablation for a patient with atrial flutter who has had prior surgery, I will initially place four vascular sheaths, two in each femoral vein. Although the case can be performed with fewer separate vascular access points, in patients with atrial tachycardia or atrial flutter with a complex medical history, placement of a multielectrode catheter in both the coronary sinus and the lateral right atrium facilitates mapping by providing two stable catheters that are kept in a relatively constant position during the entire case (Figure 13.2). The two additional venous access sites are used for a multipolar catheter that "roves" to the regions of interest within the atrium and an ablation catheter.

Just as described in the last chapter, the baseline activation pattern of the atria should be evaluated and pacing is performed (Figures 13.3–13.7) to provide some initial clues for the arrhythmia mechanism. First, notice in Figure 13.3 that the lateral wall of the right atrium and the coronary sinus appear to be activated almost simultaneously and that there is some cycle length variation in the tachycardia. Atrial pacing is first performed from the high lateral wall of the right atrium (the proximal electrodes), and consistent atrial capture is not present. It is critical to ensure atrial capture (the tachycardia is entrained) before evaluating "entrainment mapping." Although this basic concept seems obvious, it can lead many clinicians astray. Atrial pacing is performed from the proximal coronary

Understanding Intracardiac EGMs: A Patient Centered Guide, First Edition. Fred Kusumoto.
© 2015 John Wiley & Sons, Ltd. Published 2015 by John Wiley & Sons, Ltd.

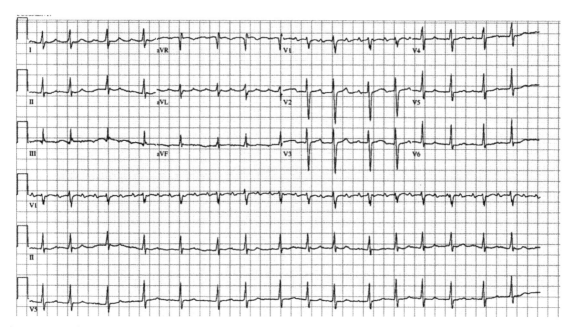

Figure 13.1 Baseline ECG.

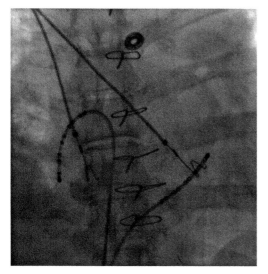

Figure 13.2 Anteroposterior fluoroscopic view of initial catheter position.

sinus (Figure 13.4), and the atrial activation pattern has changed (coronary sinus before the lateral right atrium) and the return cycle length is relatively long (369 ms) even when accounting for the tachycardia cycle length variability. Atrial pacing more distally in the coronary sinus (Figure 13.5) again changes the atrial activation pattern (left atrium before right atrium), although, interestingly, the pattern of right atrial activation during pacing matches the pattern during tachycardia. The return cycle length remains prolonged at 370 ms. As shown in Figure 13.6, pacing from the low lateral wall of the right atrium yields a much shorter return cycle length that appears to be similar to the expected cycle length and the atrial activation pattern during pacing is similar to the pattern observed during tachycardia with near simultaneous activation of the right and left atria. Another technique to use at this point of study is infusion with adenosine to better evaluate the morphology of the flutter waves (Figure 13.7).

Now that initial entrainment mapping has been performed, the findings are very suggestive of a right atrial flutter that does not involve the cavotricuspid isthmus. Although more detailed mapping of the right atrium could be undertaken, it is often more efficient to obtain left atrial access to fully map the remainder of the atria. While this initial catheter information provides a "first look" at the activation of the anterior left atrium, it does not provide any information on the activation of large portions of the left atrium including the pulmonary veins. In addition, given the near simultaneous activation of the left and right

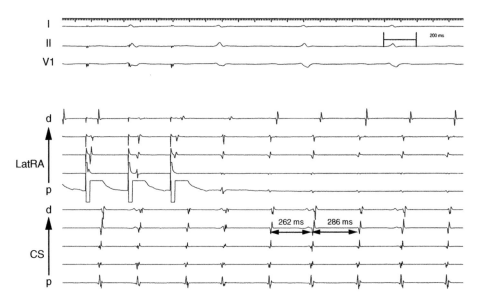

Figure 13.3 Pacing stimuli are delivered from the proximal electrodes of the right atrial catheter. However, it is important to first assess whether the tachycardia was entrained, which first requires consistent atrial capture. Pacing from the high right atrium does not result in consistent capture. Also note that the tachycardia cycle length is irregular.

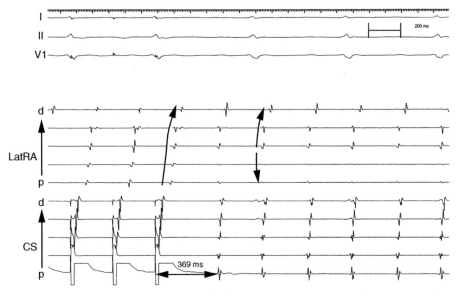

Figure 13.4 Pacing from the proximal coronary sinus completely changes atrial activation, and not surprisingly, coronary sinus activation precedes lateral right atrial activation and the right atrial activation pattern has changed. The return cycle length to the proximal coronary sinus is 369 ms.

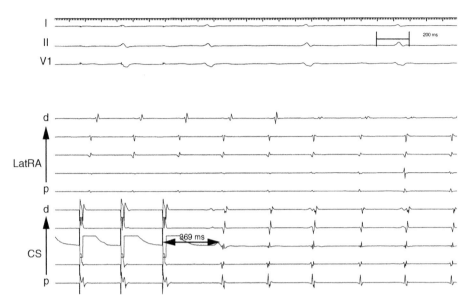

Figure 13.5 Pacing from a more distal portion of the coronary sinus also changes the atrial activation pattern (left atrium before right atrium), although interestingly, the region subtended by the right atrial catheter is activated in the same general pattern during pacing and tachycardia. The return cycle length is also 369 ms.

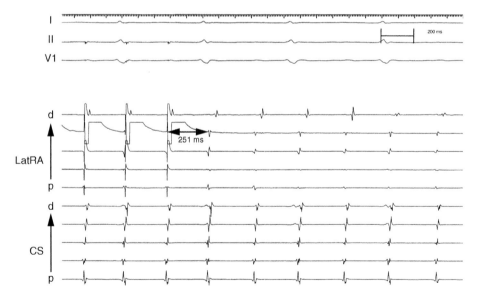

Figure 13.6 Pacing from the low lateral right atrium results in an atrial activation pattern during pacing that is similar to tachycardia and is associated with a return cycle length (251 ms) that is close to the expected cycle length of tachycardia. Both of these results suggest that the lateral wall of the right atrium is "in" or certainly close to the tachycardia circuit.

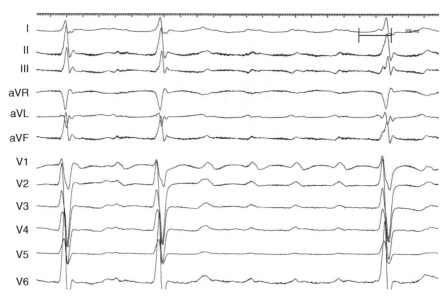

Figure 13.7 Adenosine is given to better define the morphology of atrial activation by the surface ECG. It is not entirely clear whether there is a true isoelectric period separating the waves of atrial depolarization. It does show that the major portion of the atria is activated simultaneously with a negative deflection in aVR and a positive deflection in lead II but biphasic deflections in aVF and III.

atria, it is not clear whether the tachycardia is due to automaticity rather than reentry. Entrainment mapping can only be performed in the setting of reentry, because tachycardias due to automaticity cannot be entrained by pacing but can be suppressed. Finally, left atrial access does not appear to be problematic, and once left atrial access was obtained, a multielectrode catheter was placed along the lateral wall of the left atrium and a mapping catheter in the right superior pulmonary vein (Figure 13.8). With the catheters in position, electrogram recordings demonstrate lateral left atrial activation occurring at the same time as coronary sinus activation and, in fact, the catheters only account for 91 ms of the 268 ms tachycardia cycle length (Figure 13.9). This finding essentially rules out a macroreentrant atrial flutter and suggests a more focal source – either a small reentrant circuit or automaticity. Inspection of all of the electrograms together suggests that if the tachycardia is due to automaticity, activation of the right superior pulmonary vein is either "late or early." Changing the standard multielectrode catheter to a circular mapping catheter (lasso) allows for the evaluation of the pulmonary veins (Figures 13.10–13.13). Not surprisingly, the left-sided pulmonary veins occur at the same time as the lateral wall with relatively

"early activation" at the right-sided pulmonary veins. Importantly, the right-sided pulmonary vein activity occurs almost simultaneously making reentry within the pulmonary veins less likely, although it is still theoretically possible, because there may be regions within a pulmonary vein that are not being mapped. To reduce the likelihood of this possibility, the circular mapping catheter can be moved distally and proximally within the pulmonary vein to search for fractionated electrical activity.

Unfortunately, manipulation of the circular mapping catheter within the tachycardia terminates with the transient development of more irregular activity at the posterior left atrium (Figure 13.14). This phenomenon has been well described by Waldo and colleagues. It is important to reinduce the tachycardia at this point because the underlying mechanism of the tachycardia has not been identified. Termination of the premature atrial activity (in this case, from mechanical stimulation) suggests the possibility of a reentrant mechanism; however, this behavior can also be seen with automaticity. Fortunately, in this case, atrial pacing easily reinduces the arrhythmia (Figure 13.15). With reinitiation of tachycardia, pacing is performed at the earliest electrogram site in the right inferior pulmonary

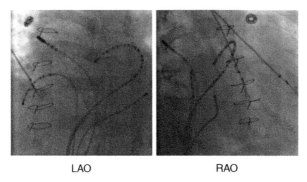

LAO   RAO

Figure 13.8 Fluoroscopic positioning of a multielectrode catheter in the left atrium and a mapping catheter in the right superior pulmonary vein.

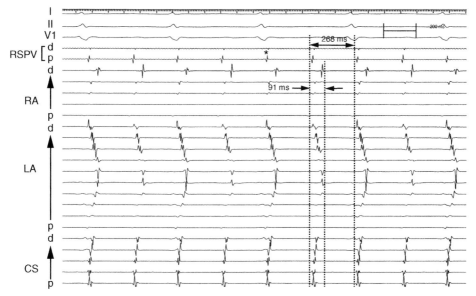

Figure 13.9 Electrograms corresponding to the catheter positions in Figure 13.7. Notice that even with multielectrode catheters placed in different regions of the heart, only a small portion of the tachycardia cycle length is "covered" (91/268 ms or 34% of the tachycardia cycle length).

vein (Figures 13.16 and 13.17). Notice that, although the activation pattern in a specific catheter remains the same (which suggests similar directions of depolarization), there are slight differences in the timing between the electrograms obtained during pacing and tachycardia. The return cycle length is shorter than the coronary sinus but not as "good" as the return cycle length from the low lateral right atrium.

Now that comprehensive left atrial mapping has been performed, it is important to again review the characteristics of the patient's tachycardia. First, from

a mechanistic standpoint, given the simultaneous activation of the left and right atria, a large macroreentrant circuit is not present. From an anatomic localization standpoint, the earliest atrial activation relative to the surface ECG has been the inferior portion of the right inferior pulmonary vein, and although pacing from this site resulted in a similar atrial activation pattern for each of the individual catheters, the timing among the different catheters was slightly different between pacing and tachycardia. If the tachycardia is due to reentry, the best return cycle length

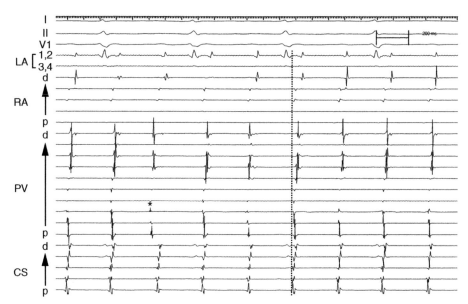

Figure 13.10 A circular mapping catheter is placed in the left superior pulmonary vein, and notice that activation is "late" and essentially simultaneous to the activation of the coronary sinus. It is important to identify consistent activation and not be misled by the single early depolarization within the left superior pulmonary vein (*).

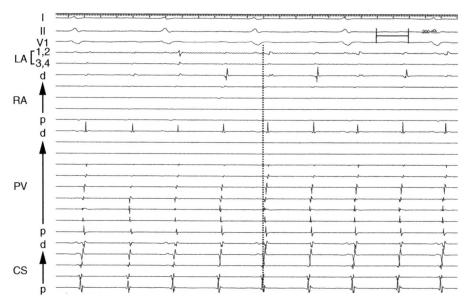

Figure 13.11 Continuation of pulmonary vein mapping. The circular mapping catheter is placed in the left inferior pulmonary vein and activation is even "later."

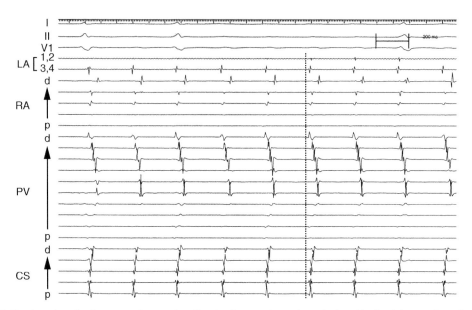

Figure 13.12 Continuation of pulmonary vein mapping. The circular mapping catheter is placed in the right superior pulmonary vein and the activation is "earlier."

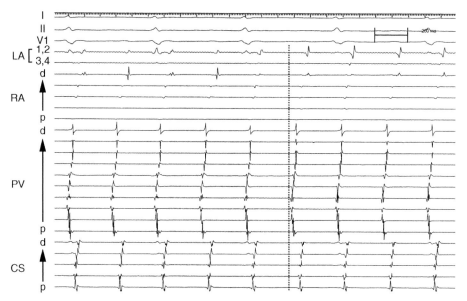

Figure 13.13 Placing the circular mapping catheter in the right inferior pulmonary vein reveals the earliest activation of all of the pulmonary veins (using the coronary sinus electrograms as a stable fiduciary point).

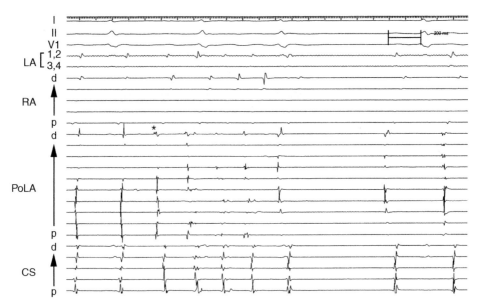

Figure 13.14 Catheter manipulation in the posterior left atrium leads to termination of the tachycardia. The tip of the circular mapping catheter appears to cause early activation that leads to termination (*).

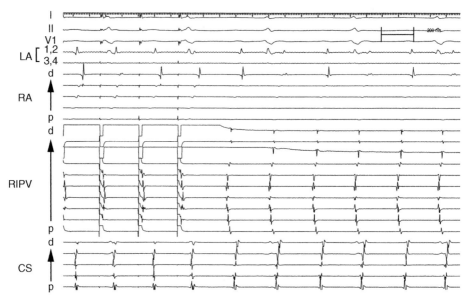

Figure 13.15 Pacing from the right inferior pulmonary vein (RIPV) leads to reinitiation of the atrial tachycardia.

was identified in the low lateral right atrium. In our experience, initial exploration of the right atrium with a multielectrode linear catheter allows larger areas of the atrium to be explored. Once a region of scar or low potential signal is identified, a circular mapping catheter can then be used to identify the potential areas that could represent isthmuses of viable tissue that are the critical pathways for perpetuation of tachycardia. Using this strategy, a circular mapping catheter is placed in the inferior and posterolateral region of the right atrium

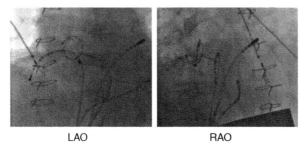

LAO   RAO

Figure 13.16 Fluoroscopy of catheter positions with a circular mapping catheter placed at the os of the right inferior pulmonary vein in the right anterior oblique (RAO) and left anterior oblique (LAO) projections. The asterisk denotes the electrode pair 13, 14 where pacing as shown in Figure 13.17 is performed.

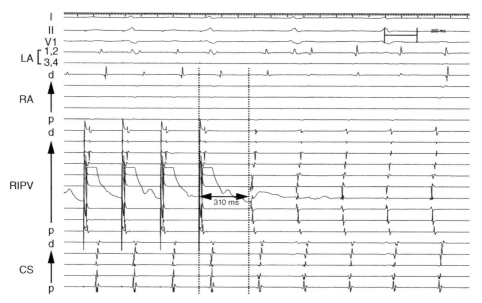

Figure 13.17 Pacing from the "earliest" electrogram in the right inferior pulmonary vein (see Figure 13.16) leads to similar activation patterns for each catheter but slight differences in timing between the different catheters, for example, during pacing, the stimulus to right atrial activation interval is ms and during tachycardia, the electrogram-to-electrogram interval is ms. The return cycle length remains prolonged (310 ms) but is shorter than the return cycle lengths from the coronary sinus.

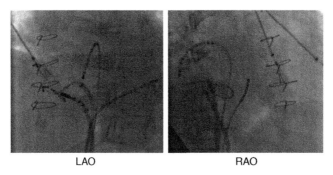

LAO   RAO

Figure 13.18 Fluoroscopic images of a circular mapping catheter placed in the inferolateral right atrium.

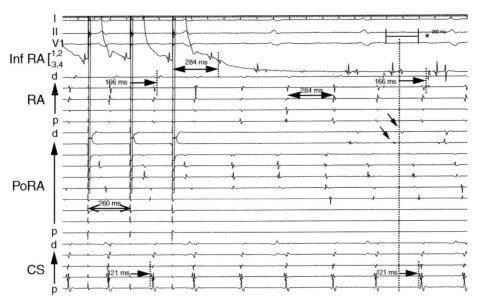

Figure 13.19 Electrograms obtained from the catheter positions shown in fluoroscopic images from Figure 13.18. Atrial pacing at a cycle length of 260 ms from the inferior and lateral right atrium at a site characterized by split potentials. First, notice that the region identified by the ablation/roving catheter and the two distal pairs of the circular mapping catheter are associated with electrograms during the isoelectric period separating the P wave identified on the surface ECG (*). Second, the electrogram pattern and timing during pacing match the pattern and timing during tachycardia (stimulus–distal RA electrogram and electrogram–distal RA electrogram intervals are both 166 ms and the stimulus–coronary sinus (CS) electrogram and the electrogram–CS electrogram intervals are both 121 ms). Finally, the return cycle length after completing the pacing is the same as the tachycardia cycle length (284 ms).

(Figure 13.18). Inspection of the electrograms from this region (Figure 13.19) reveals a region of scar subtended by the three proximal electrode pairs of the 20-electrode circular mapping catheter. Importantly, an area of electrical activity is seen in the isoelectric period separating the surface P waves. This finding strongly suggests the presence of a smaller reentrant circuit and identifies a location where electrical activity continues but is not associated with large areas of atrial depolarization. The electrograms are characterized by fractionated or double potentials. As mentioned in the previous chapter, double potentials may represent areas of partial or complete conduction block and fractionated signals may represent areas of slow conduction. Pacing at this site results in concealed entrainment. The term concealed entrainment is used because the paced depolarization pattern is exactly the same as that during tachycardia. The only sign that the tachycardia is entrained is that the electrograms occur at the paced rate rather than the tachycardia rate. When pacing is stopped, the electrogram recorded at the pacing site matches the tachycardia cycle length. These findings provide strong evidence that

pacing is being performed from within a critical isthmus used for reentry (refer back to Chapter 12, Figure 12.5, bottom schematic). Notice that the electrogram pattern is similar during both pacing and tachycardia, suggesting that the direction of atrial activation is unchanged. In addition to the pattern of activation, the timing from the pacing stimulus to the different electrograms is similar to the electrogram-to-electrogram timing during tachycardia. Both of these findings are the intracardiac electrode equivalent of similar flutter waves recorded on the surface ECG.

Ablation at this site first causes prolongation of the tachycardia cycle length, which paradoxically leads to an increase in the ventricular rate due to 1:1 AV conduction (Figure 13.20). Continued ablation leads to termination of the tachycardia. (Figure 13.21) In sinus rhythm, a region of late right atrial activation remains (Figure 13.22). This area actually depolarizes after completion of left atrial activation (estimated by the coronary sinus electrograms and the surface ECG). Additional ablation is performed here because this could represent a pathway of slow conduction.

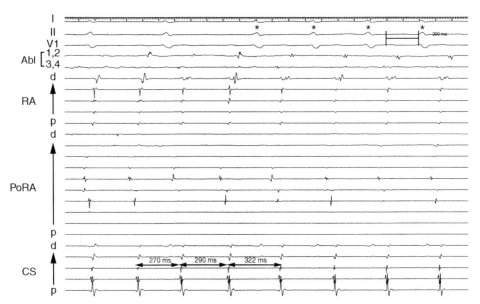

Figure 13.20 During ablation, the cycle length progressively increases from 270 ms to 322 ms, but the overall activation pattern as measured by the intracardiac electrograms remains constant. Notice that with the increase in cycle length, 1:1 AV conduction develops (*).

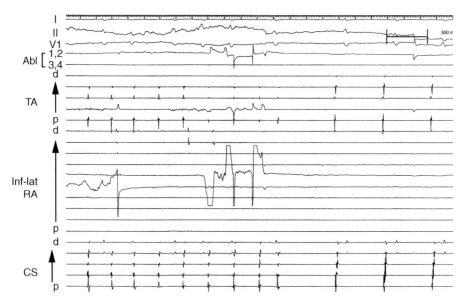

Figure 13.21 Continued ablation leads to termination of the tachycardia.

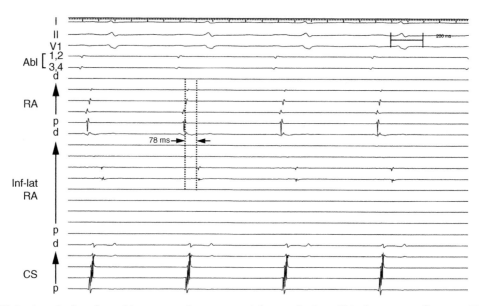

Figure 13.22 In sinus rhythm, the goal is to ensure that no areas of slow conduction within the scar are still present. The circular mapping catheter is manipulated in the region and a fairly dense scar is identified with a single region characterized by late atrial activity showing almost no electrical activity, suggesting a relatively large area of homogeneous scar. There continues to be very late activity in a small portion of the atria at the middle electrodes pairs (7,8 and 9,10) of the circular mapping catheter. Additional ablation is performed here because this area of slow conduction could facilitate the development of a stable reentrant circuit.

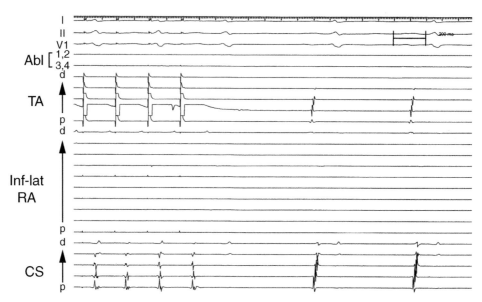

Figure 13.23 After ablation, the patient is noninducible for atrial arrhythmias and the region of interest shows a homogeneous scar.

After these ablations, the patient is noninducible for atrial arrhythmias despite aggressive pacing protocols (Figure 13.23). Had rapid atrial pacing led to the development of atrial fibrillation, in this patient, this would likely represent a nonspecific finding and should not be used as a reason to proceed with ablation of atrial fibrillation (e.g.,ablation in the pulmonary veins).

For postprocedure management of this patient, the clinician must decide between continuing oral anticoagulation with warfarin and bridging with low-molecular-weight heparin versus starting one of the "novel" oral anticoagulants that inhibit thrombin of activated Factor X. These new medicines are advantageous because adequate anticoagulation is achieved fairly quickly after an oral dose. There are no clinical data defining the relative merits and problems with each strategy; however, in general, the trend in our laboratory has been to change to one of the newer anticoagulants with increasing experience with these agents. Several single-center studies have confirmed this trend in other institutions.

KEY POINTS

- In patients with a history of cardiac surgery that required atrial incisions or prior ablation, it is often useful to have more venous access points to allow simultaneous activation of larger areas in different anatomical sites.

- Entrainment mapping is the cornerstone for identifying the critical isthmus(es) participating in the tachycardia circuit.

- Defining the location of scar is extremely useful.

- Because the critical isthmus location is often, in part, defined by unnatural history, the operative report can be useful, although even if available, sometimes they do not have enough detail to help define the potential location of scars.

CHAPTER 14

Supraventricular tachycardia case 14: atrial fibrillation

A 58-year-old woman has had several episodes of rapid heart rate and is found to be in atrial fibrillation with a rapid ventricular response (Figure 14.1). She receives intravenous diltiazem to slow her heart rate and convert to sinus rhythm in the morning. She has no other medical problems. These episodes have become progressively more frequent and now occur daily.

Atrial fibrillation (AF) is the most common tachyarrhythmia encountered in clinical medicine. Although estimates vary, approximately 4–6 million people in the United States have atrial fibrillation. Management of atrial fibrillation falls under two separate but related issues: Reduction of stroke risk and symptom management. A discussion of the risk of stroke in atrial fibrillation is beyond the scope of this chapter, and we are awaiting the results of a large randomized trial (Catheter Ablation Versus Antiarrhythmic Drug Therapy for Atrial Fibrillation (CABANA) Trial) to evaluate whether electrophysiology study and catheter ablation with drug refractory atrial fibrillation reduce the risk of stroke.

Over the past 40 years, pioneers in surgery and electrophysiology including James Cox, Michel Haissaguerre, Mel Scheinman, and many others have explored the possibility of using nonpharmacologic approaches for the treatment of atrial fibrillation. Catheter and surgical ablation for atrial fibrillation are now established treatment options for selected patients with atrial fibrillation. Although usually reserved for patients with symptomatic atrial fibrillation who have failed at least one antiarrhythmic medication, several randomized studies have suggested that catheter ablation is a reasonable first-line therapy in selected patients. The recent 2012 Heart Rhythm Society (HRS)/European Heart Rhythm Association (EHRA)/European Cardiac Arrhythmia Society (ECAS) Expert Consensus Statement on Catheter and Surgical Ablation guidelines emphasize the importance of considering multiple clinical variables such as duration of atrial fibrillation, left atrial size, and the presence of comorbid conditions but also note that patient preference must take a central role in the decision process. The current guidelines that address the use of ablation for the treatment of atrial fibrillation are summarized in Tables A8 and A9 in Appendix.

Currently, there are a number of approaches to catheter ablation of atrial fibrillation, and this field continues to evolve rapidly. We are indebted to Michel Haissaguerre and his colleagues from Bordeaux, France, who in the mid-1990s demonstrated that the pulmonary veins are often the site of ectopy that can initiate atrial fibrillation. Regardless of the technique used, for a patient with paroxysmal atrial fibrillation, the strategy is to ablate in regions around the pulmonary veins often in hopes of completely electrically isolating the pulmonary veins. In some cases, additional ablation is performed, for example, additional "lines" within the right atrium and/or the left atrium (see below).

For patients with persistent AF, the strategy varies more dramatically. Some advocate a minimalist approach ablating only the region around the pulmonary veins. Most experts note that additional lesions are usually required and also add "lines" within the left atrium and, less commonly, the right atrium. The most common "line" is a series of lesions from the mitral annulus to the left inferior pulmonary vein (LIPV). Another commonly used line is a "roof" line that connects the right superior and the left superior pulmonary veins (LSPV). In the right atrium, ablation

Understanding Intracardiac EGMs: A Patient Centered Guide, First Edition. Fred Kusumoto.
© 2015 John Wiley & Sons, Ltd. Published 2015 by John Wiley & Sons, Ltd.

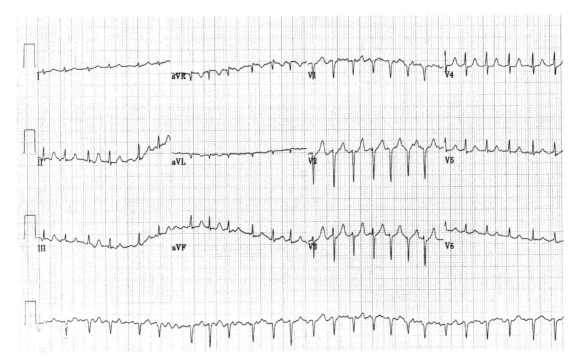

Figure 14.1 ECG showing atrial fibrillation.

is often performed in the cavotricuspid isthmus in those patients who have concomitant typical atrial flutter. Rather than doing "lines," ablation can also be performed in regions with highly fractionated electrograms with a long duration – often called complex fractionated atrial electrograms. By coupling mapping of multiple points with specialized algorithms, other investigators have identified relatively stable rotors of activation within the atria that can be ablated and appear to be important in the pathophysiology of atrial fibrillation.

In addition to evaluation of electrophysiologic properties of atrial tissue, some investigators have found imaging and identification of atrial scarring may facilitate ablation. Emphasizing that atrial fibrillation is often associated with different organs and is under complex autonomic control, several studies have reported success targeting the renal arteries and autonomic nervous system for ablation. These complex concepts are beyond the scope of this book.

For our patient with paroxysmal AF, most would first direct ablation at the left atrium just outside the pulmonary vein orifices. Figures 14.2 and 14.3

show the fluoroscopic positions of a circular mapping catheter placed within the four pulmonary veins: the left superior and inferior pulmonary veins and the right superior and inferior pulmonary veins. The LIPV is usually located below the LSPV. The main trunk of the LSPV is directed more anteriorly (best seen in the right anterior oblique (RAO) projection as shown in Figure 14.2). The main trunk of the right superior pulmonary vein (RSPV) is generally located more anteriorly (to the right in the left anterior oblique (LAO) projection: Figure 14.3) as compared to the right inferior pulmonary vein (RIPV). Anatomic variants are rather common in patients with atrial fibrillation and include a common antrum in which two pulmonary veins on one side combine before entering the left atrium, additional pulmonary veins (usually a middle branch), and the pulmonary veins are often larger and have a more trumpet-shaped orifice as compared to patients without atrial fibrillation. It is important to emphasize a final point in Figures 14.2 and 14.3. Although the circular mapping catheter has been placed into the main trunk of the pulmonary vein, it still is well within

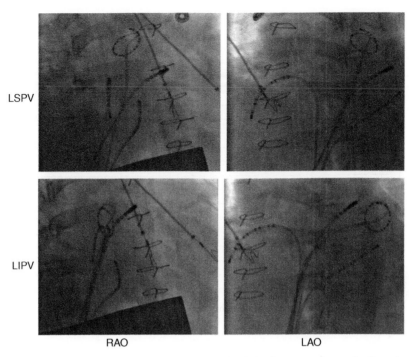

Figure 14.2 Fluoroscopic images showing the usual location of the left-sided pulmonary veins. A circular catheter is placed in the main trunk of the LSPV in the upper row and in the main trunk of the LIPV in the lower row. In the LAO projection, it looks as if the left-sided pulmonary veins "sit on top" of each other in the same plane. The RAO view shows that the main trunk of the LSPV travels anteriorly relative to the LIPV.

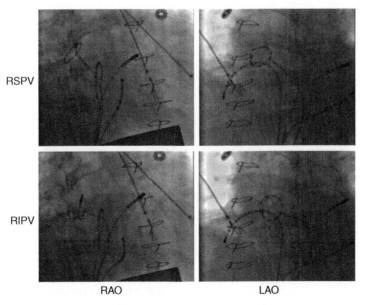

Figure 14.3 Fluoroscopic images showing the usual location of the right-sided pulmonary veins. A circular mapping catheter is placed in the main trunk of the RSPV in the top row or the RIPV in the lower row. In the RAO views, the right-sided pulmonary veins look like they are "on top of each other," but in the LAO view, it can be appreciated that the main trunk of the RSPV courses anteriorly and rightwards relative to the RIPV.

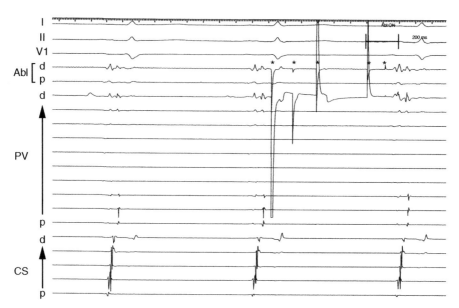

Figure 14.4 Electrograms obtained from a circular mapping catheter placed in the LSPV. The ablation catheter tip electrode must be close to electrode pair 1 and 2 on the circular mapping catheter because coincident noise can be observed (*).

the cardiac silhouette. Identifying the actual os of the pulmonary vein can be difficult and is often facilitated by intracardiac echocardiography or in comparison to preprocedure images. Another technique is to flex the catheter with the steering mechanism. Positions within the left atrium and outside the pulmonary vein are characterized by free motion of the circular mapping catheter without the "edge catching" on the lip of the pulmonary vein.

Ablation is performed by placing a series of lesions in the left atrium just beyond the pulmonary vein orifices, either ringing each of the individual pulmonary veins or ablating in a larger ring around the pulmonary vein pair on a specific side, the right-sided veins or the left-sided veins. Placement of lesions is guided by fluoroscopy or with three-dimensional mapping systems. In some cases, a circular catheter is placed at the pulmonary vein orifice and location of the ablation catheter relative to the circular mapping catheter can be inferred by "matching noise" (Figure 14.4). During ablation, electrical isolation of the pulmonary vein can be identified by loss of pulmonary vein potentials and, in some cases, dissociation (Figure 14.5).

During ablation, particularly with ablation at the anterior portions of the left pulmonary veins, a vagal response with slowing of the ventricular rate due

to either AV block or sinus pauses can be observed (Figure 14.6).

When evaluating electrograms with catheters in the pulmonary veins, it is important not to be fooled by far-field activity. In areas where there are overlapping regions of the heart in close proximity, signals will be observed that are not due to tissue adjacent to electrodes but rather due to the overlapping region. The most common situation is evaluating the LSPV and distinguishing signals from the left atrial appendage, which lies just anterior to the left superior pulmonary vein (Figure 14.7). Generally, far-field signals have lower amplitudes and lower frequencies ("rounded" rather than "spikey") but can also be evaluated by pacing maneuvers (Figure 14.8). Pacing is performed from the left atrial appendage. If the electrograms recorded in the pulmonary vein are far-field signals due to left atrial appendage activation, the signals will occur simultaneously with left atrial appendage depolarization.

Pulmonary veins have interesting electrophysiologic characteristics that may facilitate the development of sustained atrial fibrillation. First, the effective refractory period of pulmonary vein tissue is very short. Figure 14.9 shows rapid pacing within the pulmonary vein after isolation at a cycle length of 90 ms with

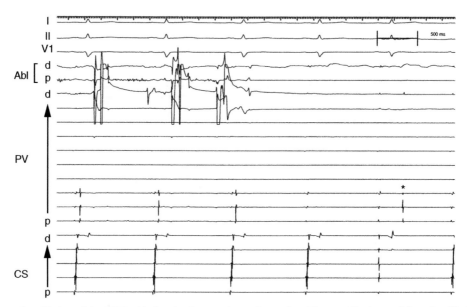

Figure 14.5 During ablation of the LSPV with the circular mapping catheter placed just outside the os of the vein, ablation leads to electrical disconnection between the pulmonary vein and the left atrium and subsequent automaticity of the pulmonary vein (*).

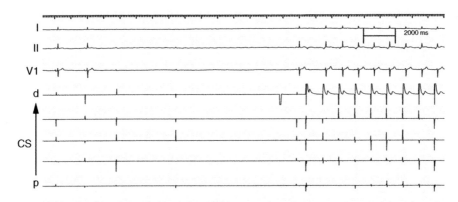

Figure 14.6 As ablation is being performed in the left-sided pulmonary vein system, significant bradycardia due to both sinus node slowing and AV block is observed. In response, atrial pacing is begun from the coronary sinus catheter, and fortunately , even with the vagal response, AV conduction continues. If the patient had continuous asystole due to AV block in the setting of atrial pacing, the decapolar catheter would have been removed from the coronary sinus and placed in the right ventricle.

1:1 capture of pulmonary vein tissue. As shown in Figure 14.10, rapid pacing leads to complex conduction patterns within the pulmonary vein and areas of apparent conduction block. As shown in Figure 14.11, rapid pacing within the pulmonary vein leads to development of a stable atrial tachycardia within the pulmonary vein that does not propagate to the atria. Short refractory periods and complex conduction within the pulmonary veins are clearly features that can facilitate perpetuation of atrial fibrillation. Although the pulmonary veins can be important in some patients for initiation and maintenance of atrial fibrillation, it is also clear that many patients with atrial fibrillation may have atrial fibrillation that is independent of pulmonary vein activity. In Figure 14.12, electrograms from another patient with recurrent atrial fibrillation 1 year after catheter ablation are shown. In the presence of persistent atrial fibrillation, all four pulmonary veins remained isolated

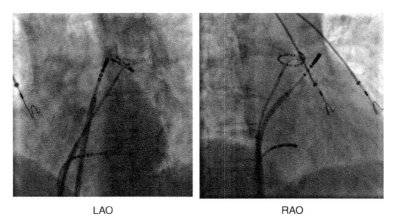

LAO   RAO

Figure 14.7 Fluoroscopic images showing the close anatomic relationship between the left atrial appendage and the LSPV. The quadripolar large-tipped ablation catheter is placed in the left atrial appendage and the circular mapping catheter within the LSPV. In the LAO projection, the catheters appear to be in the same region. However, the true position of the catheters can be identified by the RAO projection with the more anterior left atrial appendage and posterior LSPV.

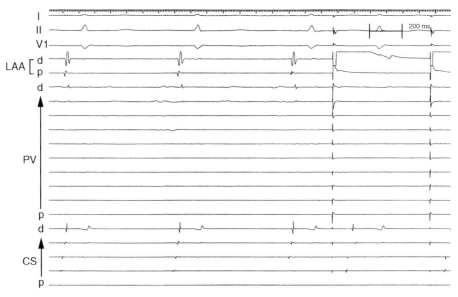

Figure 14.8 Recordings from a circular mapping catheter placed in the LSPV. In this case, low-frequency signals suggestive of recording a far-field signal from the left atrial appendage are recorded distal two electrode pairs. With pacing from the left atrial appendage, the far-field signals in the circular mapping catheter are obscured by the pacing stimuli, confirming that these signals were due to left atrial appendage activity rather than the activity within the pulmonary vein.

and two pulmonary veins exhibited slow but dissociated activity. This emphasizes that the pathophysiologic mechanism for atrial fibrillation is complex and will vary from patient to patient. Although patients will have a common "phenotype" of atrial fibrillation, the "genotype" will vary. When we are able to understand patient-specific causes for atrial fibrillation, it is likely that ablation will become a far more successful form of therapy.

Although the "point-by-point" process has been shown to be effective, every manufacturer is trying to develop techniques that can ablate larger areas of the region around the pulmonary veins with a "single shot." For example, one method is to place a balloon at

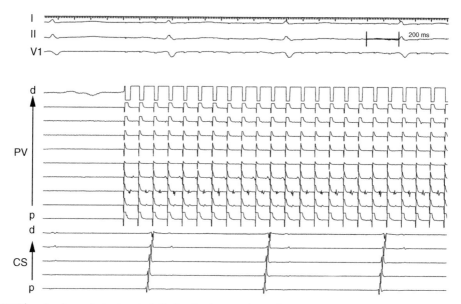

Figure 14.9 Rapid pacing from electrode pair 1, 2 of a circular mapping catheter at a cycle length of 90 ms is associated with 1:1 capture, best seen in electrode pairs 15,16 and 17,18. Notice that the pulmonary vein remains isolated with no change in the sinus rate.

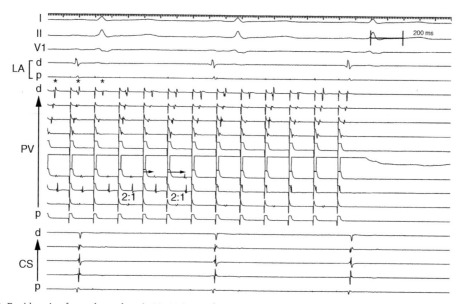

Figure 14.10 Rapid pacing from electrode pair 11, 12 in another patient at a cycle length of 140 ms results in complex conduction patterns within the pulmonary vein. A 1:1 relationship between stimulus and conduction is noted in electrode pairs 1,2 and 3,4, and 5,6, and 7,8 (marked by the asterisks), a constant 2:1 relationship in electrode pair 17,18 (marked by "2:1"), and development of block with gradual prolongation of the stimulus–to–electrogram interval in electrode pairs 13,14 and 15,16 (marked by the arrows).

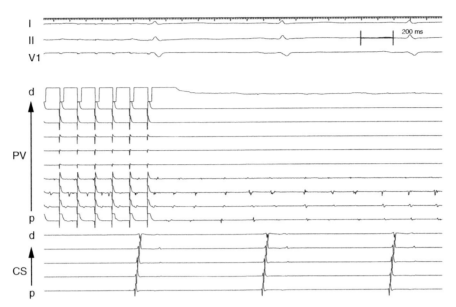

Figure 14.11 Rapid pacing from the distal pair of electrodes within the pulmonary vein at a cycle length of 120 ms induces a sustained tachycardia within the pulmonary vein with discrete electrograms occurring at varying cycle lengths.

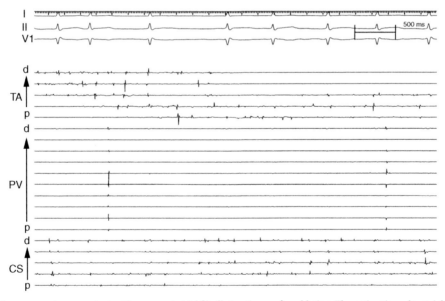

Figure 14.12 Electrograms from a patient with recurrent atrial fibrillation 1 year after ablation. The patient is under atrial fibrillation (as noted by the irregular coronary sinus (CS) and tricuspid annulus (TA) electrograms but has slow dissociated activity within the RSPV. In this patient who had durable isolation of the pulmonary veins, recurrent atrial fibrillation was "pulmonary vein independent" and due to another unidentified mechanism.

the atrial wall with the nose of the catheter and a wire within the pulmonary vein (Figure 14.13). Cryoenergy leads to destruction of the cardiac tissue, and early experience suggests that this ablation technique is more effective as compared to antiarrhythmic medications in patients with recurrent paroxysmal atrial fibrillation. Effective ablation using the cryoballoon requires near-complete occlusion of the pulmonary veins that can be confirmed fluoroscopically with contrast (Figure 14.13) or by recording a "reverse wedge pressure" (Figure 14.14), where a pulmonary artery tracing is recorded from the tip of the catheter. Another emerging technology for ablation is shown in Figure 14.15. This balloon incorporates a small endoscope and ablation with laser can be performed on the atrial tissue with direct visual evaluation. Although these new technologies are extremely promising, and small nonrandomized studies have suggested that one

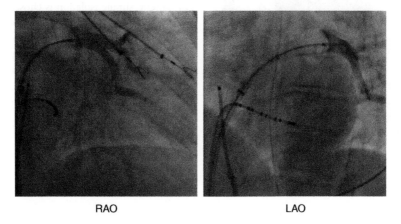

RAO   LAO

Figure 14.13 A cryoballoon catheter is placed in the LSPV and contrast injection leads to contrast "hang-up," confirming the presence of an excellent occlusion and increasing the likelihood that an effective ablation lesion will be produced. Notice the relatively anterior course of the LSPV.

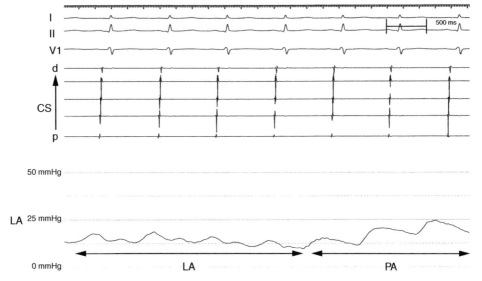

Figure 14.14 Another sign of occlusion when using a cryoballoon ablation technique is the presence of a pulmonary artery (PA) pressure tracing rather than a left atrial (LA) pressure tracing with effective balloon occlusion of the pulmonary vein. This is called a "reverse wedge" waveform.

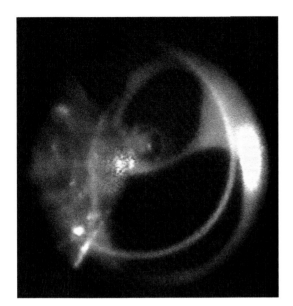

Figure 14.15 Another balloon-based catheter design uses a balloon to occlude the pulmonary vein and allow direct visualization using an endoscope. With this catheter design, lesions are produced with laser.

technique may be superior to another, the data comparing the effectiveness of different ablation techniques are scant and incomplete.

Ablation is performed in our patient by placing a series of lesions in the left atrium around the right-sided and left-sided pulmonary veins. One of the problems with ablation for atrial fibrillation is identification of the best endpoint(s) for successful ablation. Endpoints for supraventricular tachycardia are reasonably well defined (noninducibility after ablation, loss of preexcitation in those patients with anterograde accessory pathway conduction); although they still vary among clinicians, for example, after ablation for AVNRT, is a residual single echo reasonable (as discussed in Chapter 2)? For atrial flutter, once the critical isthmus has been identified, proof of bidirectional conduction block in the isthmus is an important indicator and a reasonable endpoint for predicting success. In contrast, the appropriate endpoint after atrial fibrillation

ablation is not known. Most clinicians would agree that it is important to achieve electrical isolation if the pulmonary veins are targeted. Some investigators use noninducibility with or without isoproterenol as endpoints after ablation, while others argue that many induced arrhythmias are nonclinical and do not predict future success. A more detailed discussion of ablation techniques and endpoints is available in the 2012 HRS/EHRA/ECAS Expert Consensus Statement on Catheter and Surgical Ablation of Atrial Fibrillation. In our patient, simple isolation is chosen as the endpoint, and she has remained atrial fibrillation free after 1-year follow-up. Unfortunately, the recurrence rate after ablation remains high, 20–60%, depending on study, and our understanding of the role of atrial fibrillation ablation, particularly in those patients with persistent atrial fibrillation, remains in its nascent stage. The array of arrhythmias that can occur after ablation for atrial fibrillation is quite diverse, and some possibilities will be covered in the next five cases.

KEY POINTS

- Ablation of atrial fibrillation is a rapidly evolving field with different strategies for ablation that have been described by multiple investigators.

- Patient input is essential for determining whether catheter ablation is appropriate.

- For patients with paroxysmal atrial fibrillation, it appears that ablation within the left atria around the pulmonary vein ostia can be successful for reducing episodes of atrial fibrillation, particularly those that are symptomatic.

- The pulmonary veins have complex electrophysiologic properties that may be important in facilitating the development of atrial fibrillation.

- New tools are emerging that can facilitate ablation in the left atrium near the pulmonary vein ostia.

- Our understanding (and thus our ability to successfully treat) of atrial fibrillation remains in its infancy and will continue to evolve rapidly.

CHAPTER 15

Supraventricular tachycardia case 15: atrial tachycardia after atrial fibrillation ablation

A 68-year-old man underwent catheter ablation for atrial fibrillation 2 years ago and had done well until the last month when he had had episodes of rapid heart rate associated with exercise. After a discussion on treatment options, the patient opts for repeat electrophysiology study and catheter ablation.

When the patient arrives at the electrophysiology laboratory, he is in an obvious atrial flutter or atrial tachycardia (Figure 15.1). Because recurrent pulmonary vein conduction is a common cause of recurrent atrial tachycardia after prior ablation for atrial fibrillation, four venous access sites are obtained and a decapolar catheter is placed in the coronary sinus, a second decapolar catheter is placed at the lateral right atrium, and a 20-electrode circular mapping catheter is placed in the left superior pulmonary vein. The baseline electrograms are shown in Figure 15.2. He is in an atrial tachycardia with a cycle length of 270 ms characterized by near simultaneous activation of the right and the left atrium. In this case, there is continued activity within at least one of the four pulmonary veins that is suspicious for providing a region of slow conduction necessary for the maintenance of atrial flutter. Notice that electrograms within the pulmonary vein can account for 170 ms or more than 60% of the tachycardia cycle length. Although hard to measure accurately, given the low-amplitude flutter waves, left atrial (as defined by the coronary sinus) and right atrial activation (as defined by the lateral right atrial catheter) occur during the flutter wave, and pulmonary vein activity recorded on the distal electrodes of the circular mapping catheter occurs during the isoelectric period separating the

flutter waves. Although together these findings provide strong evidence that the left superior pulmonary vein is critically involved in the reentrant circuit, it is important to evaluate the atrial flutter with a standardized method because the recurrent pulmonary vein conduction could be a bystander to the cause for atrial flutter. Similar to the evaluation of any atrial flutter, pacing from different regions of the right and left atria is performed (Figures 15.3–15.5). As expected, pacing from the low lateral right atrium (the tip of the right atrial catheter) is associated with a change in the direction of depolarization of the right atrium. Importantly, notice that it is unclear whether the pacing interacted with the tachycardia circuit. This is one of the problems associated with pacing at a relatively long cycle length close to the tachycardia cycle length. When pacing from the mid-portion of the coronary sinus, the right atrial and coronary sinus electrograms are consistently "reeled in" to the paced cycle length, but only one interval in the left superior pulmonary vein matches the paced cycle length. Although pacing maneuvers did not capture and entrain all of the recorded electrograms, some beneficial information has been obtained. Even if pacing does not interact with a reentrant circuit, a long return cycle length would not be observed if the pacing site was relatively near the reentrant circuit, and the general concept "the longer the return cycle length the farther away the pacing site is to the from the circuit" holds true.

At this point, it is useful to evaluate the results of these pacing maneuvers. Because the return cycle lengths are shorter in the left atrium when compared to the right atrium, the results are consistent with a left atrial flutter. In addition, although shorter than the right atrium, the return cycle lengths from the coronary

Understanding Intracardiac EGMs: A Patient Centered Guide, First Edition. Fred Kusumoto.
© 2015 John Wiley & Sons, Ltd. Published 2015 by John Wiley & Sons, Ltd.

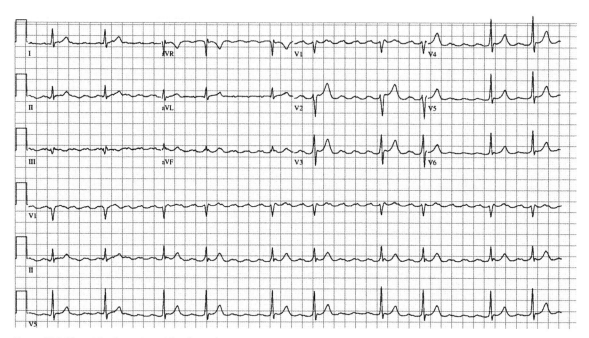

Figure 15.1 The 12-lead ECG in atrial tachycardia.

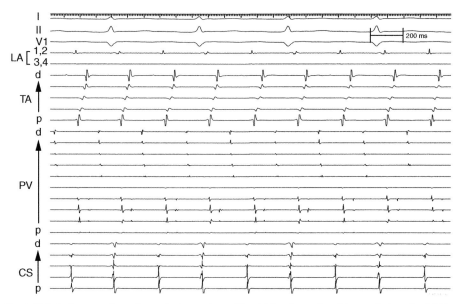

Figure 15.2 The initial electrograms from the patient reveal a stable atrial tachycardia with a cycle length of 260 ms. Decapolar catheters are placed in the coronary sinus (CS) and the tricuspid annulus (TA). A twenty-electrode circular mapping catheter is placed in the left superior pulmonary vein, and a quadripolar catheter is placed in the left atrial (LA) appendage.

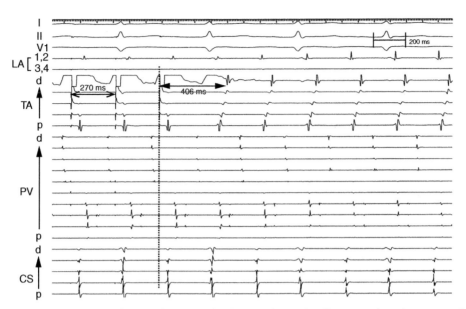

Figure 15.3 Pacing at a cycle length of 270 ms from the inferolateral right atrial wall captures the right atrium and left atrium (confirmed by the shorter cycle length) but does not entrain the electrograms in the left superior pulmonary vein (PV). This is one problem with pacing at relatively slow pacing rates. Even without capture of the underlying reentrant circuit, the prolonged return cycle length (407 ms) on cessation of pacing suggests that the lateral right atrium is far from the circuit of interest.

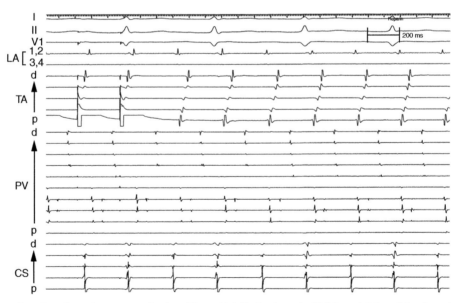

Figure 15.4 Continuation of entrainment mapping from Figure 15.3. Pacing from the high lateral right atrial wall results in a shorter return cycle length but still does not interact with the tachycardia.

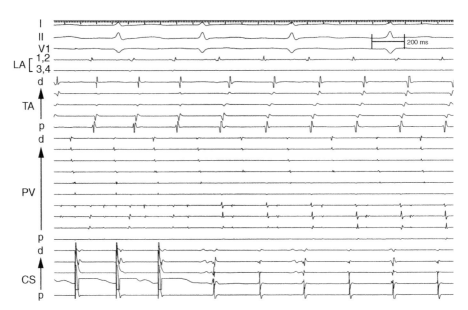

Figure 15.5 Continuation of entrainment mapping from Figures 15.3 and 15.4. Pacing from the proximal coronary sinus finally entrains the pulmonary vein electrograms, but the return cycle length remains prolonged.

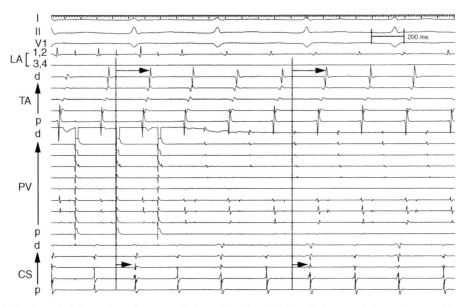

Figure 15.6 Pacing from the left superior pulmonary vein from electrode pair 1,2 results in concealed entrainment with a return cycle length that matches the tachycardia cycle length on cessation of pacing. The stimulus–to-coronary sinus electrograms and right atrial electrograms match the electrogram-to-electrogram intervals during tachycardia (solid and dashed arrows, respectively), confirming an exact match of atrial depolarization during pacing and tachycardia and concealed entrainment.

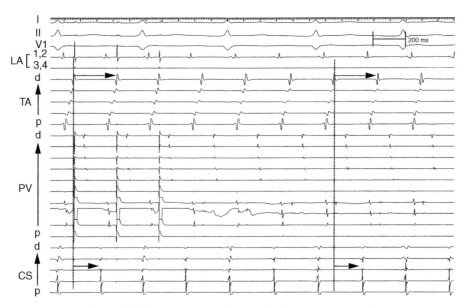

Figure 15.7 Continuation from Figure 15.6. Pacing from electrode pair 15, 16 shows results similar to those of electrode pair 1,2; however, concealed entrainment is characterized by longer stimulus-to-coronary sinus and stimulus-to-right atrial activation intervals. This suggests that electrode pair 15,16 is located closer to the "entrance" of the protected critical isthmus and electrode pair 1,2 closer to the "exit."

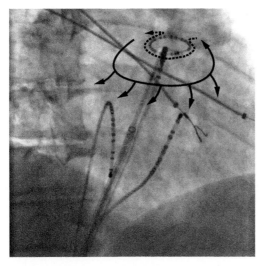

Figure 15.8 Fluoroscopy in the right anterior oblique projection of the catheter positions in Figure 15.6 and 15.7 with the likely course of the reentrant circuit. Dashed arrow denotes the reentrant circuit within the left superior pulmonary vein, and the solid arrow denotes depolarization of the atria.

sinus (which represents activation of the anterior mitral annulus) were still relatively long, and the posterior wall becomes the most likely site for slow conduction that is responsible for maintaining atrial flutter.

Only now after initial pacing results have directed the clinician to the posterior left atrium, pacing from the pulmonary veins is performed. My staff laughs at me because I have always called this "not opening your Christmas presents early," but on a serious note, this strategy forces a careful and systematic evaluation of atrial arrhythmias. Pacing from the left superior pulmonary vein reveals a return cycle length that is equal to the tachycardia cycle length but more critically is associated with an activation pattern for all of the catheters subtending different regions of the heart that is the same as during tachycardia (Figures 15.6–15.8). Pacing from both electrode pairs 1,2 (Figure 15.6) and 15,16 (Figure 15.7) are characterized by concealed entrainment. The fluoroscopic position of the catheters is shown in Figure 15.8. At this point, the more general classification of atrial tachycardia can be replaced by the

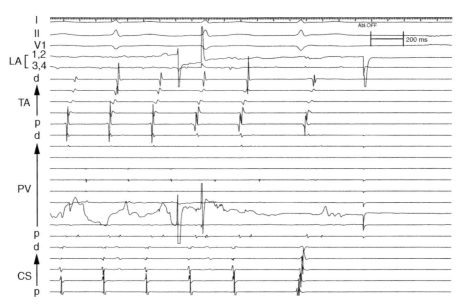

Figure 15.9 Catheter ablation at electrode pair 15,16 leads to termination of the atrial flutter, although conduction into the pulmonary vein remains.

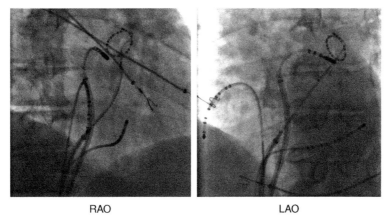

RAO   LAO

Figure 15.10 Fluoroscopy of catheter positions from Figure 9. Flexing the ablation catheter will reduce the likelihood of applying radio-frequency energy within the vein.

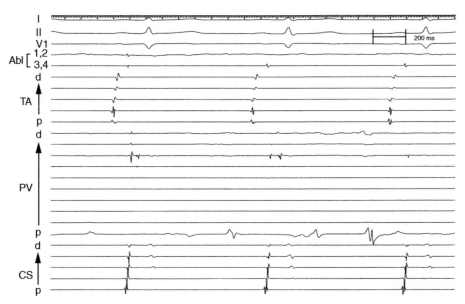

Figure 15.11 Additional ablation at electrode pair 19,20 results in loss of all pulmonary vein potentials.

more specific classification of atrial flutter because the tachycardia mechanism is now well defined. It appears that electrode pair 13,14 represents the entrance into the isthmus ("earliest" depolarization), the wave of depolarization travels around the circular mapping catheter and exits at around electrode pair 9,10 ("latest" depolarization). Prior ablation of the left superior pulmonary vein likely contributed by artificially producing relative electrical isolation of the left pulmonary vein from the left atrium to facilitate the development of a stable reentrant circuit. Application of radio-frequency energy at electrode pairs 13,14 and 15,16 terminates the tachycardia (Figures 15.9 and 15.10). Although the tachycardia has been terminated, additional ablation is performed and leads to loss of pulmonary vein potentials (Figure 15.11). The other pulmonary veins did not have recurrent conduction. The patient has remained tachycardia free for 2 years with significant improvement in symptoms.

KEY POINTS

- After prior ablation for atrial fibrillation, in patients with recurrent arrhythmia, it is often helpful to evaluate the pulmonary veins and determine whether the veins remain isolated and confirm the absence of pulmonary vein potentials.

- Mapping requires careful evaluation of the atrial electrograms and the methodical use of entrainment mapping.

- Catheter ablation can be proarrhythmic by producing electrically isolated regions within the pulmonary vein with one barrier produced by the ablation line and the other barrier formed by the more distal portion of the pulmonary vein.

CHAPTER 16

Supraventricular tachycardia case 16: atrial tachycardia after atrial fibrillation ablation

A 71-year-old woman has a 9-year history of atrial arrhythmias. Over the past 7 years, she has had five catheter ablations for atrial fibrillation at another institution; however, she continues to have drug refractory atrial tachyarrhythmias. She has undergone several recent cardioversions but continues to have recurrent persistent atrial flutter associated with profound tiredness and fatigue. Currently, she is being managed with a rate control strategy with high doses of beta-blockade and diltiazem. She has a history of hypothyroidism (currently euthyroid found by blood testing), hypertension, and diabetes mellitus. In her physical examination, a paradoxically split second heart sound is noted, but no significant mumurs are present. Her ECG is shown in Figure 16.1. A recent echocardiogram shows normal left ventricular function.

At this point, certainly the decision must be made whether to pursue AV nodal ablation and pacing or another attempt at catheter ablation. Multiple studies have shown the utility of AV node ablation for achieving rate control. In the AIRCRAFT trial, AV nodal ablation and permanent pacing were associated with significant improvement in left ventricular function. One problem with AV nodal ablation is that it is "irreversible" and some patients will remain symptomatic even with the strict rate control that this strategy provides. After careful discussion of the options, the patient opts for a sixth ablation.

Inspection of her ECG shows a regular rapid rhythm and biphasic flutter waves in the inferior leads. It can be extremely difficult to localize the mechanism of atrial flutter after prior ablation or MAZE surgery.

In the electrophysiology laboratory, catheters are placed in standardized initial positions with multi-electrode catheters placed in the coronary sinus, the tricuspid annulus, and the pulmonary veins. All four pulmonary veins are explored and "are clean" as shown in Figure 16.2 (it is good to know after five prior ablations, the veins can be made electrically inert). Initial inspection of the electrograms shows alternating activation of the coronary sinus and the lateral wall of the right atrium. Now that it has been convincingly shown that the pulmonary veins are not involved, a multipolar catheter is placed along the mitral annulus (Figure 16.3).

When confronted with an atrial flutter or atrial tachycardia, I believe that it is important to perform pacing from distal and proximal locations of catheters, regardless of any clinical suspicion of the type of atrial flutter that is present. This standardized approach is extremely useful for reducing the likelihood of "finding what you want to find." As in our discussion in Chapter 12, response to pacing is evaluated by evaluating what portions of the atrium are activated in the same or different fashion as in tachycardia (called orthodromic or antidromic capture respectively) and the postpacing interval ("longer *usually* equals farther" from the circuit). Pacing from the low lateral right atrium is associated with antidromic capture of the right atrium and a long return cycle length (Figure 16.4). Also note that, although the general pattern of activation observed in the coronary sinus, the decapolar catheter and the 20-electrode catheter placed in the left atrium are the same for both pacing and tachycardia, the timing between right atrial and eft atrial activation are very different. When a region of the atria is activated similarly during pacing and tachycardia, it is common to say that portion of the atrium is being activated orthodromically. Pacing from the high right atrium is associated with the same general direction of activation in the right atrium, left atrium, and coronary sinus (Figure 16.5). Again, the timing of the sequences is

Understanding Intracardiac EGMs: A Patient Centered Guide, First Edition. Fred Kusumoto.
© 2015 John Wiley & Sons, Ltd. Published 2015 by John Wiley & Sons, Ltd.

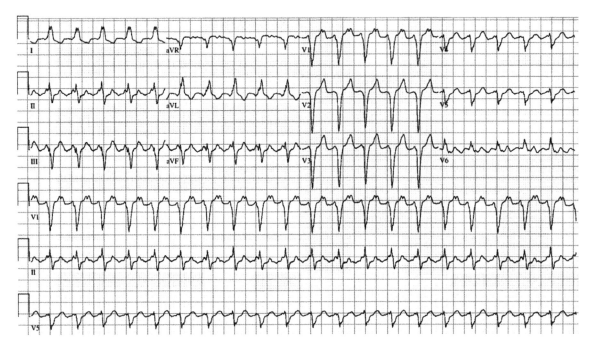

Figure 16.1 Baseline ECG shows atrial flutter associated with a rapid and regular ventricular response.

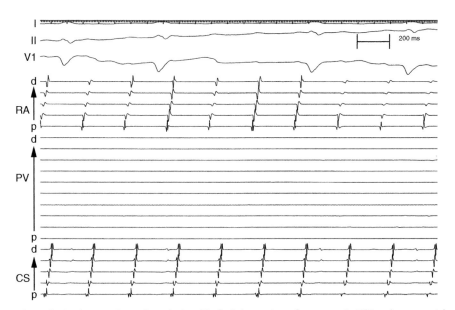

Figure 16.2 A 20-electrode circular mapping catheter is placed in the left superior pulmonary vein (PV) and no potentials are observed. Similarly, when the circular mapping catheter is placed in the other three pulmonary veins, no electrical activity is observed. RA, right atrium; CS, coronary sinus;

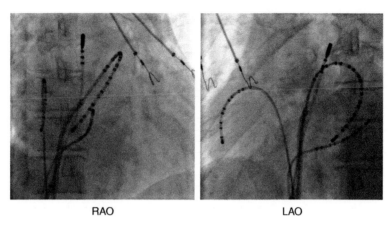

RAO   LAO

Figure 16.3 Fluoroscopy in the left anterior oblique imaging plane with a decapolar catheter placed in the right atrium, a decapolar catheter in the coronary sinus, and a 20-electrode catheter in the left atrium along the mitral annulus.

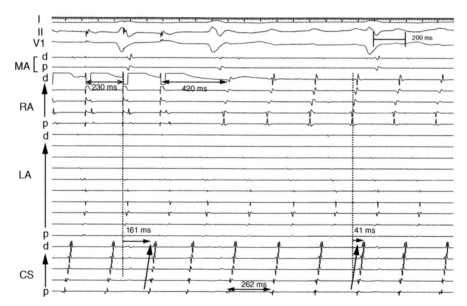

Figure 16.4 The tachycardia cycle length is 262 ms. Pacing is performed at a cycle length of 230 ms (longer cycle lengths required a significant amount of time to entrain the tachycardia). Notice that the pattern of activation in the 20-electrode catheter in the left atrium and the decapolar catheter placed in the coronary sinus (curved arrows) are the same during pacing and during tachycardia. However, the timing of activation is very different. For example, the stimulus-to-distal coronary sinus electrogram interval is 161 ms during pacing and the electrogram-to-distal coronary sinus electrogram interval is only 41 ms during tachycardia.

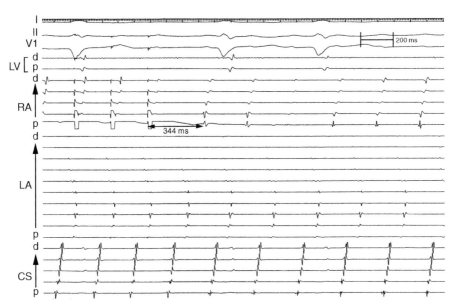

Figure 16.5 Pacing from the high right atrium is associated with a shorter return cycle length of 344 ms than the low lateral right atrium, suggesting this electrode pair is "closer" to the tachycardia circuit.

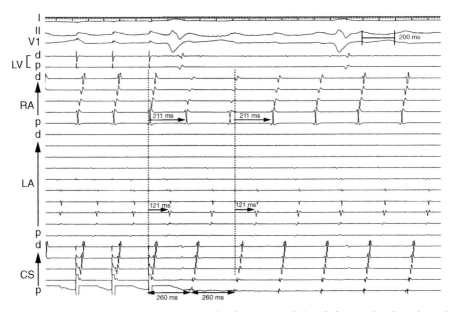

Figure 16.6 Pacing from the proximal coronary sinus is associated with a return cycle length that matches the tachycardia cycle length (260 ms) and the stimulus to electrogram intervals during pacing and the electrogram–to-electrogram intervals match, whether measured in the high right atrium (211 ms) or the left atrium (121 ms). These findings represent "concealed entrainment" and provide strong evidence that the proximal coronary sinus is "in the circuit."

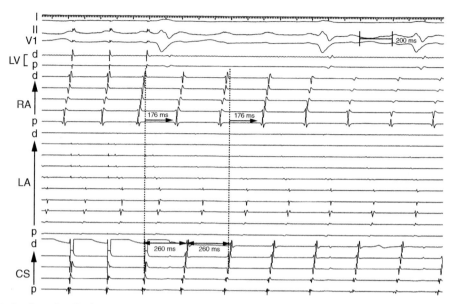

Figure 16.7 Pacing from the distal coronary sinus (CS) is also associated with a return cycle length after the last paced beat that matches the tachycardia cycle length (260 ms), and the stimulus-to-electrogram and electrogram-to-electrogram intervals match.

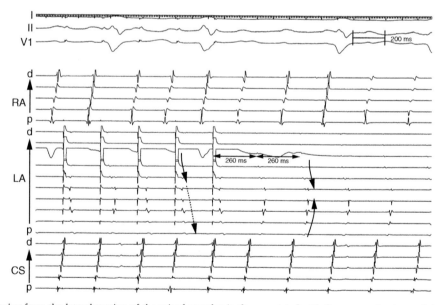

Figure 16.8 Pacing from the lateral portion of the mitral annulus is also associated with first postpacing interval that matches the tachycardia cycle length, but a portion of the left atrium is now activated antidromically (dashed line) or in a direction opposite to the activation of that region during tachycardia.

completely changed and the return cycle length remains long but is shorter than the low lateral right atrium. Pacing from the proximal coronary sinus and the distal coronary sinus both show a perfect match of direction and timing of atrial activation and a return cycle length that matches tachycardia (Figures 16.6 and 16.7). With both the distal and the proximal coronary sinus "in the circuit," it makes an atrial flutter rotating around the mitral annulus extremely likely. This is confirmed by pacing from the lateral left atrium (Figure 16.8). Notice the return cycle length is "spot on," although there is antidromic capture of a portion of the left atrium.

Figure 16.9 is a schematic of a reentrant circuit and the effects of pacing. If the reentrant circuit has a large excitable gap, when pacing is performed at faster rates, more of the tachycardia circuit is captured antidromically (or in the opposite direction of depolarization during tachycardia), and if enough tissue is capture antidromically to cause the orthodromic wavefront to encounter refractory tissue, the tachycardia will terminate.

Now that the mechanism of the arrhythmia has been determined, attention is shifted to deciding on the best ablation strategy. For mitral annular flutters,

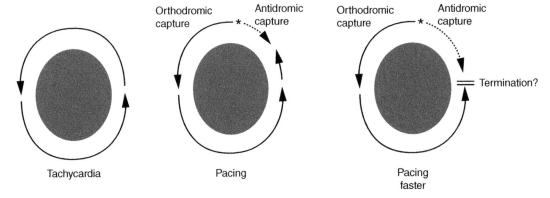

Figure 16.9 Schematic of antidromic versus orthodromic capture. When pacing from within a tachycardia circuit, orthodromic capture are those portions of the circuit that are depolarized in the same way both during tachycardia and during pacing, while antidromic capture are those portions that are activated in the opposite direction. Pacing faster will often lead to more antidromic capture of the circuit and, in some cases, lead to termination if antidromic capture leads to refractory tissue and block of the orthodromic wavefront.

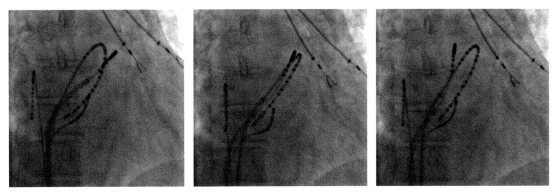

Figure 16.10 Sequential fluoroscopic images of the ablation in the right anterior oblique view. Ablation was started at the mitral annulus, and the ablation catheter was slowly moved more posteriorly until the anterior portion of the roof scar.

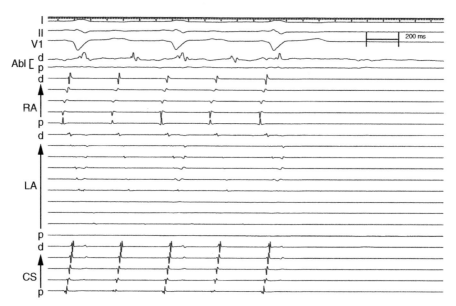

Figure 16.11 With completion of the roof line, the tachycardia is terminated. Abl, ablation catheter; CS, coronary sinus; RA, right atrium; LA, left atrium.

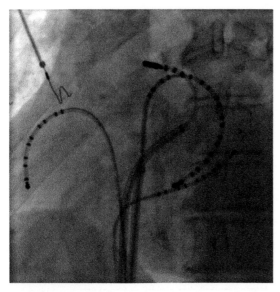

Figure 16.12 Fluoroscopy of catheter positions to evaluate the block across the anterior roof line in the left anterior oblique projection. The ablation catheter is placed on the medial aspect of the anterior roof line.

ablation is traditionally performed from the mitral valve to the left inferior pulmonary vein, generally trying to make a linear lesion set just inferior to the left atrial appendage. Oftentimes, patients will have large areas of scar, particularly those who have had prior ablation. These areas of scar can be proarrhythmic because they facilitate development of reentrant circuits. In this case, a large area of scar was found on the roof with a relatively narrow isthmus of tissue separating the roof scar and the mitral annulus. The clinician should try to identify the narrowest isthmus of tissue that would require the least amount of ablation and most likely be associated with long-term success. As shown in Figures 16.10 and 16.11, ablation was performed superiorly from the mitral annulus to the anterior edge of the roof scar and with completion of the "line" the tachycardia terminated.

It is imperative to confirm a block across the newly created ablation line. After the ablation line is completed, pacing is performed on either side of the ablation line. The easiest way to confirm bidirectional block

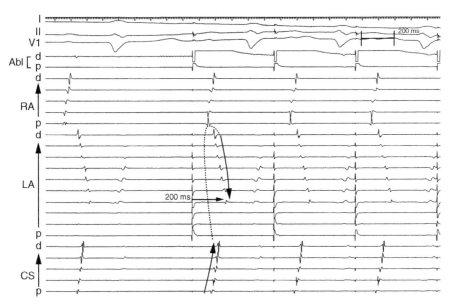

Figure 16.13 Pacing from the Abl on the medial side of the anterior roof line with the catheter positions shown in Figure 16.12 leads to proximal-to-distal activation of the CS followed by inferolateral-to-superior activation of the lateral left atrium (LA). The interval from the pacing stimulus to electrode pair 13,14 on the 20-electrode catheter is 200 ms. RA, right atrium.

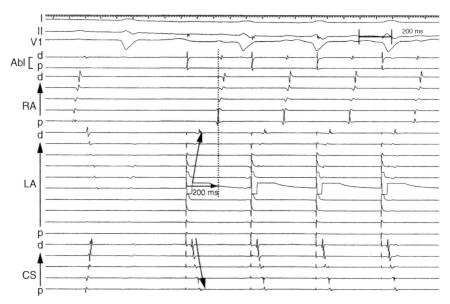

Figure 16.14 Continuation of Figures 16.12 and 16.13. Pacing from the lateral side of the anterior roof line (electrodes 11,12) leads to superior-to-inferior activation of the lateral left atrium (LA) and distal-to-proximal activation of the coronary sinus (CS), and the interval from the pacing stimulus to the distal electrodes of the ablation catheter (Abl) is 200 ms. RA, right atrium.

across an ablation line is to place a catheter across the putative site of block, pace from either side, measure the conduction time, and evaluate the direction of activation (Figures 16.12–16.14). As shown in Figure 16.13, pacing from the medial side of the line of block leads to a long conduction interval to electrode pair 13, 14, which is located on the lateral side of the ablation line. Conversely, pacing from electrode pair 13, 14 on the lateral side of the line of block results in a long conduction interval to the distal electrode pair of the ablation catheter located on the medial side of the line of block.

Because of ablation, the patient has remained arrhythmia free for the past 1 year, and hopefully "the sixth time will be the charm."

- A macroreentrant circuit is characterized by a number of areas with return cycle lengths similar to the tachycardia cycle lengths during entrainment mapping.
- Mitral annular flutter is a relatively commonly observed flutter after ablation for atrial fibrillation and is confirmed when the regions around the mitral annulus are all within the circuit.
- Regardless of the type of atrial flutter, the clinician must define an ablation strategy usually by identifying a critical isthmus that is formed by electrically inert structures – valvular annuli, venous structures, scars, and so on.

KEY POINTS

- Response of the tachycardia to pacing from different sites in the atria should focus first on defining in order: which atria, what regions are within the circuit, and finally, what critical isthmus is being used.

CHAPTER 17

Supraventricular tachycardia case 17: atrial tachycardia after atrial fibrillation ablation

A 77-year-old painter first developed exertional tachy-cardia 8 years ago and underwent electrophysiology study and AV node modification for atypical AVNRT. He was well until 2 years ago when he developed atrial fibrillation and underwent catheter ablation for atrial fib-rillation. He had recurrent atrial flutter (Figure 17.1) and underwent cardioversion with initiation of dofetilide. Although he has done reasonably well on dofetilide, he continues to have arrhythmia when he swims.

This patient remains symptomatic despite his ablation, and electrophysiology study is a reasonable option. His baseline electrograms are shown in Figure 17.2. Unlike the previous case, the patient is in sinus rhythm; how-ever, the first order of business is still to evaluate the pulmonary veins. In this case, there is no recurrent con-duction in the pulmonary veins and any inducible tachy-cardia must be pulmonary vein independent.

The patient then undergoes programmed stimulation in an attempt to induce his clinical atrial arrhythmia. Rapid atrial pacing induces a stable atrial tachycardia with a cycle length of 405 ms. The patient undergoes entrainment mapping as shown in Figures 17.3–17.8. Initial pacing is performed at the high lateral wall of the right atrium. The return cycle is prolonged at 517 ms (Figure 17.4). As shown in Figure 17.5, pacing is performed from the low lateral wall of the right atrium. As shown in Figures 17.6 and 17.7, pacing is performed from the proximal and distal coronary sinus, respectively. Of the four sites, notice that the best return cycle length is observed with pacing from the distal coronary sinus but that the pacing associated with a different pattern of activation of the distal portion of

the left atrial catheter when compared to tachycardia. In electrophysiologic terminology, this region of the left atrium is being activated "antidromically" or in the opposite direction compared to tachycardia. Finally, pacing is performed from the roof of the left atrium, and the electrogram activation and the return cycle length are the best among the five pacing sites.

Since the critical portion of the tachycardia has been localized to the roof of the left atrium, exchang-ing catheters may be useful. The linear 20-electrode catheter is extremely valuable in the initial portions of the study because large areas of activation (or scar) can be evaluated quickly. However, once a region of interest is identified, a catheter with multiple electrodes in a smaller area is often more useful because it can provide more accurate mapping. Some sites use a multispline catheter for this; however, we have found that a simple circular mapping catheter is generally sufficient. As shown in Figure 17.9, a lasso catheter is placed in the roof of the left atrium. The catheter is manipulated within different areas of the roof to provide informa-tion on the presence and location of large areas of scar and potential critical regions of electrical activity participating in tachycardia.

Placement of the lasso identifies a large area of scar with activity only at three electrode pairs (1,2; 17,18; 19,20). Pacing from these three sites shows excellent return cycle lengths and electrogram activation pat-terns that suggest that this region is within the circuit (Figures 17.10, 17.11, and 17.12). Not shown is the movement of the lasso to a more medial aspect of the roof, which shows a region of scar on the septal side of these electrode pairs. These results suggest that the best ablation strategy would target this relatively narrow

Understanding Intracardiac EGMs: A Patient Centered Guide, First Edition. Fred Kusumoto.
© 2015 John Wiley & Sons, Ltd. Published 2015 by John Wiley & Sons, Ltd.

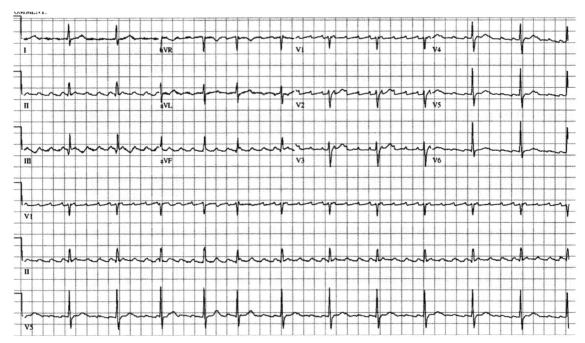

Figure 17.1 ECG of atrial flutter. Flutter waves are positive in the anterior leads and show relatively continuous atrial activation in the inferior leads.

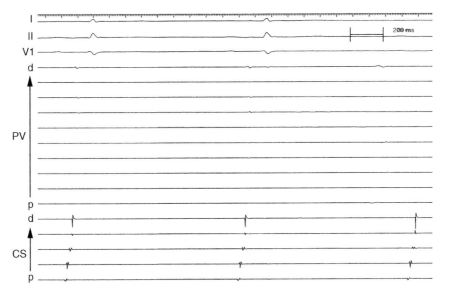

Figure 17.2 A circular mapping catheter is placed in the left superior pulmonary vein and no electrical activity is observed within the pulmonary vein.

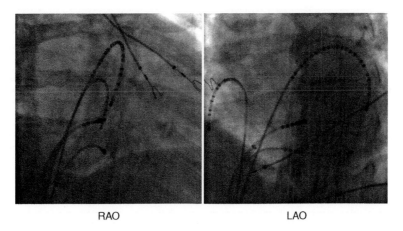

RAO   LAO

Figure 17.3 Atrial flutter is induced with atrial pacing, and to explore the mechanism of atrial flutter, decapolar catheters are placed in the lateral wall of the right atrium and the coronary sinus. A 20-electrode catheter is placed at the superior, lateral, and inferior walls of the left atrium and the mapping catheter is placed within the left atrial cavity, which does not record the electrical activity.

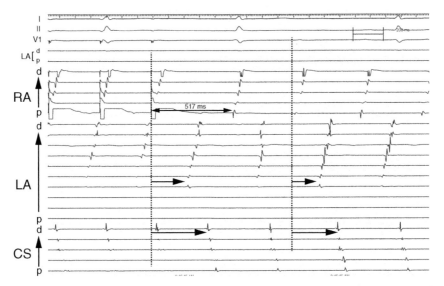

Figure 17.4 Pacing is first performed at the high lateral right atrium with a return cycle length of 517 ms. Notice that although the general direction of depolarization in all three catheters is similar during both pacing and tachycardia, the stimulation to the earliest activation of the left atrial catheter or the distal coronary sinus (CS) is longer during pacing when compared to tachycardia. When deciding "what goes to what," it is important to evaluate within a set of electrograms recorded from the catheter what was entrained and what was from tachycardia. In the case of the coronary sinus electrograms, there is significant delay to the last entrained "set of signals."

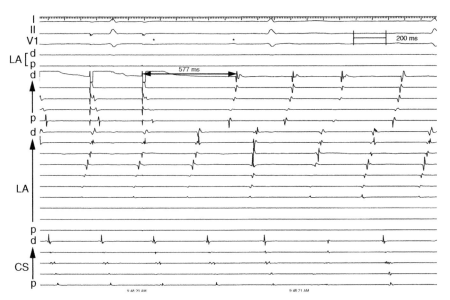

Figure 17.5 Pacing is performed from the low lateral right atrium with a very long return cycle length of 577 ms. In addition, notice how different the entrained P wave and the spontaneous P wave morphologies are (*).

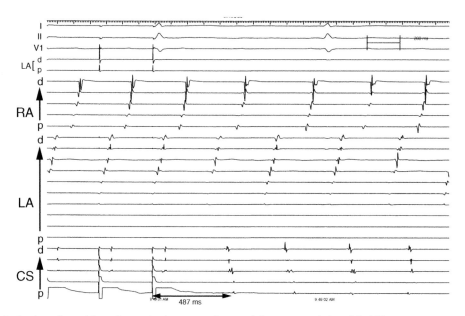

Figure 17.6 Pacing is performed from the proximal coronary sinus, and the return cycle length is 487 ms.

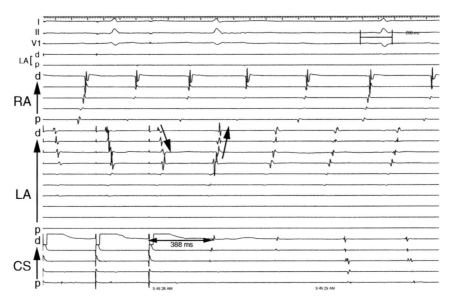

Figure 17.7 Pacing is performed from the distal coronary sinus, and the return cycle length is much shorter (388 ms) suggesting that this site is nearer the tachycardia circuit as compared to the proximal coronary sinus or the right atrium. However, as shown by the arrows, notice that depolarization of the left atrium catheter is completely changed (or that large areas of the left atrium are activated "antidromically" when compared to tachycardia).

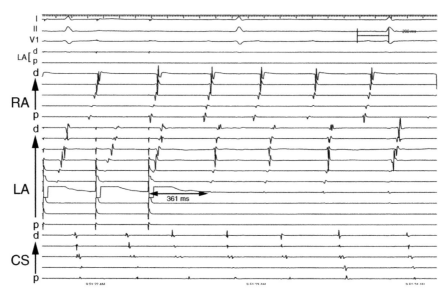

Figure 17.8 Pacing is performed from the roof and the return cycle length is 361 ms, and the pattern and timing of atrial activation are similar for both during pacing and during tachycardia.

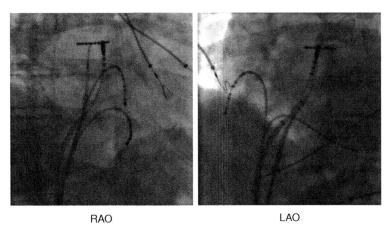

RAO   LAO

Figure 17.9 As the tachycardia appears to be emanating from the roof, a circular mapping catheter is placed in the roof to provide more detailed electrophysiologic evaluation from the region of interest.

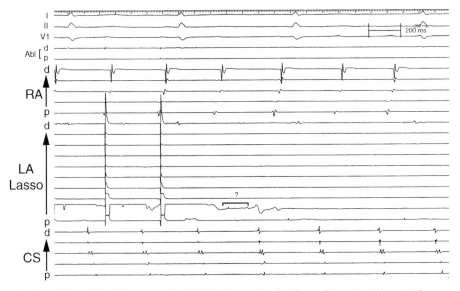

Figure 17.10 Pacing is performed from lasso electrodes 17,18. First, notice that the roof is a site with a significant amount of scar and with very little recordable electrical activity. Very low amplitude signal is recorded on electrode pairs 17,18 and 19,20. Although pacing captures the atrium and entrains the tachycardia, it is very difficult to identify low-frequency electrograms to measure the return cycle length (?).

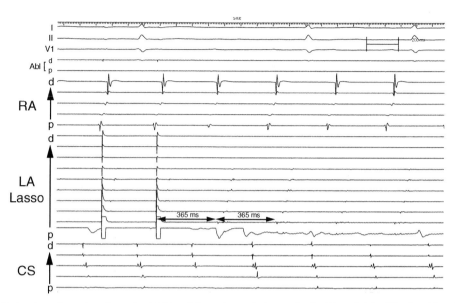

Figure 17.11 Pacing is performed at electrodes 19,20 and the tachycardia is entrained. Although it is difficult to identify signals on electrode pair 19,20, notice that the electrograms recorded on adjacent electrode pair 17,18 has a return cycle length (365 ms) that matches the tachycardia cycle length.

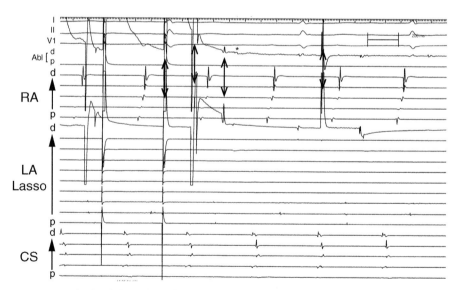

Figure 17.12 Pacing nearer to the distal electrodes of the lasso leads to entrainment. The tachycardia has slowed to 420 ms, and pacing is now performed at 390 ms. It can often be difficult to decide what signals represent the artifact (double-headed open arrows) as compared to a true low-frequency electrogram (*).

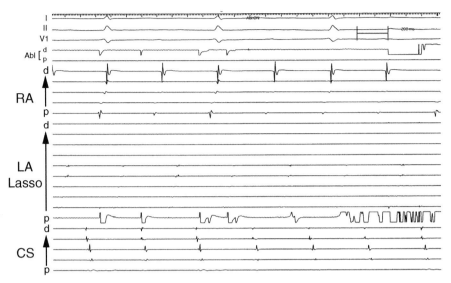

Figure 17.13 Although no signal can be recorded, pacing was successful and the matching noise ("Catheter clang") on the distal electrode pair of the ablation catheter and the distal electrodes of the circular mapping catheter confirm this to be the position of the catheter.

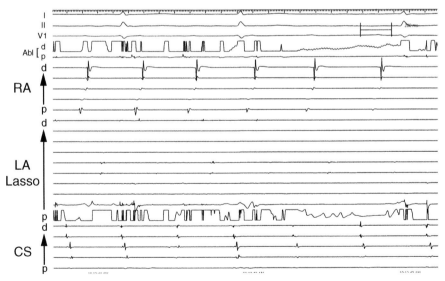

Figure 17.14 Ablation at this site initially leads to cycle length slowing.

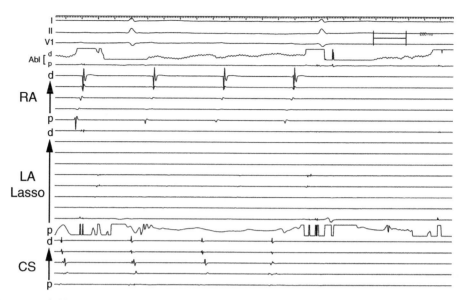

Figure 17.15 Continued ablation leads to termination of the tachycardia.

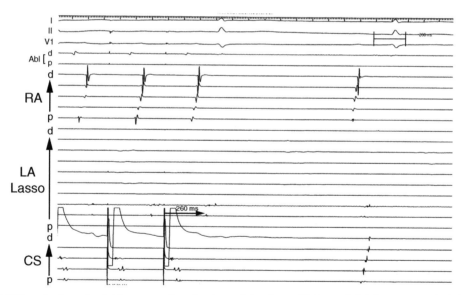

Figure 17.16 With pacing from the distal coronary sinus, fractionated signals are still observed slightly more posteriorly in electrodes 17,18 with a stimulus-to-electrogram interval of 260 ms.

isthmus, and ablation is planned to begin anteriorly at electrode pair 1,2 on the circular mapping catheter and move posteriorly to electrode pair 17,18.

Although no signal is recorded on the ablation electrodes, the presence of "matching noise" on the ablation electrograms and the distal pair of electrodes of the circular mapping catheter along with fluoroscopy suggest that the ablation catheter is located in the correct position (Figure 17.13). As ablation is performed, the tachycardia cycle length slows and then the tachycardia terminates (Figures 17.14 and 17.15). After ablation, pacing is performed from the distal coronary sinus, and highly delayed activation to the roof (260 ms) implies block (Figure 17.16). Despite aggressive atrial pacing protocols, the patient has no inducible atrial flutter. After ablation, the patient has had no recurrent arrhythmias and has stopped taking dofetilide.

KEY POINTS

- It is often beneficial to use different catheter types depending on the stage of the procedure.
- Catheters with more electrodes in a smaller area can be extremely useful for localizing a critical isthmus participating in tachycardia.

CHAPTER 18

Supraventricular tachycardia case 18: atrial tachycardia after atrial fibrillation ablation

A 68-year-old man has undergone two catheter ablation procedures for atrial fibrillation at another hospital. The details of the ablations are not available. Unfortunately, he has had continued episodes of atrial flutter associated with profound fatigue. He has hypertension but otherwise has no medical problems. His current medical regimen is metoprolol 50 mg twice daily and anticoagulation with warfarin. His physical examination does not reveal any significant abnormalities, and his baseline ECG is shown in Figure 18.1.

His baseline ECG reveals atrial flutter with 2:1 atrioventricular conduction. The flutter waves are negative in the inferior leads and have multiple components in lead V1. As the patient has had multiple catheter ablations in the past, four venous sheaths are placed and initially, catheters are placed in the right atrium near the tricuspid annulus and the coronary sinus. As catheters are placed in the atrium, his tachycardia terminates with mechanical stimulation.

The patient has had prior ablations for atrial fibrillation and has likely had ablation to isolate the pulmonary veins. The strategy in this case is to evaluate the pulmonary veins first to identify any areas of recurrent conduction. A circular mapping catheter is placed in all four pulmonary veins and recurrent activation is identified in the left inferior pulmonary vein (LIPV) (Figure 18.2). Ablation is performed with loss of pulmonary vein potentials (Figure 18.3). The other pulmonary veins do not display electrical activity.

Now that the pulmonary veins have been electrically isolated, atrial pacing is performed and atrial tachycardia with atrial activation matching the patient's clinical atrial tachycardia is induced. The tachycardia has a cycle length of 350 ms and is characterized by near simultaneous activation of the lateral wall of the right atrium and the coronary sinus and is evaluated by pacing from two sites in the right atrium and two sites in the coronary sinus (Figures 18.4–18.7). This results in better return cycle lengths from the right atrial sites as compared to the left atrial sites; however, large areas of the atria have not been studied.

A 20-electrode catheter is first placed along the mitral annulus and pacing is performed (Figures 18.8–18.10). The return cycle lengths and the activation sequences are all poor. The posterior left atrium has still not been evaluated; therefore, the 20-electrode catheter is placed more posteriorly and pacing is performed again (Figures 18.11–18.13). Collectively, none of the sites are consistent with a critical tachycardia site. The "best" pacing site remains the high right atrium with a return cycle length of 387 ms, and capture sequences during pacing that are similar to tachycardia for each catheter, but the time intervals between stimulus to electrogram and electrogram to electrogram (Figure 18.4) are different.

At this point, the clinician "knows" that the pulmonary veins are not part of the circuit and the best electrograms, whether by activation or by return cycle length, are from the right atrial sites. At this point, it is extremely useful to place the 20-electrode catheter within the right atrium anteriorly and the decapolar catheter is placed more posteriorly. In addition, it is often useful to evaluate the cavotricuspid isthmus (Figure 18.14).

Pacing from the anterolateral right atrial wall is associated with an excellent return cycle length (if the tachycardia mechanism is reentry); however, the activation sequence is incorrect in the right atrial catheters

Understanding Intracardiac EGMs: A Patient Centered Guide, First Edition. Fred Kusumoto.
© 2015 John Wiley & Sons, Ltd. Published 2015 by John Wiley & Sons, Ltd.

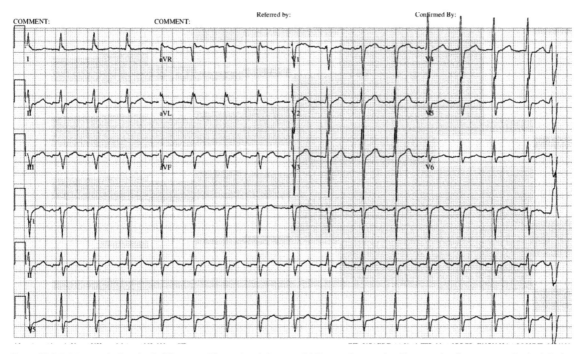

Figure 18.1 ECG on arrival to the holding area. The patient is in an atrial flutter characterized by negative flutter waves in the inferior leads and multiphasic but predominantly positive in lead V1.

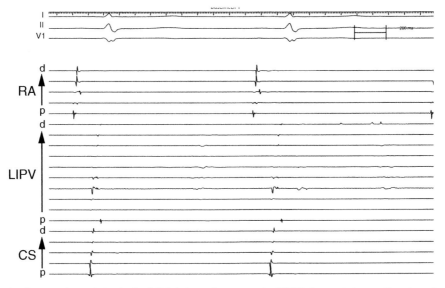

Figure 18.2 A circular mapping catheter in the left inferior pulmonary vein (LIPV) demonstrates continued conduction into the pulmonary vein. Earliest activation is observed in electrode pair 13,14.

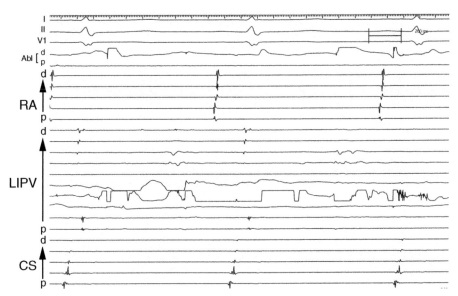

Figure 18.3 Ablation at electrode pair 13,14 (confirmed fluoroscopically and by the presence of matching artifact) leads to loss of pulmonary vein potentials.

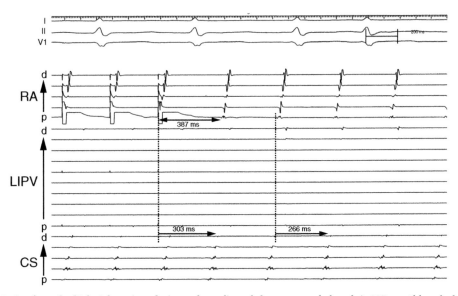

Figure 18.4 Pacing from the high right atrium during tachycardia and the return cycle length is 387 ms. Although the pattern of activation is similar during tachycardia and pacing, the stimulus-to-electrogram (266 ms) and electrogram-to-electrogram intervals (303 ms) differ, confirming change in the timing of the right atrial and coronary sinus activation.

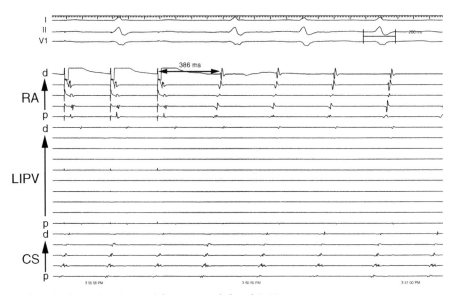

Figure 18.5 Pacing from the low right atrium and the return cycle length is 386 ms.

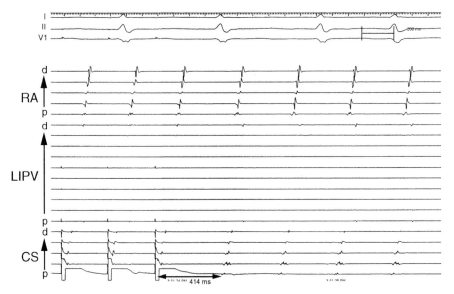

Figure 18.6 Pacing from the proximal coronary sinus is associated with a return cycle length of 414 ms.

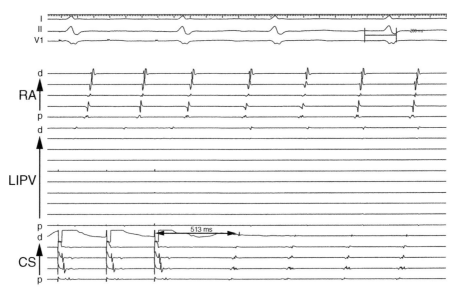

Figure 18.7 Pacing from the distal coronary sinus results in a very long return cycle length of 513 ms and completely opposite activation of the coronary sinus electrograms.

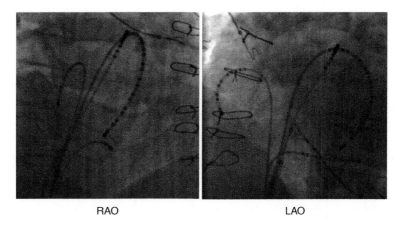

RAO   LAO

Figure 18.8 Right anterior oblique (RAO) and left anterior oblique (LAO) fluoroscopic projections showing a 20-pole catheter placed along the left atrial wall.

(Figure 18.15). However, the stimulus-to-proximal coronary sinus electrogram interval exactly matches the electrogram-to-electrogram interval. Taken together, the data suggest that the critical portions of the tachycardia circuit are located in the inferior portion of the right atrium near the cavotricuspid isthmus. To better explore the area, the 20-electrode catheter is placed

more inferiorly to "cover" this region with the tip just posterior to the coronary sinus os (Figure 18.16 and 18.17). Notice the very large area devoid of electrograms in the cavotricuspid isthmus at electrode pairs 5,6, and 7,8, and 9,10 (notice the low-frequency "far-field" atrial and ventricular signals). Pacing from the distal electrode entrains the tachycardia; while it is difficult to

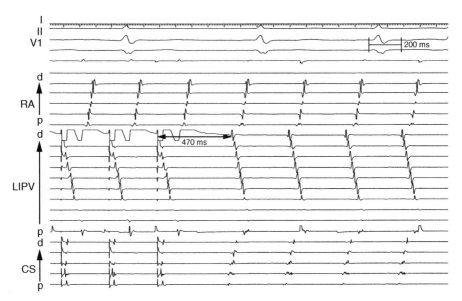

Figure 18.9 Pacing from the endocardial surface of the mitral annulus results in a return cycle length of 470 ms. Also notice that coronary sinus activation is completely different as is the timing between left atrial and right atrial activation.

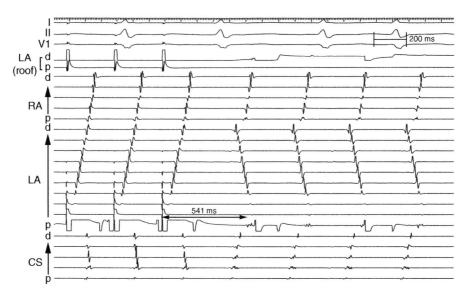

Figure 18.10 Pacing from the superior portion of the mitral annulus results in a very long return cycle length (541 ms) and completely changes the left atrial activation as measured by the coronary sinus and mitral annular catheters.

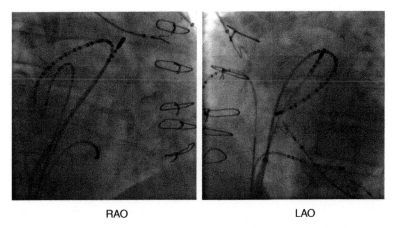

RAO   LAO

Figure 18.11 Fluoroscopic images showing that the 20-electrode catheter has been moved to the tricuspid annulus anterior to the crista terminalis while the decapolar catheter is placed in the posterior right atrium.

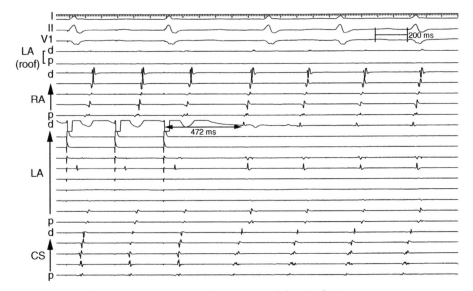

Figure 18.12 Pacing from the inferoposterior left atrium yields a return cycle length of 472 ms.

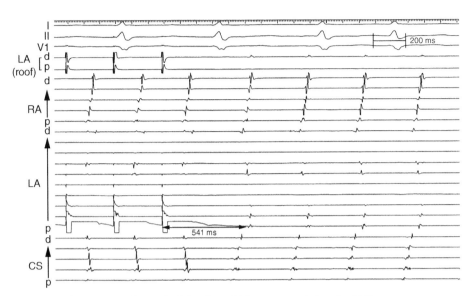

Figure 18.13 Pacing from the superior and posterior left atrium yields a return cycle length of 541 ms.

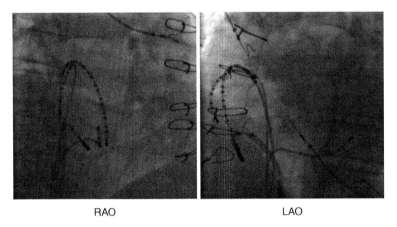

RAO   LAO

Figure 18.14 Two multielectrode catheters are placed in the right atrium: A decapolar catheter more posteriorly and a 20-electrode catheter placed more anteriorly near the tricuspid annulus. The crista terminalis travels vertically on the lateral wall of the right atrium between the decapolar catheter and the 20-electrode catheter.

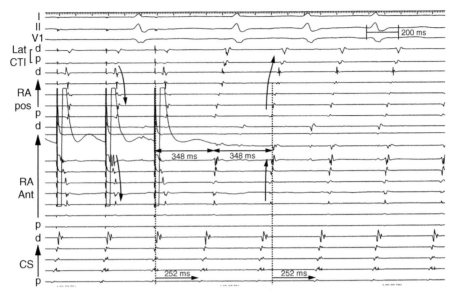

Figure 18.15 Pacing from electrode pair 5,6 shows a return cycle length that matches the tachycardia cycle length, but activation of the posterior right atrium and the more superior part of the right atrium is completely changed. Notice that the stimulus–to-proximal coronary sinus intervals exactly match the electrogram-to-electrogram intervals. Taken together, these findings suggest a localized reentrant circuit in the inferior and anterior portions of the right atrium.

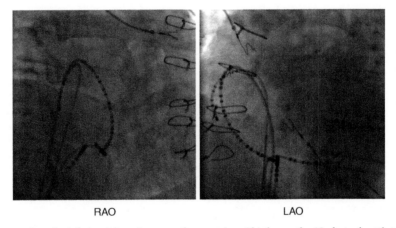

RAO   LAO

Figure 18.16 To better explore the inferior right atrium near the cavotricuspid isthmus, the 20-electrode catheter is repositioned to this region with the distal electrode near the coronary sinus os.

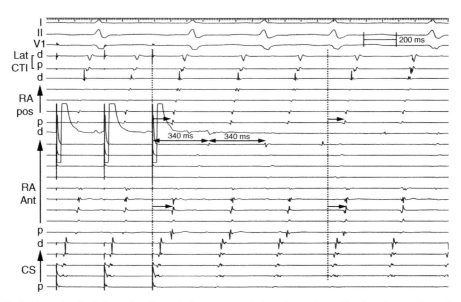

Figure 18.17 Pacing from the distal electrode pair results in a return cycle length as estimated by the adjacent electrode pair matches the tachycardia cycle length. Importantly, the stimulus-to-electrogram intervals (as measured on all of the catheter electrode pairs) are very close to the corresponding electrogram-to-electrogram intervals during tachycardia, suggesting that this area is associated with concealed entrainment. This region would be described as "near the exit site" because of the short stimulus-to-proximal coronary sinus electrogram interval.

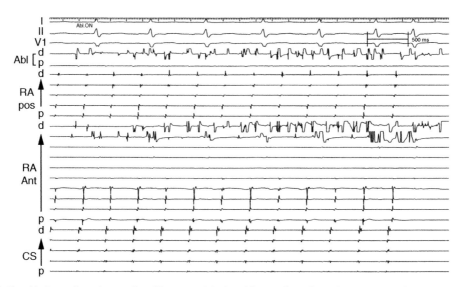

Figure 18.18 The ablation catheter is moved to this area, and during ablation, the tachycardia terminates after 4 s of radio-frequency energy delivery.

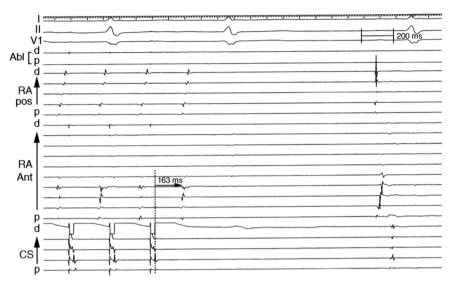

Figure 18.19 After ablation, there is evidence for cavotricuspid isthmus block with a conduction time of 163 ms from the proximal coronary sinus to the lateral right atrium.

evaluate the low-frequency electrograms on the distal electrode pair, the return cycle length to electrode pair 3,4 appears to be close to the tachycardia cycle length (Figure 18.17). Although the electrograms are difficult to evaluate on the distal electrode pair, notice that the intervals of stimulus-to-right atrial electrograms and the stimulus-to-coronary sinus electrograms exactly match the corresponding electrogram to electrogram intervals during tachycardia. It appears that this tachycardia involves the prior ablation scar, and although it appears to be dependent on cavotricuspid isthmus, it is not a typical atrial flutter because only the lateral portion of the anterior right atrium is "in the circuit."

Ablation posterior to the Eustachian ridge and between the ridge and the inferior vena cava leads to prompt termination of the tachycardia within 4 s of radio-frequency energy (Figure 18.18). After this, there appears to be a block across the cavotricuspid isthmus (Figure 18.19). The patient has been arrhythmia-free for the past 1 year.

KEY POINTS

- Atrial flutter can be due to a number of different mechanisms and a methodical approach is essential
- Prior ablation can facilitate the development of unusual arrhythmia circuits due to the production of protected slowly conducting isthmuses.

CHAPTER 19

Supraventricular tachycardia case 19: atrial tachycardia after atrial fibrillation ablation

A 67-year-old woman had undergone catheter ablation for atrial fibrillation several years ago and now has recurrent rapid heart rates associated with shortness of breath and tiredness. Her ECG is shown in Figure 19.1.

The patient is in an obvious regular supraventricular tachycardia. There appears to be discrete positive P waves just after the T waves in leads V1 and V2. The P waves might be upright in the inferior leads; however, often, when the P wave is associated with the T wave, it can be difficult to assess the exact morphology.

The patient is taken to the electrophysiology laboratory and evaluation of all four pulmonary veins demonstrates no recurrent conduction. Attention is turned to evaluating the atrial tachycardia and a 20-electrode catheter is placed in the left atrium near the mitral annulus, in addition to decapolar catheters placed in the coronary sinus and the lateral wall of the right atrium (Figure 19.2). Figure 19.3 shows the baseline atrial tachycardia with a cycle length of 262 ms and 2:1 AV conduction. Although the clinician cannot be sure at this point whether the tachycardia is due to reentry (where continuous activation is present) or automaticity, it is often helpful to arbitrarily decide what is "early" versus "late" by comparing activation to the P waves recorded on the surface ECG. In this case, lateral wall activation of the left atrium appears to precede the distal-to-proximal activation of the coronary sinus, which is then followed by superior-to-inferior activation of the lateral wall of the right atrium. Evaluation of the electrograms shows that left atrial electrograms are characterized by low-frequency and low-amplitude

signals suggesting the presence of a significant left atrial myopathy. In contrast, the right atrial electrograms have a higher amplitude and higher frequency (they are "sharper and spikier").

Atrial pacing is first performed at the distal coronary sinus (Figure 19.4). Not surprisingly, coronary sinus depolarization is similar during pacing and tachycardia, whereas right atrial depolarization is different during pacing when compared to tachycardia. In Figure 19.5, pacing is performed from the "earliest" recorded electrogram (electrode pair 15,16 of the 20-electrode left atrial catheter), and the return cycle length on cessation of pacing (275 ms) is similar to the tachycardia cycle length (268 ms). Pacing is associated with a subtle change in the coronary sinus activation; however, generally, the electrograms recorded during pacing match the electrograms recorded during tachycardia. The mapping catheter is moved to electrode pair 15,16 and suddenly depolarization of the atrium changes (Figure 19.6), particularly evident in the coronary sinus electrograms where activation of the proximal-mid coronary sinus (electrode pairs 5,6 and 7,8) precedes depolarization of the distal coronary sinus.

At this point, it is often easy to become frustrated by the complexity and apparent changing arrhythmias, but it is often instructive to evaluate the transition between the "two" tachycardias. The electrograms recorded at electrodes 15,16 are now "late" and appear to occur at the terminal portion of the P wave recorded on V1 rather than before the P wave. Interestingly, notice that although the pattern of coronary sinus activation has changed, the interval between the electrogram recorded at the proximal coronary sinus and the lateral wall of the right atrium is similar for "both" tachycardias. There are

Understanding Intracardiac EGMs: A Patient Centered Guide, First Edition. Fred Kusumoto.
© 2015 John Wiley & Sons, Ltd. Published 2015 by John Wiley & Sons, Ltd.

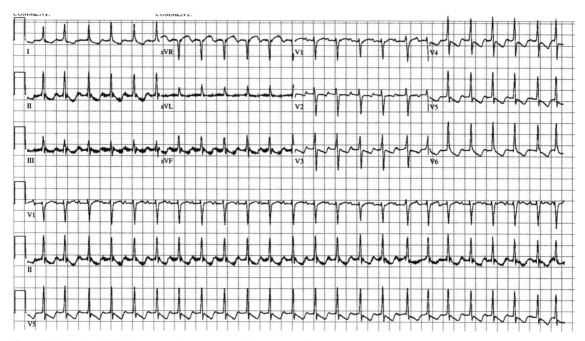

Figure 19.1 Baseline ECG shows a regular supraventricular tachycardia.

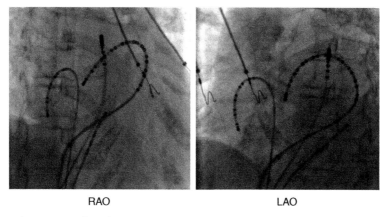

RAO   LAO

Figure 19.2 Once the pulmonary veins have been ruled out as a source of tachycardia, a 20-electrode catheter is placed along the mitral annulus along with decapolar catheters in the coronary sinus and the lateral right atrium.

basically two general possibilities here. First, there could be one underlying tachycardia, and catheter trauma led to local block and a change in the atrial activation pattern. Second, there could be two tachycardias simultaneously present (with one entrained by the other) or two tachycardias that develop sequentially (perhaps local block led to the development of another reentrant tachycardia through another critical isthmus). Although

at this point, it is impossible to distinguish between the two general possibilities, the similar tachycardia rates and the constant interval between proximal coronary sinus depolarization and right atrial depolarization make one underlying tachycardia and a local block an intriguing possibility.

Again, as emphasized throughout this book, it is important to maintain a methodical approach to

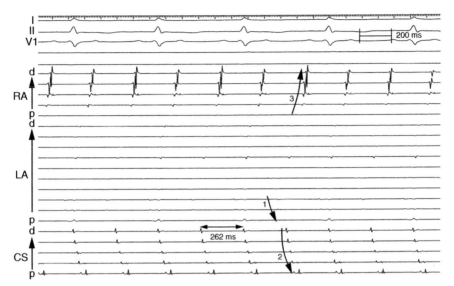

Figure 19.3 Baseline electrograms reveal a tachycardia with a cycle length of 262 ms with "initial" activation in the lateral wall of the left atrium (arrow 1), followed by distal-to-proximal activation of the coronary sinus (arrow 2), and, finally, by superior-to-inferior activation of the lateral wall of the right atrium (arrow 3 – from the proximal to the distal electrodes). The atrial deflections recorded on the surface ECG appear to coincide with right atrial depolarization.

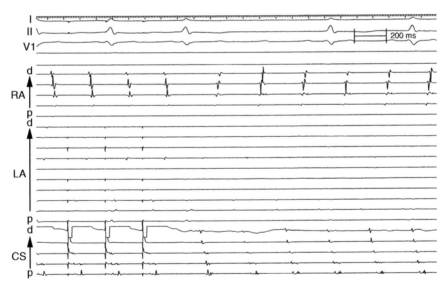

Figure 19.4 Pacing from the distal coronary sinus is associated with a different pattern of right atrial activation when compared to tachycardia.

tachycardia evaluation. Pacing is performed again from electrode pair 15,16, and this time, atrial activation is completely different and the return cycle length after cessation of pacing is prolonged (Figure 19.7). Importantly, notice that the second postpacing electrogram-to-electrogram interval is very

prolonged (472 ms), essentially ruling this area out as a critical region for the current tachycardia. Now the "earliest" electrograms are in electrode pair 7,8 of the coronary sinus, and pacing is performed at this site. Although this is the earliest site of the current electrograms being evaluated, the postpacing interval

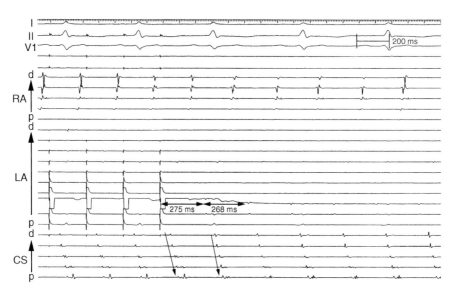

Figure 19.5 Pacing from the lateral left atrium at electrode pair 15,16 is associated with a postpacing interval (275 ms) that is close to the tachycardia cycle length (268 ms). Importantly, the electrograms recorded during pacing are similar to the electrograms recorded during tachycardia with some subtle differences such as in the coronary sinus (arrows).

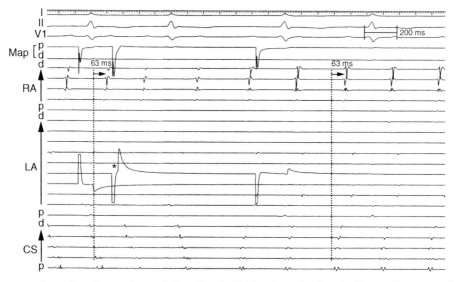

Figure 19.6 The mapping catheter is moved toward electrode pair 15,16 as shown by the coincident artifact (*) noted on the distal electrodes of the mapping catheter and electrode pair 15,16. This is associated with a sudden change in the activation pattern observed in the coronary sinus. Interestingly, the interval between the electrograms recorded on electrode pair 7,8 and on the coronary sinus and distal right atrial electrodes remains the same (63 ms).

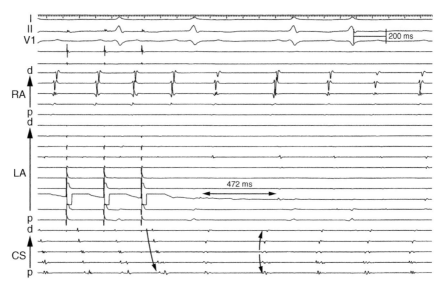

Figure 19.7 Pacing from electrode pair 15,16 is now associated with a completely different pattern of atrial depolarization in the coronary sinus and the left atrium (compare electrograms in electrode pair 7,8 and electrode pair 15,16 during pacing and tachycardia). Also notice the apparent long interval between electrograms in electrode pair 15,16 in the second postpacing interval (472 ms), which rules out this region as a critical area for the current tachycardia.

is prolonged and activation of the right atrium and the left atrium is completely different during pacing when compared to tachycardia (Figure 19.8). Clearly, if this tachycardia is due to automaticity, the coronary sinus is not near the site of origin, and if the tachycardia is due to re-entry, the coronary sinus is not near the exit site. In reentry, the "head" of activation meets the "tail," and it is useful to pace from a site characterized by a late electrogram at the terminal portion of the P wave or in the immediate isoelectric period after the P wave. Pacing from electrode pair 7,8 of the 20-electrode left atrial catheter results in a very long postpacing interval and a complete change in the activation pattern observed in the coronary sinus (Figure 19.9). If a site is near the entrance site to a slow area of conduction, the return cycle length will be close to the tachycardia cycle length and often some portions of the atrium (usually the "earliest" recorded electrogram) will be activated in the same way for both during pacing and tachycardia ("orthodromic" capture). In this case, the electrogram recorded at coronary sinus electrode pair 7,8 is completely different during pacing when compared to tachycardia.

Pacing from the posterior left atrium and the lateral wall of the right atrium (Figure 19.10) is also associated with a change in the atrial activation pattern and long postpacing intervals. Collectively, the data suggest that the tachycardia arises from the atrial septum. In order to evaluate the atrial septum more carefully (particularly the His bundle region), the 20-electrode catheter is repositioned to straddle the tricuspid valve (Figure 19.11).

At this point, it is useful to decide whether the underlying mechanism of a tachycardia is reentry or automaticity. This distinction is important because of the two very different strategies for effective ablation: ablation of an isthmus to cause block versus ablation of a specific site of abnormal rapid depolarization. Evaluating the tachycardia response to different pacing rates can sometimes help the clinician to make this distinction. In this case, pacing from the superior portion of the left atrial side of the septum is performed at a more rapid cycle length (Figure 19.12). More rapid pacing is associated with a longer pause before the first beat of tachycardia. Although this response can be observed in reentry due to slower conduction through a critical isthmus, an exaggerated response as shown

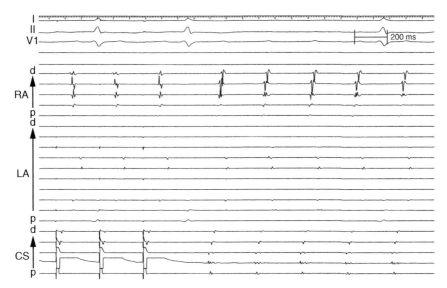

Figure 19.8 Electrode pair 7,8 is the earliest recoded electrograms with the current catheter positioning. Pacing from this site is associated with a prolonged postpacing interval and completely different activation of the coronary sinus (arrows), left atrium (compare the relative electrogram timing of electrode pairs 7,8 and 15,16), and the right atrium (compare relative electrogram timing of the distal and proximal electrode pairs).

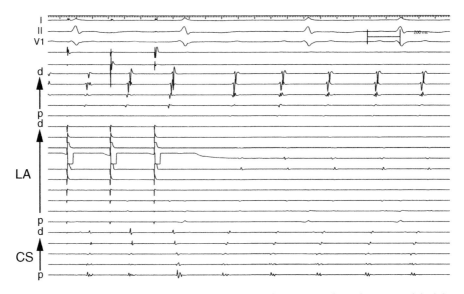

Figure 19.9 Pacing from one of the "latest" electrograms relative to the surface P wave (electrode pair 7,8 of the left atrial catheter) results in a long postpacing interval and a complete change in the depolarization pattern recorded in the coronary sinus.

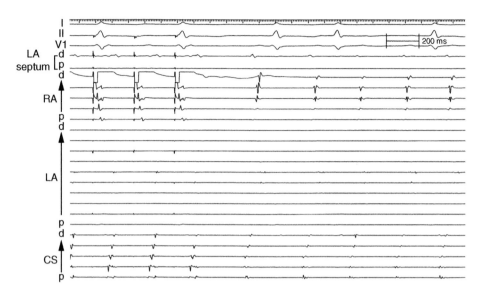

Figure 19.10 Pacing from the lateral wall of the right atrium is associated with a long postpacing interval and a complete change in atrial activation: pacing depolarizes the right atrium before the coronary sinus, whereas during tachycardia, the proximal coronary sinus activation precedes the right atrial activation.

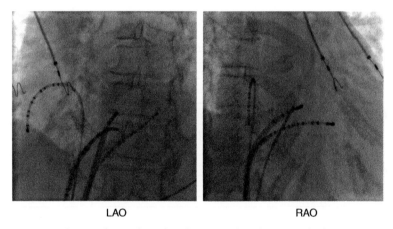

LAO   RAO

Figure 19.11 Fluoroscopic images showing the 20-electrode catheter straddling the tricuspid valve.

here with relatively similar electrogram patterns during pacing and tachycardia would be more consistent with automaticity. The mapping catheter is carefully manipulated in this region and a site characterized by a very early electrogram, and an electrogram pattern that is the same during tachycardia and pacing is identified (Figure 19.13). The mapping catheter is carefully

moved to the immediate surrounding area, and no earlier electrograms can be identified. This provides strong evidence that a site characterized by abnormal automaticity is responsible for the tachycardia. The site is on the left atrial side of the septum and superior to the 20-electrode catheter straddling the tricuspid valve (Figure 19.11). Notice that as this site is near

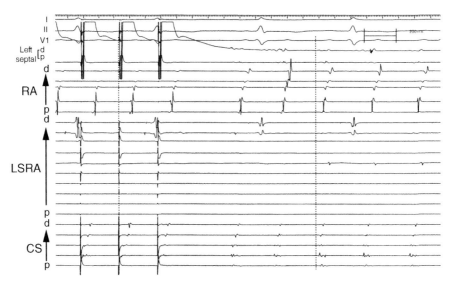

Figure 19.12 Pacing from the superior portion of the left side of the interatrial septum at a cycle length of 250 ms. There is a longer pause from cessation of pacing to the first beat of tachycardia. Notice that although the interval between the mapping electrode electrogram and the right atrial electrogram is longer during tachycardia when compared to pacing, generally the activation patterns are similar.

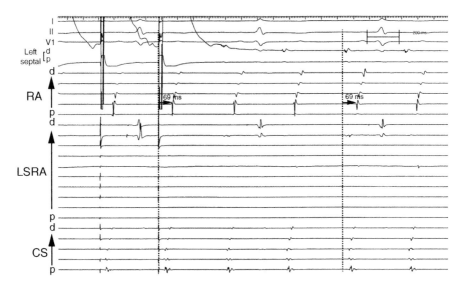

Figure 19.13 Pacing from a site associated with an early electrogram results in an activation pattern that is similar during pacing when compared to tachycardia.

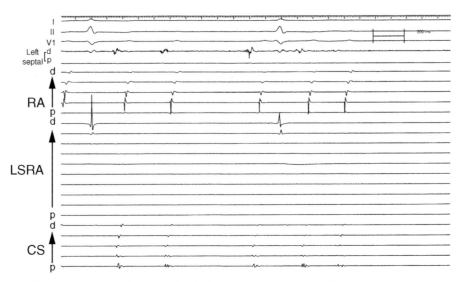

Figure 19.14 Radio-frequency energy application at this site led to termination of the tachycardia.

the AV node, the 8 mm tip ablation catheter has been exchanged for a 4 mm tip (compare the catheter tips in Figures 19.2 and 19.11). Application of radio-frequency energy at this site leads to termination of the tachycardia within several seconds (Figure 19.14). During ablation, the PR interval is carefully monitored and the total energy application is limited to 40 s. The patient has been tachycardia-free for several years off medications.

- It is important to take a methodical approach to electrophysiology evaluation.
- Recurrent arrhythmias are relatively common after ablation of atrial tachycardias including atrial fibrillation and often have very different mechanisms and evaluation must be approached with persistence and an "open mind."

KEY POINTS

- Multiple atrial tachycardias or atrial flutters may be present in an individual patient.

CHAPTER 20

Wide complex tachycardia case 1

A 47-year-old woman has palpitations and light-headedness while playing tennis. She does not lose consciousness but is found by paramedics to be in a wide complex tachycardia. Her blood pressure is 100/60, and she complains of rapid heart rate and light-headedness. She is given amiodarone 150 mg, which converts her to sinus rhythm, and is brought to the emergency room. Her ECG from the paramedics is shown in Figure 20.1.

One of the important functions of electrophysiologic testing is the evaluation of the patient with wide complex tachycardia with an unknown mechanism. Recall from Chapter 1 that there are only four anatomic types of tachycardia. All four types can be associated with a wide complex tachycardia; however, clinically, it is usually first important to differentiate ventricular tachycardia from "everything else" because ventricular tachycardia is more likely to be life-threatening. There are a number of ECG algorithms that can be useful for determining whether wide complex tachycardia is due to ventricular tachycardia; however, in some cases, the diagnosis is unclear and an electrophysiologic test is indicated to determine the underlying cause.

Once the tachycardia has been corrected, the main issue is to ascertain whether or not "structural heart disease" is present. Any condition that can lead to the development of scar in the ventricles makes ventricular tachycardia more likely because the presence of scar can lead to the development of reentrant circuits. In the Western world, by far and away, the most common form of ventricular scarring is the presence of a prior myocardial infarction. However, it is important for the clinician to remember that many other conditions (e.g., dilated cardiomyopathy, hypertrophic cardiomyopathy, prior ventriculotomy for surgical treatment of congenital heart disease, or arrhythmogenic right ventricular cardiomyopathy or ARVC) can be associated with ventricular scarring and the development of reentrant ventricular arrhythmias. In addition, some genetic disorders such as the long QT syndrome and Brugada syndrome (often collectively referred to as "channelopathies" because they involve a genetic defect of a critical ion channel involved in cardiac depolarization or repolarization) and conditions such as coronary artery spasm can lead to ventricular arrhythmias and sudden cardiac death in the absence of "structural heart disease" (Table 20.1).

The baseline ECG is shown in Figure 20.2. The patient undergoes transthoracic echocardiography that demonstrates an LVEF of 0.62 and no valvular or other structural abnormalities.

The baseline ECG shows no abnormalities suggestive of a cause for ventricular tachycardia such as long QT syndrome or Brugada syndrome. An echocardiogram demonstrates no structural abnormalities. She is taken to the electrophysiology laboratory for evaluation.

Although in the setting of evaluation of wide complex tachycardia, it is easy to focus first on identifying whether or not ventricular tachycardia is the cause of a wide complex tachycardia, it is always important to take a methodical approach to electrophysiology testing, particularly in the setting of normal left ventricular function (as this reduces the pretest probability for ventricular tachycardia).

Just as in a patient with documented supraventricular tachycardia, quadripolar catheters are placed in the right atrium, the His bundle position, and the right ventricle and a decapolar catheter is placed in the coronary sinus. Baseline cardiac intervals are shown in Figure 20.3 and are normal. However, atrial pacing

Understanding Intracardiac EGMs: A Patient Centered Guide, First Edition. Fred Kusumoto.
© 2015 John Wiley & Sons, Ltd. Published 2015 by John Wiley & Sons, Ltd.

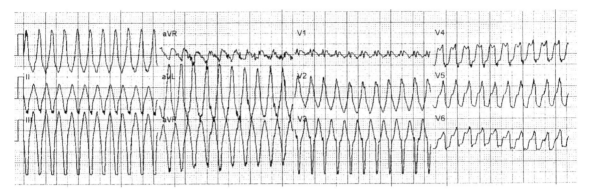

Figure 20.1 A 12-lead ECG during tachycardia recorded by the paramedics.

Table 20.1 Baseline ECG clues in the patient with wide complex tachycardia.

Condition	ECG findings:
Prior myocardial infarction	• Abnormal Q waves
Dilated cardiomyopathy	• Widened QRS complex due to bundle branch block • Low QRS voltage
Hypertrophic cardiomyopathy	• Prominent QRS voltage • Abnormal septal depolarization (Large septal R wave) in V1 • Abnormal repolarization
Wolff–Parkinson–White syndrome	• Delta waves
Long QT syndrome	• Prolonged QT interval
Brugada syndrome	• Characteristic "shark fin" in V1 due to ST segment elevation in the right-sided chest leads
ARVC	• Epsilon waves • Inverted anterior T waves

at a cycle length of 500 ms leads to a change in the QRS complex (Figure 20.4). Pacing-associated change in the QRS complex can be due to either development of bundle branch block or the presence of an antero-gradely conducting accessory pathway. In this case, the beginning of the QRS complex precedes the His bundle deflection and the presence of an accessory pathway is confirmed. Shortening the pacing rate cycle length to 350 ms is associated with 2:1 AV block due to block in both the accessory pathway and the AV node (Figure 20.5).

Now that the AVBCL has been determined, atrial premature stimuli are delivered at progressively shorter coupling intervals (Figures 20.6–20.8). At a drive cycle length of 600 ms, a premature atrial extrastimulus delivered at a coupling interval of 2390 ms is associated with a more abnormal appearing QRS complex as most of the ventricle is depolarized by the accessory pathway when compared to the normal AV node and His Purkinje system (Figure 20.6). Shortening the coupling interval to 380 ms causes block in the accessory pathway and is associated with a long AH interval and an apparent atrial "echo" due to dual AVN node physiology (Figure 20.7). The QRS complex is "normal and narrow" due to complete depolarization of the ventricle via the His Purkinje system. As shown in Figure 20.8, the premature atrial extrastimulus is delivered 10 ms earlier, and block in the AV node ensues.

Ventricular pacing demonstrates 1:1 VA conduction with a concentric pattern of retrograde atrial activation until the cycle length is shortened to 350 ms (Figure 20.9). Ventricular premature stimuli reveal normal response and ventricular effective refractory period of 280 ms (Figures 20.10 and 20.11). Decremental VA conduction is observed, presumably via the His bundle and AV node and definitive retrograde activation via the accessory pathway cannot be elicited. Unfortunately, para-Hisian pacing is unsuccessful because a narrow QRS complex cannot be elicited despite maximal outputs and catheter manipulation.

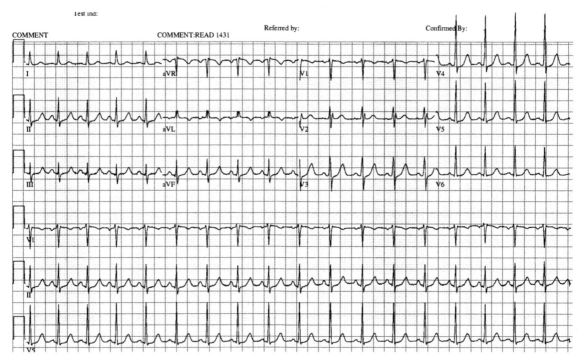

Figure 20.2 Baseline ECG appears normal.

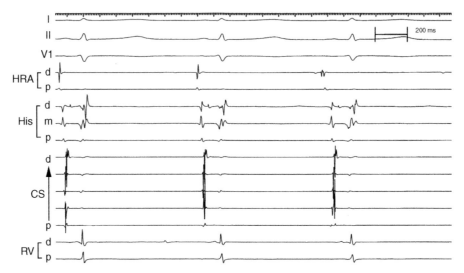

Figure 20.3 Baseline electrograms are normal with an AH interval of 44 ms and an HV interval of 50 ms.

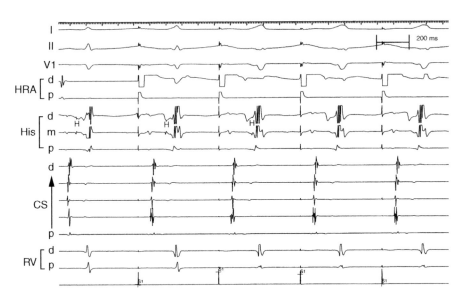

Figure 20.4 Atrial pacing is started at a cycle length of 500 ms, and there is a change in the QRS complex with His electrogram (H) being "driven into" the QRS complex. Although difficult to assess with the presence of only three leads, the accessory pathway appears to be inferior due to the negative delta wave observed in lead II.

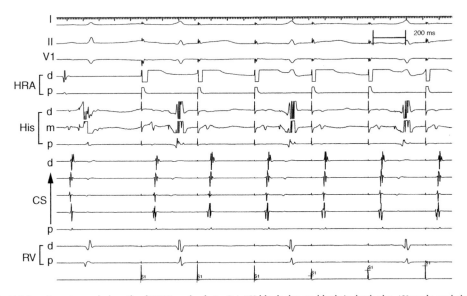

Figure 20.5 Atrial pacing at a cycle length of 2350 ms leads to 2:1 AV block due to block in both the AV node and the accessory pathway.

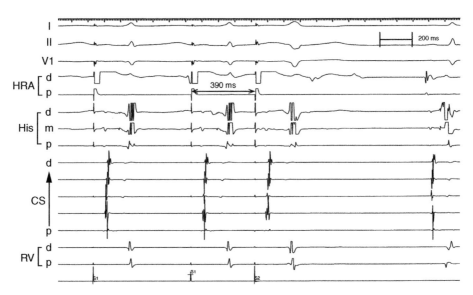

Figure 20.6 At a basic pacing cycle length of 600 ms, a premature atrial extrastimulus is delivered at a coupling interval of 390 ms. Notice the more prominent preexcitation evident in the QRS complex as most of the ventricles are activated via the accessory pathway when compared to the AV node.

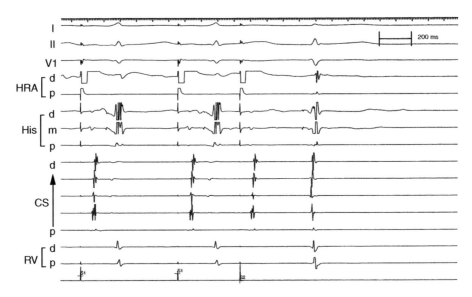

Figure 20.7 Continued from Figure 20.6. Shortening the coupling interval to 380 ms leads to block in the accessory pathway, thus defining the accessory pathway effective refractory period or APERP. With block in the accessory pathway, there is prolonged conduction via the AV node and a long AH interval, followed by a normal QRS complex because the ventricles are activated solely by the His Purkinje system. Interestingly, there appears to be a retrograde atrial "echo" due to dual pathway physiology.

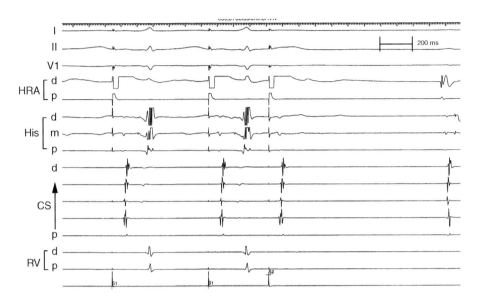

Figure 20.8 Continued from Figure 20.7. Shortening the coupling interval to 370 ms leads to block in the AV node.

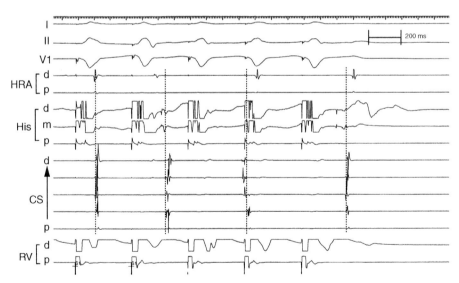

Figure 20.9 Ventricular pacing at a cycle length of 350 ms is associated with variable VA conduction. Notice that each of the four atrial electrograms has a subtly different electrogram pattern suggesting different forms of atrial activation (a fiduciary line is placed on coronary sinus electrode pair 7,8 to allow comparison).

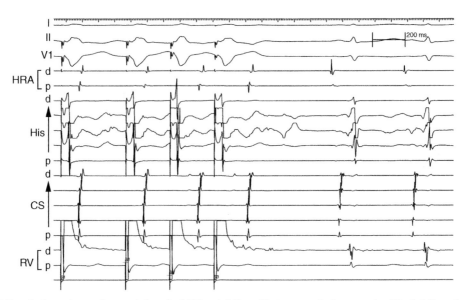

Figure 20.10 Ventricular pacing at a base cycle length of 400 ms is followed by two ventricular extrastimuli both delivered at a coupling interval of 270 ms. Decrement in VA conduction is observed, and comparison of retrograde activation patterns does not reveal any differences.

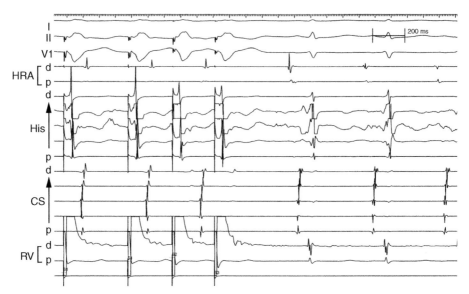

Figure 20.11 Continuation of Figure 20.10. Shortening the ventricular extrastimuli coupling intervals to 270 ms and 260 ms results in VA block and the retrograde ventriculoatrial effective refractory period (VAERP).

As the patient shows evidence for an anterogradely conducting accessory pathway, adenosine is given to cause block in the AV node and maximize preexcitation (Figure 20.12). Evaluation of the 12-lead ECG with adenosine infusion is extremely helpful (Figure 20.13). Close inspection of the ECG shows negative delta waves in V1 and in the inferior leads (II, III, and aVF) and an unusual precordial transition with an RSr' complex in lead V2 and an RS complex in V3. As mentioned in Chapter 7, left-sided accessory pathways have an early transition and relatively prominent R waves in leads V1 and V2 because the left ventricle is a posterior structure and right-sided accessory pathways have a later transition because the right ventricle is an anterior structure. An excellent sign for the presence of a septal accessory pathway is a negative delta wave in lead V1. Taken together, the ECG data suggest that the patient has an inferoseptal accessory pathway. In addition, preexcitation in the setting of AV node block provides strong evidence that the patient has an AV accessory pathway rather than a nodoventricular accessory pathway.

At this point, it is now evident that the patient has an accessory pathway that can conduct anterogradely and is suspicious as the underlying mechanism of her wide complex tachycardia. The QRS recorded on the ECG during her clinical event is grossly similar in appearance to the QRS associated with preexcitation (compare Figure 20.1 and 20.13). At this point, it would be reasonable to proceed with mapping and ablation as in Chapter 7. Unlike in Chapter 7, in this case, we also have evidence that the patient has dual AV node physiology and wide QRS tachycardia; while arrhythmia such as AVNRT is far less likely that an accessory pathway has been identified, it is still a possibility as a cause for her wide complex tachycardia. A decision is made to begin isoproterenol in hopes of inducing clinically sustained wide complex tachycardia.

In order to help define the pattern of atrial depolarization, the quadripolar catheter is removed and replaced by a decapolar catheter placed along the tricuspid annulus. Atrial pacing initiates a wide complex tachycardia with a cycle length of 245 ms (Figure 20.14). The tachycardia is characterized by a 1:1 relationship between atrial and ventricular activation; while it is difficult to accurately define the pattern of retrograde conduction, it does appear to be concentric with the earliest atrial depolarization in the His bundle region. There are no visible His bundle electrograms preceding the QRS complexes and the QRS complexes do not have the appearance of aberrant conduction (QS complex with a notch on the downstroke in lead V1). Both of

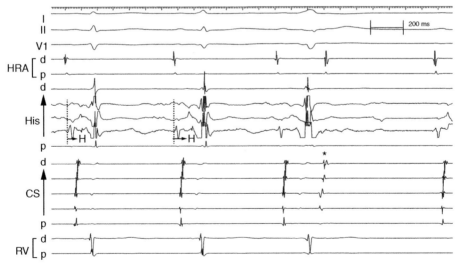

Figure 20.12 Adenosine during sinus rhythm leads to progressive AV nodal conduction delay and block (notice the progressive delay in the His (H) bundle electrogram denoted by the arrows) and maximal preexcitation. Adenosine is associated with premature atrial contractions (*) and has also been associated with the development of atrial fibrillation.

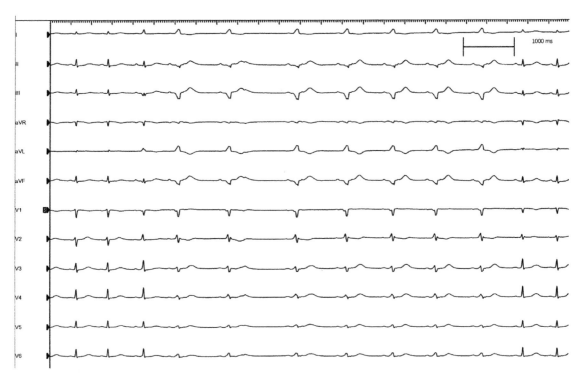

Figure 20.13 A 12-lead ECG during adenosine infusion shows progressive PR interval prolongation in conjunction with increasing preexcitation. At maximal preexcitation, the negative delta waves observed in leads V1, II, III, and aVF suggest that the accessory pathway is in the inferoseptal region. As the effects of adenosine resolve, the QRS complex normalizes due to the return of normal AV node conduction.

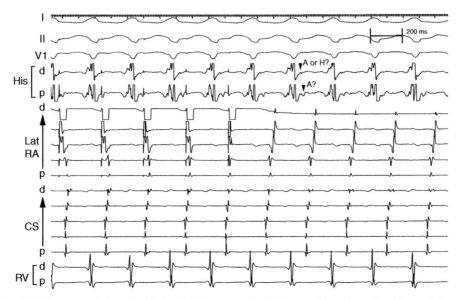

Figure 20.14 Atrial pacing at a cycle length of 260 ms initiates a sustained wide complex tachycardia with a cycle length of 250 ms and an LBBB pattern and superior axis. There is a 1:1 relationship between the atrial and the ventricular activity. It is often extremely hard to assess the electrograms in the His bundle recordings, particularly differentiating the His bundle electrograms from the atrial electrograms (arrowheads); however, it does appear that atrial depolarization in the His bundle region precedes the earliest atrial activity observed in the coronary sinus.

these findings "rule out" supraventricular tachycardia with left bundle branch block morphology aberrancy. It is vital to confirm hemodynamic stability of any tachycardia, but it is particularly critical in wide complex tachycardia. In this case, the patient has a systolic blood pressure in the 85–90 mm Hg range and on questioning, denies any symptoms other than the sensation of a rapid heart rate. In our laboratory, we have one team member who is solely responsible for assessing the patient's comfort and symptoms (if awake) during tachycardia. After confirming the clinical stability, the tachycardia can be evaluated. A 12-lead ECG confirms that the morphology of the tachycardia is similar to that of the clinical tachycardia (Figure 20.15). Changes in the precordial QRS morphology are probably due to differences in lead placement. Notice that the V2 morphology of the induced tachycardia is very similar to the V1 morphology of the spontaneous tachycardia.

Importantly, in the frontal leads, which are less prone to lead placement issues, QRS complexes match exactly.

As supraventricular tachycardia with aberrant conduction has been effectively ruled out and a 1:1 VA relationship is present, the differential diagnosis for the wide complex tachycardia is antidromic tachycardia (using either the AV node or another accessory pathway as the retrograde limb), a condition where the accessory pathway activates the ventricles but is not involved in the underlying tachycardia mechanism (atrial tachycardia with anterograde accessory pathway conduction or AVNRT with anterograde accessory pathway conduction), or ventricular tachycardia. Of these possibilities, ventricular tachycardia is the least likely possibility because the QRS complex in tachycardia matches maximal preexcitation that was previously measured (the QRS complexes associated with atrial pacing exactly match the QRS complexes in tachycardia shown in Figure 20.10). Before the tachycardia can

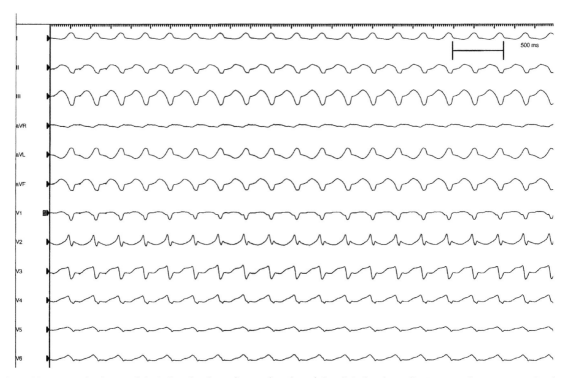

Figure 20.15 A 12-lead ECG of the induced tachycardia matches that of the clinical tachycardia. Importantly, accounting for the vagaries of electrode position in the precordial leads, the Rsr morphology of the QRS complex in lead V2 is almost an exact match to that of the QRS complex in lead V1 in the clinical tachycardia. The frontal plane ECG leads (where there is less variability due to lead position) are an exact match when comparing the induced and clinical tachycardias.

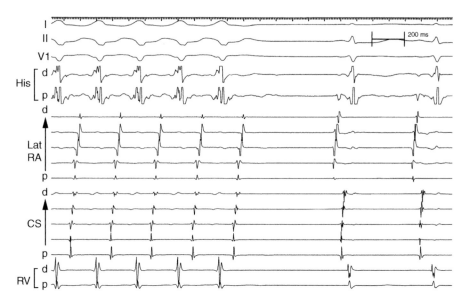

Figure 20.16 Spontaneous termination of the tachycardia on an atrial electrogram. This finding provides very strong evidence that anterograde conduction via the accessory pathway is necessary for perpetuation of tachycardia.

be evaluated with pacing maneuvers, the tachycardia terminates spontaneously (Figure 20.16). Spontaneous termination on an atrial electrogram is extremely helpful. This finding implies that maintenance of tachycardia is dependent on ventricular depolarization via the accessory pathway and makes any tachycardia where the accessory pathway is a "bystander" extremely unlikely (atrial tachycardia with a bystander accessory pathway or AVNRT with a bystander accessory pathway, both of which on termination would be associated with AV conduction via the bystander accessory pathway).

As discussed in Chapter 8, once wide complex tachycardia is induced, it can be very helpful to scan with premature atrial stimuli to help decipher the underlying mechanism of tachycardia. In addition, atrial overdrive pacing can provide important information; while, generally, less fruitful in the setting of wide complex tachycardia, ventricular stimuli (either with scanning diastole or with overdrive pacing) can provide additional information on patients with wide complex tachycardia, a 1:1 AV relationship, and no visible His deflection (Table 20.2). Figure 20.17 shows the effects of ventricular pacing during tachycardia. The tachycardia is entrained and appears to terminate with VA block. Although suggestive that perpetuation of tachycardia depends on VA conduction, ventricular pacing can

also terminate ventricular tachycardia (antitachycardia pacing in implantable cardioverter defibrillators).

Tachycardia is reinitiated again, and premature atrial stimuli induce atrial fibrillation (Figure 20.18). Notice the ECG hallmarks of atrial fibrillation in the setting of an accessory pathway: a very rapid irregular, wide complex tachycardia (Figure 20.19). In addition, notice that in broad terms, there is only one abnormal QRS complex morphology, which provides indirect evidence that only one accessory pathway is present. The shortest R–R interval during tachycardia is 230 ms, which places the patient in a higher risk category. Fortunately, the patient's atrial fibrillation converts spontaneously. With reinitiation of tachycardia, atrial fibrillation is again induced with atrial pacing protocols, and after 5 min, the patient's atrial fibrillation again spontaneously converts.

Although one could continue the electrophysiologic evaluation at this point, we now have strong evidence that accessory pathway conduction is the anterograde component of her clinical wide complex tachycardia. In addition, the patient has had episodes of atrial fibrillation during the procedure that preclude atrial stimulation during tachycardia, and it is possible that the patient might develop sustained atrial fibrillation requiring cardioversion with continued attempts at

Table 20.2 Diagnostic yield of pacing maneuvers in wide complex tachycardia with 1:1 ventricular and atrial relationship and no visible His electrogram.

Maneuver	Response
Premature atrial extrastimulus when the septal atrial region has been depolarized or "committed."	• Termination of tachycardia increases the likelihood that the accessory pathway is the anterograde limb of the circuit. • Advancing ventricular depolarization with the same QRS and the subsequent atrial electrogram confirms that an accessory pathway is the anterograde limb of the circuit. • Advancing ventricular depolarization with the same QRS complex without affecting the subsequent atrial electrogram increases the likelihood that a bystander accessory pathway is present. • Advancing depolarization with a different QRS morphology "rules in" a bystander accessory pathway.
Atrial pacing entrains the ventricles during tachycardia.	• If the QRS normalizes or AV block develops, and on cessation of pacing, tachycardia continues, then atrial tachycardia with a bystander accessory pathway is "ruled in." • If a different wide QRS morphology is observed, then either a bystander accessory pathway or ventricular tachycardia is present. • If the QRS does not change and on cessation of pacing, if a V-V-A response is identified, ventricular tachycardia is "ruled in." • If the QRS does not change and a V-A-V response is observed, antidromic tachycardia or supraventricular tachycardia with a bystander accessory pathway can be present.
Premature ventricular stimulus when the His bundle has been depolarized or is "committed."	• Advancing atrial depolarization identifies the presence of an accessory pathway (whether as a bystander or as the retrograde limb of the tachycardia circuit).
Premature ventricular stimulus	• Advancing atrial depolarization without resetting the tachycardia makes ventricular tachycardia the most likely diagnosis.
Ventricular pacing and entrainment of tachycardia	• Termination usually does not help • VV-A-A-V response makes atrial tachycardia the most likely diagnosis • VV-A-V response is not helpful.

atrial pacing during tachycardia. While cardioversions have a very small absolute risk, it is reasonable to avoid performing them during electrophysiologic tests if possible.

As a first step for mapping and ablation, as the accessory pathway is in the inferoseptal region, a coronary sinus angiogram is performed, which demonstrates no abnormalities such as an anomalous vein or coronary sinus diverticulum. The right atrial septum is mapped using an anterograde mapping strategy to identify the earliest ventricular electrogram on an annular site (large atrial and ventricular electrograms). Atrial pacing often facilitates anterograde mapping by producing a delay in AV node conduction. Identifying the exact onset of the QRS complex can sometimes be difficult because of fusion between the P wave and the QRS complex. Pacing from a site that is relatively far from the accessory pathway insertion point can minimize

but does not eliminate this problem. Atrial pacing from the distal coronary sinus is performed at a cycle length of 500 ms and a septal site just above the coronary sinus is identified (Figures 20.20 and 20.21). As this septal accessory pathway is relatively far from the His bundle region (compare Figure 20.21 with Figure 5.25 in Chapter 5), radio-frequency energy application is performed in sinus rhythm, and with ablation, preexcitation disappears and a His bundle electrogram appears (Figure 20.22).

After ablation, the patient is noninducible for any sustained arrhythmias although an intermittent single AV node echo remains. The patient is given adenosine, and block in the AV node results in a "naked" P wave (Figure 20.23). Although the patient has a single AV node echo, slow pathway modification should not be performed because sustained AVNRT is not present. The patient has been arrhythmia-free for the past 2 years.

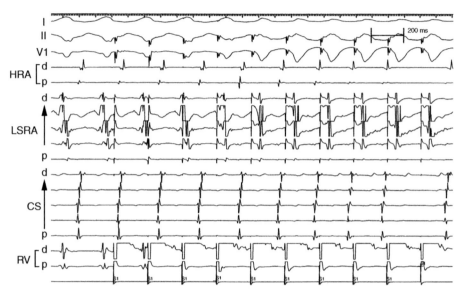

Figure 20.17 Ventricular pacing at a cycle length of 220 ms (the tachycardia cycle length is 240 ms) entrains the atrium, and tachycardia appears to terminate with the development of VA block. Although this finding suggests that perpetuation of tachycardia is dependent on VA conduction, this response could also be observed in ventricular tachycardia.

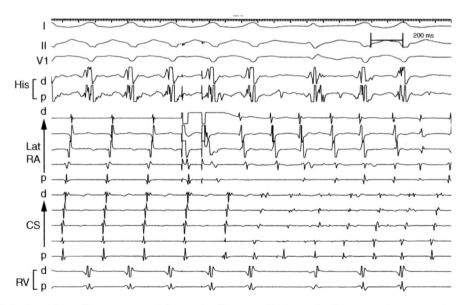

Figure 20.18 During tachycardia, premature atrial extrastimuli at a coupling intervals of 180 ms and 120 ms result in initiation of atrial fibrillation. Notice that the second QRS complex in atrial fibrillation has a right bundle branch block due to anterograde block in the accessory pathway.

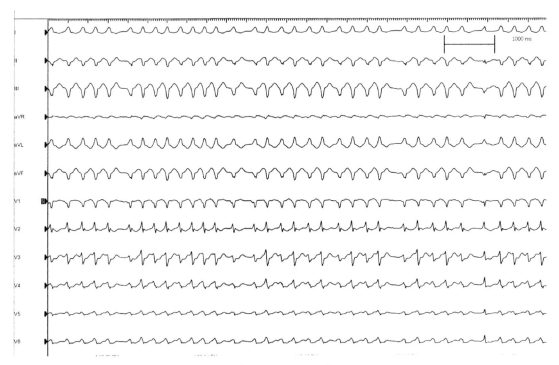

Figure 20.19 Surface ECG of preexcited tachycardia. The shortest R–R interval is 232 ms.

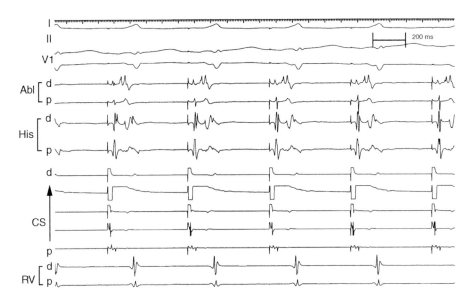

Figure 20.20 During pacing from the distal coronary sinus at a cycle length of 500 ms, a site with an early ventricular electrogram relative to the QRS complex is identified.

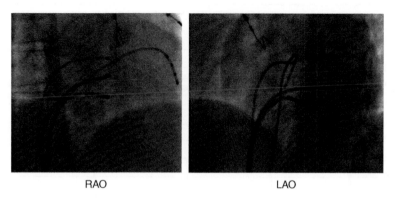

RAO   LAO

Figure 20.21 Fluoroscopy of the ablation catheter and other catheters shown in Figure 20.18.

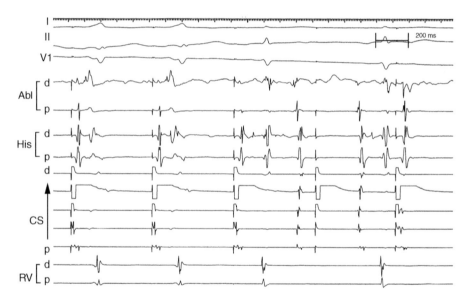

Figure 20.22 During application of radio-frequency energy, preexcitation disappears and a His bundle electrogram emerges, suggesting successful ablation of the accessory pathway.

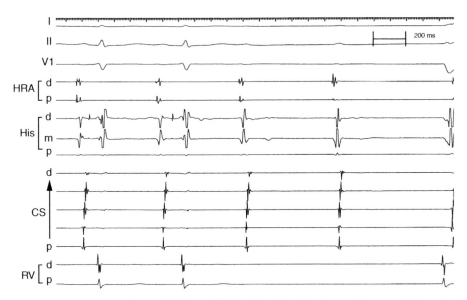

Figure 20.23 After ablation, intravenous adenosine leads to AV block and confirms the absence of anterogradely conducting accessory pathway.

KEY POINTS

- Electrophysiologic testing is an important diagnostic tool for the evaluation of a wide complex tachycardia with an unknown mechanism.
- Although ventricular tachycardia is the most common cause of wide complex tachycardia in a patient with structural heart disease, diverse causes for wide complex tachycardia can be identified in patients without structural heart disease.
- When wide complex tachycardia with a 1:1 AV relationship is induced without a visible His electrogram, atrial pacing – either with scanning premature atrial stimuli or with atrial overdrive pacing – is generally the best electrophysiologic maneuver for evaluating the etiology of the tachycardia.

CHAPTER 21

Wide complex tachycardia case 2

A healthy 23-year-old man was working in the yard, and he noted that with exertion he began having episodes of rapid heart rate punctuated by short periods of a normal heart rate. The rapid heart rate episodes were associated with dizziness and light-headedness but no true syncope. He called emergency services and was found to have frequent ventricular ectopy and was admitted to the hospital. Otherwise, he has no prior medical history and is not on any medications. His physical examination is normal. Initial ECGs from the paramedics and his baseline ECG on arrival to the hospital are shown in Figures 21.1 and 21.2.

The ECGs from the paramedics show salvos of ventricular tachycardia. His baseline ECG shows early repolarization and anterior T wave inversion with no evidence of preexcitation. At this point, it is important to evaluate the patient for structural heart disease. Particularly, in the presence of anterior T wave inversion, arrhythmogenic right ventricular cardiomyopathy must be an important consideration in this young man with wide complex tachycardia. An initial echocardiogram is performed and reveals no significant abnormalities. Although echocardiography provides an important first look for the identification of structural heart disease, advanced imaging techniques to evaluate coronary anatomy and better identify any myocardial abnormalities may sometimes be required. In this case, a cardiac magnetic resonance imaging study is performed and reveals normal left and right ventricular anatomy without scarring and normal coronary artery anatomy. Treadmill testing is also normal.

Given the wide complex tachycardia of uncertain etiology, as in the previous case, electrophysiologic testing to better delineate the mechanism of the wide complex tachycardia is a reasonable next step. It is important to make a decision on whether the cardiac function is normal or abnormal and, in many cases, whether or not coronary ischemia is present before performing an electrophysiology study. Although an electrophysiology study is often the most definitive test for evaluating the patient with wide complex tachycardia, knowing what underlying abnormalities are present is important for planning the specific strategy during the electrophysiologic study.

During electrophysiologic testing, initially, catheters are placed in the His bundle region, the coronary sinus, and the right ventricular outflow tract. Atrial pacing induces a wide complex tachycardia (Figure 21.3). The 12-lead ECG of the wide complex tachycardia is shown in Figure 21.4. During wide complex tachycardia, AV dissociation is an excellent indicator that ventricular tachycardia is present. There are a few very rare types of tachycardia that can be associated with AV dissociation. For example, a tachycardia with antero-grade activation of the ventricles via a nodoventricular accessory pathway and retrograde activation via the His Purkinje system and retrograde block from the AV nodal region to the atria would be associated with AV dissociation. The finding that definitively defines ventricular tachycardia is the presence of dissociation of His bundle activity from ventricular activity (Figure 21.5). However, unless there is a clinical suspicion otherwise, the presence of AV dissociation is usually sufficient to confirm the presence of ventricular tachycardia. Spontaneous termination of the tachycardia is shown in Figure 21.6. Notice that during the tachycardia, the patient developed 2:1 retrograde VA conduction. This is an interesting electrophysiologic finding that is of no clinical consequence in this patient.

In this case, the patient likely has abnormal automaticity as the cause for his arrhythmia rather than reentry because there is no underlying heart disease (myocardial infarction, cardiomyopathy, etc.) that

Understanding Intracardiac EGMs: A Patient Centered Guide, First Edition. Fred Kusumoto.
© 2015 John Wiley & Sons, Ltd. Published 2015 by John Wiley & Sons, Ltd.

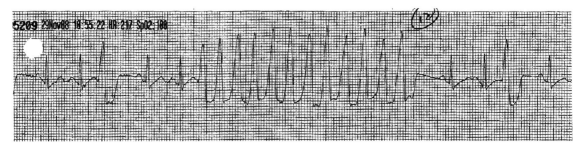

Figure 21.1 ECG from the paramedics showing salvo of rapid wide complex tachycardia.

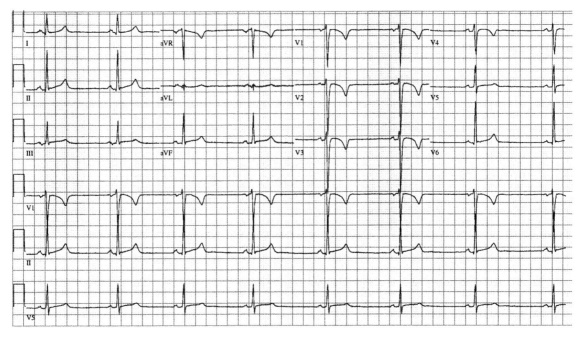

Figure 21.2 ECG shows anterior T wave inversion.

would lead to scar formation and allow reentry. There are two ways to ablate an automatic focus. One option is to identify the site of the earliest ventricular electrogram during ventricular tachycardia. The second method is to "pacemap," identifying a site where pacing results in a QRS complex that is similar to that in tachycardia.

For pacemapping, the catheter is moved carefully in the area of interest and a site with a pacing morphology that matches the QRS morphology in tachycardia is identified. Pacemapping is more successful when smaller tipped catheters are used because the area paced is smaller and the pacing threshold is lower. Conversely, this can sometimes be problematic because a larger

tipped catheter may facilitate successful ablation by producing a larger lesion. Unipolar pacing is generally better than bipolar pacing because anodal capture can change the QRS morphology particularly with high pacing outputs. When pacemapping, it is important that pacing produces a QRS complex that *exactly* matches the QRS of interest including every deflection and notch. Pacemapping has important limitations including capture of the contralateral chamber when evaluating the septal sites.

For electrogram mapping in the patient with normal cardiac structure, the patient must be with a wide complex tachycardia (or at a minimum, premature

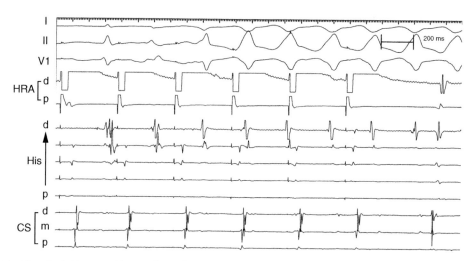

Figure 21.3 Atrial pacing initiates a wide complex tachycardia with obvious AV dissociation.

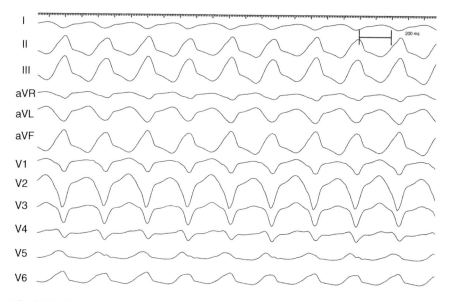

Figure 21.4 A 12-lead ECG of the sustained ventricular tachycardia shows a left bundle branch block and inferior axis morphology.

ventricular contractions with the same morphology as that of sustained tachycardia), and the catheter is manipulated to identify the earliest ventricular electrogram. If possible, electrogram mapping is preferred because it is generally able to localize the site of origin to a smaller area. However, electrogram mapping requires the presence of continued tachycardia, whereas pacemapping can be performed in the absence of tachycardia. The two techniques are not mutually exclusive,

and often, successful ablation requires the use of both techniques.

As the patient is now in sinus rhythm, pacemapping is performed in the right ventricular outflow tract (Figures 21.7 and 21.8). As shown in Figure 21.7 the QRS morphologies in the limb leads are similar during pacing and ventricular tachycardia; while the precordial QRS complexes are similar, differences remain (compare lead V5 in both). A good pacemap that will be associated

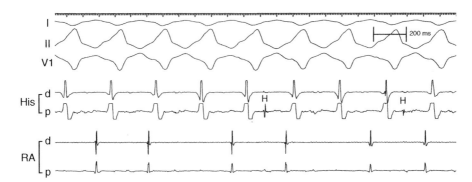

Figure 21.5 During tachycardia, AV dissociation and dissociation of ventricular activity from His bundle activity (H) are present.

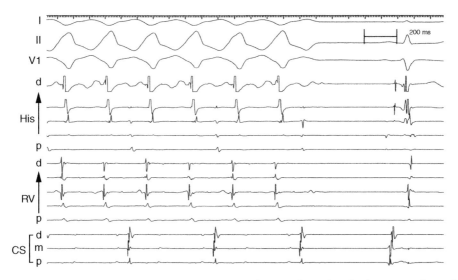

Figure 21.6 Spontaneous termination of wide complex tachycardia. In this case, the His bundle electrogram observed in the distal electrodes of the His catheter is likely obscured within the ventricular electrograms. Notice that the patient has developed retrograde 2:1 VA conduction, probably due to reduced refractoriness in the His Purkinje system.

with a successful ablation often requires an exact match. In idiopathic ventricular tachycardia where ventricular tissue is often relatively normal, pacing is generally effective for capturing the ventricle; however, as shown in Figure 21.8, intermittent capture can be observed. In this case, when the ventricle is captured, a completely different QRS complex is produced in lead I during pacing when compared to tachycardia.

It is often easier to map in the presence of sustained tachycardia because electrogram mapping can be performed. Of course, this requires hemodynamic stability during tachycardia. In order to produce sustained tachycardia, isoproterenol infusion is begun

and sustained tachycardia with stable blood pressure is induced. For electrogram mapping in ventricular tachycardia, the catheter is moved to different sites in the right ventricular outflow tract looking for the earliest electrogram relative to the onset of the QRS complex. Electrogram mapping is shown in Figures 21.9–21.11. As shown in Figure 21.11, it is often extremely helpful to increase the gains in the surface ECGs such that the earliest deflection of the QRS complex can be identified. Unipolar mapping is another technique that can be extremely helpful for identifying an automatic focus. Generally, mapping is performed using a bipolar electrode configuration that measures the electrical

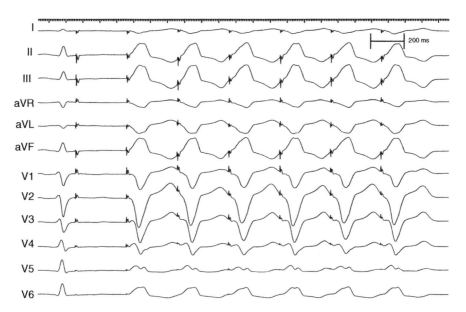

Figure 21.7 Pacemapping from the right ventricular outflow tract. The QRS morphology during pacing is compared to the QRS morphology in tachycardia (Figure 21.4). The better the match, the closer the mapping catheter is to the site of the tachycardia.

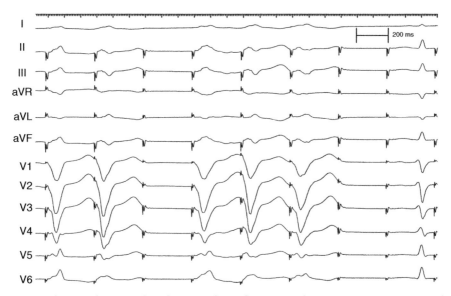

Figure 21.8 Pacemapping from another site in the right ventricular outflow tract. In this case, intermittent capture is observed, which can be a problem with pacemapping. Regardless, the QRS morphology when the ventricle is captured is different than the QRS morphology during tachycardia.

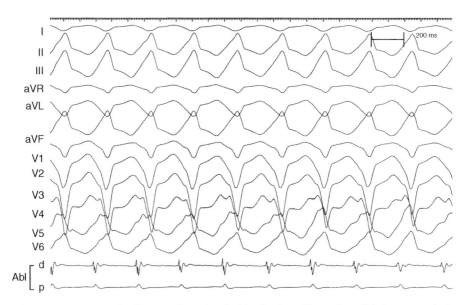

Figure 21.9 An alternative to pacemapping is to map the regions looking for the earliest endocardial electrogram during tachycardia. This approach is generally more effective as compared to pacemapping but requires a stable tachycardia that is also hemodynamically stable.

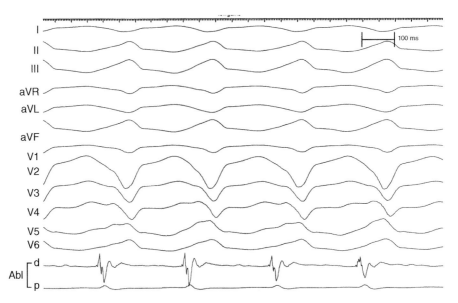

Figure 21.10 When electrogram mapping, it is often useful to increase the sweep speed to better measure the potentially small differences in the interval between electrogram and the onset of the QRS complex.

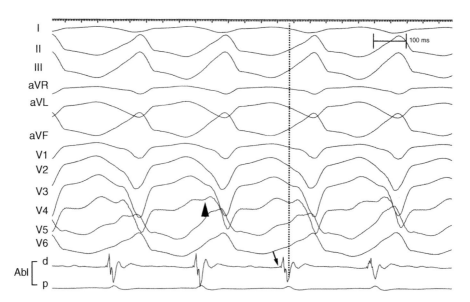

Figure 21.11 One of the problems when mapping at faster sweep speeds is that the onset of the QRS complex can be difficult to identify. Just as in our discussion of atrial tachycardia, it is very helpful to increase the gains to consistently identify the earliest QRS deflection (arrowhead and dashed line) and measure the interval between electrogram onset (small arrow) and the QRS.

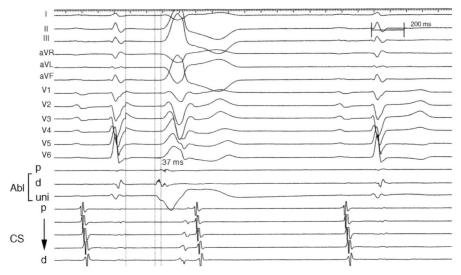

Figure 21.12 Bipolar and unipolar electrograms from a patient with frequent premature ventricular contractions and nonsustained ventricular tachycardia arising from the right ventricular outflow tract. The bipolar electrogram is 37 ms before the onset of the QRS complex. The unipolar electrogram has an initial negative downstroke providing additional supporting evidence that the distal electrode is directly over the focus. (Courtesy K.L. Venkatachalam).

fields underneath the distal and penultimate electrodes. In unipolar mapping, the electrogram is measured from the distal tip to a distant electrode that is usually located in the inferior vena cava. Unipolar is a misnomer because measurement of electrical activity requires both a cathode and an anode. In unipolar recording, only the cathode is located in the heart and the recorded electrogram measures the activity from a smaller area (the anode can be Wilson's central terminal or an electrode located in the inferior vena cava). Figure 21.12 shows the bipolar electrogram and unipolar electrograms from another patient with premature ventricular contractions from a right ventricular outflow tract site.

The bipolar electrogram is 37 ms before the onset of the QRS complex, and the unipolar recording has a characteristic QS complex that is completely negative with a relatively sharp downstroke. When recording unipolar electrograms, it is important to open the recording window by decreasing the high-pass filter such that low-frequency components of the electrogram can be measured.

Returning to our patient, a site is found as shown in Figure 21.13 by fluoroscopy. Application of radio-frequency energy leads to termination of the tachycardia (Figure 21.14). The patient was noninducible after the ablation, despite aggressive atrial

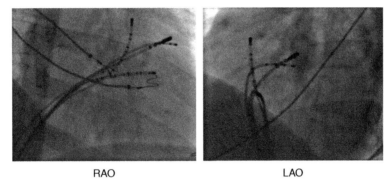

RAO   LAO

Figure 21.13 Fluoroscopic view of the ablation catheter recording the earliest endocardial electrogram in the right anterior oblique (RAO) and left anterior oblique (LAO) imaging planes.

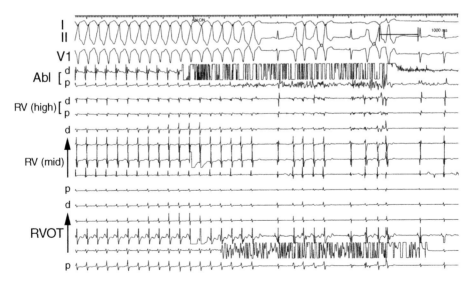

Figure 21.14 Radio-frequency energy application at the site of earliest ventricular signal results in prompt termination of the ventricular tachycardia in several seconds followed by a short salvo of nonsustained ventricular tachycardia.

pacing protocols and high doses of isoproterenol. He has been arrhythmia-free since his ablation. Repeat cardiac imaging has not demonstrated the development of any structural heart disease.

KEY POINTS

- The presence of AV dissociation or fewer atrial electrograms as compared to ventricular electrograms is sufficient to make the diagnosis of ventricular tachycardia.
- The most common location for idiopathic ventricular tachycardias is from the right ventricular outflow tract and must be differentiated from arrhythmogenic right ventricular cardiomyopathy and Brugada syndrome.
- Mapping can be performed by pacemapping (matching the paced QRS complex and the tachycardia QRS complex) or by identifying the earliest electrogram relative to the onset of the QRS complex during tachycardia.

CHAPTER 22

Wide complex tachycardia case 3: premature ventricular contractions

A 75-year-old man has had a 2-year history of exertional shortness of breath. An echocardiogram demonstrated global hypokinesis with an estimated left ventricular ejection fraction (LVEF) of 0.30. He underwent cardiac catheterization and did not have any significant coronary artery disease. He was started on carvedilol and lisinopril and continues to complain of shortness of breath and fatigue. His LVEF has improved to 0.35, and his ECG is shown in Figure 22.1. A 24h ambulatory ECG monitor shows 49,870 premature ventricular beats during a 24h period. He is referred for evaluation.

Frequent premature ventricular contractions can lead to symptoms of palpitations, fatigue, and shortness of breath, and, in some cases, development of cardiomyopathy. Generally, a threshold of 15,000–25,000 per 24h is required for the development of cardiomyopathy; however, given the normal variability in a 24h sample, it is not surprising that cardiomyopathy has also been reported in patients with a smaller PVC burden (e.g., 10,000/24h). There are also some data that the more left ventricular dyssynchrony associated with a premature ventricular contraction, the more likely that an associated cardiomyopathy will be observed. Retrospective single-center studies have suggested that PVCs from the right ventricle (functional left bundle branch block) can be associated with reduced LVEF with a lower PVC burden (≥10%) when compared to PVCs from the left ventricle (≥20%). The decision on whether an invasive approach is used depends on the magnitude of symptoms and LVEF. In patients with symptoms and no structural heart disease, a trial of medical therapy can sometimes be useful to determine the symptoms associated with the PVCs. Class IC drugs, such as propafenone and flecainide, are often reasonable choices for this approach.

The morphology of the premature ventricular contractions can give some guidance of the most likely source of the premature ventricular contractions. Premature ventricular contractions from the right ventricle have a left bundle branch block morphology. As the aortic valve and left ventricular outflow tract are behind, lower, and course rightward as compared to the anterior, leftward-directed right ventricular outflow tract, premature ventricular contractions from the left ventricular outflow tract can also have a left bundle branch block pattern but exhibit an earlier transition (Figure 22.2).

It is often useful to first evaluate the QRS axis in the frontal plane, because the right and left ventricular outflow tracts are such common sites for PVC foci. PVCs from the outflow tract will have an inferior axis and be positive in the inferior leads II, III, and aVF. In this setting, a right bundle branch block morphology is generally from the more lateral aspects of the aortic root (left coronary cusp) or the mitral annulus. As mentioned earlier, the left bundle branch block morphology can be observed in lead V1 from both left ventricular outflow and right ventricular outflow sites. In this case, the precordial transition helps, with a later transition (V3, V4) more consistent with the right ventricular outflow tract and an earlier transition (V2) more consistent with a left ventricular outflow tract site. As the area near the confluence of the mitral and aortic valves (called the aortomitral continuity) is the most posterior structure of the left ventricular outflow tract, PVCs from this region are often characterized by a prominent R wave in V1 (Figure 22.3).

Although there are many ECG criteria that have been developed to localize specific locations of PVCs within the outflow tracts, there are several anatomic issues that make identification of the site without

Understanding Intracardiac EGMs: A Patient Centered Guide, First Edition. Fred Kusumoto.
© 2015 John Wiley & Sons, Ltd. Published 2015 by John Wiley & Sons, Ltd.

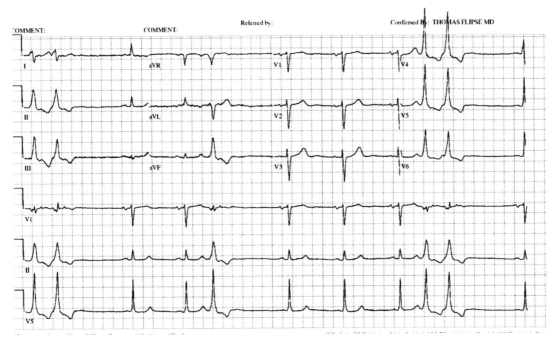

Figure 22.1 Baseline ECG showing frequent PVCs.

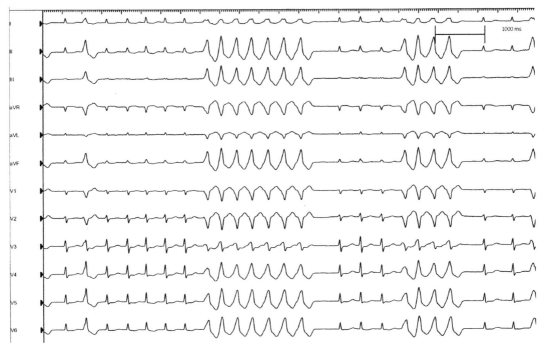

Figure 22.2 Patient with salvos of nonsustained ventricular tachycardia that was found to be arising from the right coronary cusp of the aortic valve. ECG findings consistent with this location include precordial transition at lead V3 and an R wave in lead I. Compare this ECG to Figure 22.4. In that case, as the ventricular tachycardia arose from a right ventricular outflow tract site, the transition occurs in V4 and lead I has a QS complex (because the septal portion of the right ventricular outflow tract is anterior and directed leftward.

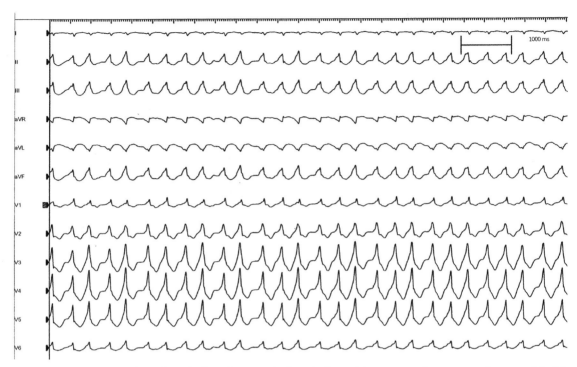

Figure 22.3 Sustained ventricular tachycardia from the aortomitral continuity. As it is more posterior as compared to most of the left ventricular outflow tract sites, an early transition (positive R wave in lead V1) is observed.

endocardial mapping difficult. First, the outflow tracts are adjacent to each other, and the septal portions of the outflow tracts are very close to each other. Second, the two outflow tracts not only are located directly anterior and posterior to one another but also "criss-cross" with the pulmonic trunk directed from right to left and the aortic trunk from left to right. Third, superior sites anatomically located above the aortic and pulmonic valves may have different exit sites that initiate ventricular depolarization. Couple these issues with individual anatomic variability, and it is easy to see why it is difficult to identify specific ECG findings (Figure 22.4). However, there are some findings that can guide initial "guesses" (Table 22.1) that will then need to be confirmed during the electrophysiology study. Sites that are more superior tend to have more positive QRS complexes. Sites near the His Purkinje tissue often have narrower QRS complexes because the ventricles are depolarized in part by the His Purkinje

system. Conversely, epicardial sites often have relatively wide QRS complexes with a slurred upstroke and a "pseudo delta wave."

The ablation strategy for premature ventricular contractions arising from the left ventricle will be dependent on the likely site of origin. For sites arising from the aortic cusp, a retrograde approach through the femoral artery is preferred. For sites "below" the aortic valve, either retrograde or transseptal approaches can be successful, and the choice often depends on personal preference. The shortcomings of a retrograde approach include catheter stability in the outflow tract and possible injury to the coronary arteries or aortic valve. For a transseptal approach, the longer sheath may provide additional support but it may be more difficult to get to certain sites. In addition to endovascular approaches, a pericardial approach can access the epicardial sites and, sometimes, ablation within the coronary sinus is successful.

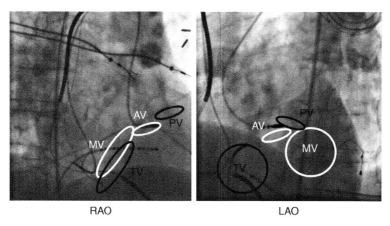

RAO   LAO

Figure 22.4 Fluoroscopic anatomy showing the complex relationship of the right-sided (black) and left-sided (white) valvular annuli in the right anterior oblique (RAO) and left anterior oblique (LAO) projections. TV, Tricuspid valve; PV, Pulmonic valve; MV, Mitral valve; AV, Aortic valve.

Table 22.1 ECG "pearls" for localization of PVCs/VT in the outflow tracts.

Anatomic characteristics	ECG
RVOT is more anterior as compared to the LVOT, and AMC is most posterior	Transition V3 or later for RVOT, V2/V3 transition for the right coronary cusp, V1/V2 transition for the left coronary cusp, and V1 or earlier transition for the AMC
In the LVOT: left coronary cusp most lateral, right coronary cusp most medial, AMC intermediate and lower than the left coronary cusp	In lead I: left coronary cusp: QS or rS right coronary cusp: larger R wave AMC: Rs or rs
Epicardial sites as compared to endocardial sites	Slower upstroke and initial notching (pseudo delta wave)
Septal versus free-wall sites	Narrower QRS complexes due to partial activation of the His Purkinje system

Once a basic approach to ablation has been selected, as in the previous chapter, ablation can be performed either by pacemapping or by identifying the earliest electrogram. Generally, in patients with frequent PVCs, an electrogram mapping strategy is the easiest and most fruitful. Returning to our patient, the premature ventricular contraction has a left bundle branch block pattern in lead V1, and unfortunately, the exact transition cannot be determined because of the absence of a

PVC in leads V2 or V3. Notice that the QRS complex in V1 has an unusual configuration with a qrS morphology (for the first PVC in a couplet). This morphology is often associated with PVCs from the junction of the right and left coronary cusp, in part because this region is the most anterior aspect of the aortic valve. As there is a high likelihood that the site will be above the aortic valve, a retrograde aortic approach is chosen and the aortic cusps are explored to identify a site with an

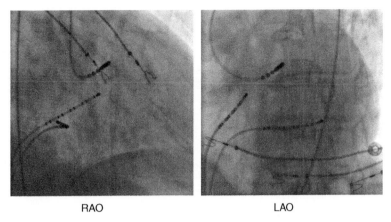

RAO   LAO

Figure 22.5 Ablation catheter is located at the junction between the left and the right coronary cusp. This location is "just behind" the right ventricular outflow tract.

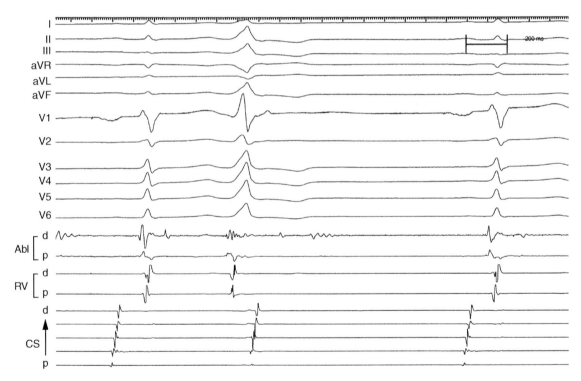

Figure 22.6 Electrograms from the fluoroscopic location in Figure 22.4 showing an early fractionated ventricular electrogram associated with the premature ventricular contraction.

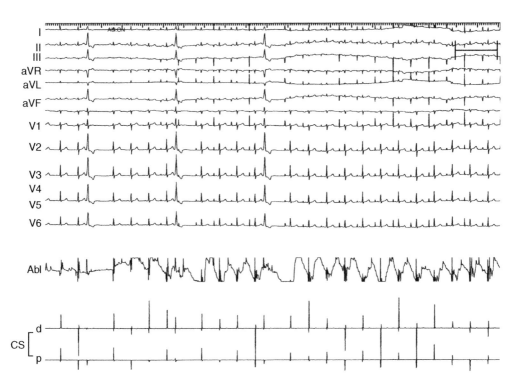

Figure 22.7 Ablation at this site leads to elimination of premature ventricular contractions.

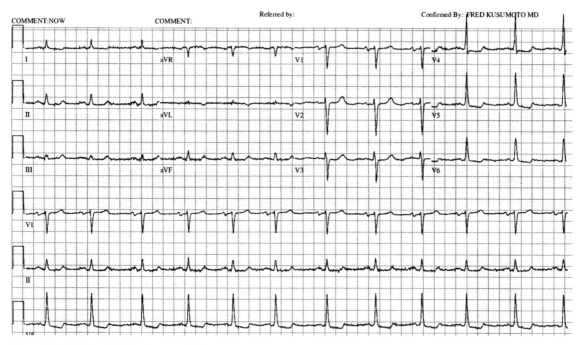

Figure 22.8 ECG after ablation shows no PVCs.

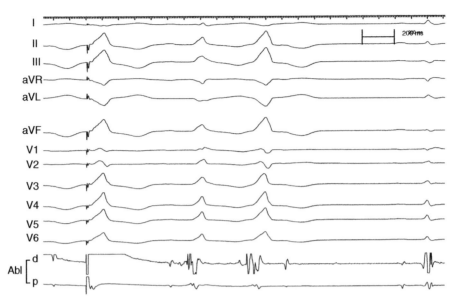

Figure 22.9 In another patient with frequent premature ventricular contractions, the earliest electrograms associated with the premature ventricular contraction were located at the junction of the coronary sinus and the great cardiac vein. Pacing from this site (first QRS complex) is an exact match to the clinical PVC (third QRS complex). The second QRS complex is a fusion beat from sinus rhythm and a PVC.

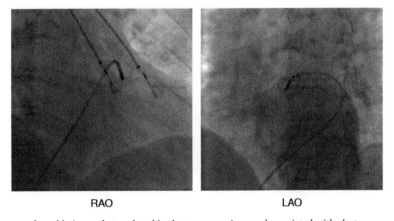

RAO   LAO

Figure 22.10 Fluoroscopy of an ablation catheter placed in the coronary sinus and associated with electrograms from Figure 22.8.

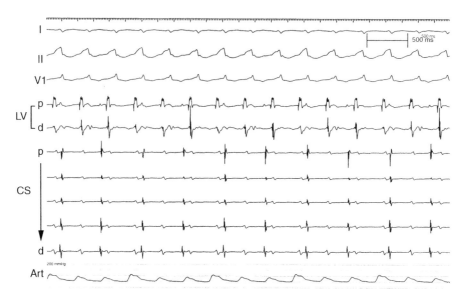

Figure 22.11 Electrograms from the patient shown in Figure 22.3 with the earliest ventricular electrograms located at the aortomitral continuity. Notice the small atrial electrogram on the ablation catheter.

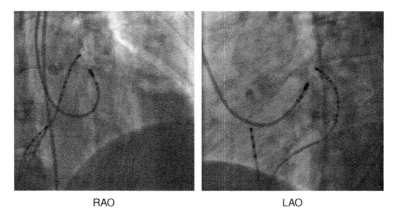

RAO   LAO

Figure 22.12 Fluoroscopic location of the aortomitral continuity. Application of radio-frequency energy led to termination of ventricular tachycardia in 3 s.

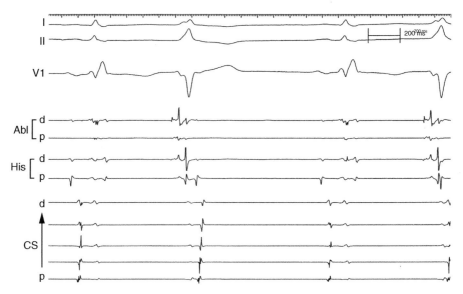

Figure 22.13 A patient with frequent premature ventricular contractions arising from just above the His bundle region. Notice that the QRS width of the premature ventricular contraction is relatively narrow, consistent with a septal site. A discrete high frequency signal can be observed before the QRS complex of the PVC (2nd and 4th QRS complexes).

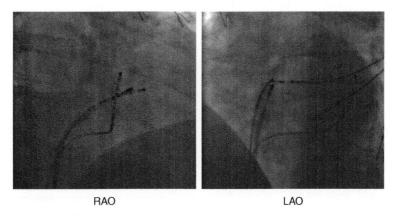

Figure 22.14 Fluoroscopy of catheter positions from the electrogram recordings shown in Figure 22.13. The ablation catheter is located just superior and distal to the His bundle.

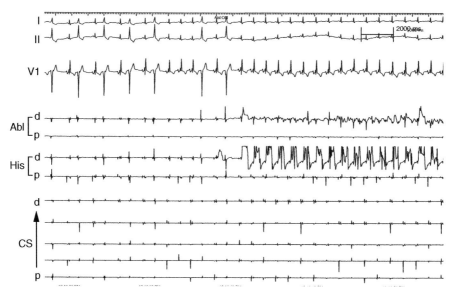

Figure 22.15 Continuation of Figures 22.12 and 22.13. Judicious application of radio-frequency energy leads to prompt elimination of premature ventricular contractions.

early ventricular electrogram. A site near the junction of the left and right coronary cusps (Figures 22.5) is found with an early ventricular electrogram relative to the QRS complex (Figure 22.6). Application of radio-frequency energy here leads to elimination of the premature ventricular contractions (Figure 22.7).

The patient's ECG 1 month later demonstrates no PVCs (Figure 22.8), which is confirmed on 24 h ambulatory ECG monitoring. Echocardiography shows LVEF improvement to 0.50–0.55. Single-center studies have suggested that among the selected patients, 80–100% of patients with frequent PVCs and reduced LVEF will have improvement and often normalization of their left ventricular function after successful ablation.

Figures 22.9 and 22.10 show the electrograms and fluoroscopy of another patient in whom the earliest electrogram was identified at the junction of the coronary sinus and the great cardiac vein. Figures 22.11 and 22.12 show the intracardiac electrograms and fluoroscopic position of an ablation catheter placed at the aortomitral continuity in the patient with the ECG from Figure 22.3. To complete our discussion of premature ventricular contractions, Figures 22.13 and 22.14 show another patient with frequent premature

ventricular contractions that arose from just above the His bundle in the right ventricular outflow tract. Obviously, careful application of radio-frequency energy (often with pulses at low powers) using small-tipped catheters to avoid collateral damage is essential in this region. With radio-frequency energy application, the premature ventricular contractions were eliminated quickly and there was no worsening of AV conduction (Figure 22.15).

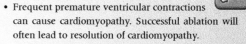

KEY POINTS

- Frequent premature ventricular contractions can cause cardiomyopathy. Successful ablation will often lead to resolution of cardiomyopathy.

- Although the right ventricular outflow tract is the most common site for premature ventricular contractions, they can also arise from the left ventricular outflow tract.

- Although pacemapping can be performed, generally, endocardial mapping is more efficient but requires the presence of frequent PVCs (or ventricular tachycardia).

CHAPTER 23

Wide complex tachycardia case 4

A 66-year-old man has a history of ventricular tachycardia and underwent ICD placement 3 years ago at another institution after an episode of syncope. He is now referred for evaluation because of recurrent symptomatic episodes of ventricular tachycardia that has required frequent treatment by the ICD. He has no history of heart disease. A recent echocardiogram demonstrates normal left ventricular function. His ECG is shown in Figure 23.1, and a nonsustained episode of tachycardia recorded by the ICD is shown in Figure 23.2.

The implantable cardioverter-defibrillator (ICD) is an important treatment option for reducing the likelihood of sudden cardiac death due to ventricular arrhythmia. In the large trials completed a decade ago, implantation of an ICD improved survival in patients with reduced left ventricular ejection fraction (LVEF) (<0.30) due to myocardial infarction and in patients with Class II or III heart failure symptoms and an LVEF less than or equal to 0.35 (MADIT-II and SCD-HeFT trials, respectively). In addition, ICD implantation is an option for selected patients with other forms of structural heart disease (e.g., hypertrophic cardiomyopathy) or genetic conditions that increase the risk of sudden cardiac death (e.g., Brugada syndrome and long QT syndrome). The use of an ICD in this type of patient with no structural heart disease or other identifiable high-risk conditions is less clear but may have been implanted for secondary prevention in the setting of ventricular tachycardia.

It is reasonable to consider electrophysiology study at this point, given the frequent symptomatic episodes of ventricular tachycardia requiring treatment by the ICD (Tables A12 and A13). Baseline electrograms are shown in Figure 23.3. The HV interval is at the upper limit of normal (35–55 ms); but otherwise, the baseline electrograms are normal.

Atrial pacing from the distal coronary sinus induces a wide complex tachycardia with a right bundle branch block (RBBB), right superior axis morphology with 1:1 ventriculoatrial relationship (Figure 23.4 and 23.5). The 12-lead ECG is shown in Figure 23.5. Although the right superior axis makes ventricular tachycardia the most likely diagnosis, the absence of His bundle electrogram during atrial pacing prevents definitive electrogram diagnosis of ventricular tachycardia. However, initiation of the tachycardia with two consecutive ventricular signals without an intervening atrial electrogram also makes ventricular tachycardia far more likely. A finding that confirms the presence of ventricular tachycardia is shown in Figure 23.6. A premature ventricular stimulus at a coupling interval of 340 ms preexcites the right and left atria in the same pattern without affecting the tachycardia. This finding provides strong evidence that retrograde activation of the atria (most likely via the His bundle and AV node) does not occur in the tachycardia circuit. Earlier premature ventricular stimuli lead to termination of the tachycardia (Figure 23.7).

At this point, now that ventricular tachycardia has been induced and terminated, it is important to consider the findings and assess the possible diagnoses and therapeutic options. We now have convincing evidence that the clinical arrhythmia is the monomorphic ventricular tachycardia with an RBBB and superior axis morphology in a patient without structural heart disease. The tachycardia was initiated with atrial pacing and likely has a reentrant mechanism, given termination by the ventricular stimuli.

One possible specific diagnosis is verapamil-sensitive fascicular ventricular tachycardia. This unusual ventricular tachycardia is due to reentry in the Purkinje network and left fascicles, is often induced by atrial pacing, and is verapamil sensitive. The most common form

Understanding Intracardiac EGMs: A Patient Centered Guide, First Edition. Fred Kusumoto.
© 2015 John Wiley & Sons, Ltd. Published 2015 by John Wiley & Sons, Ltd.

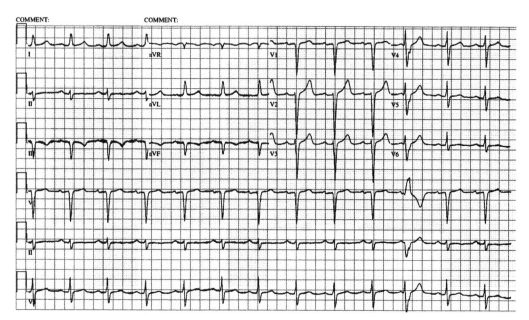

Figure 23.1 Baseline ECG shows a leftward axis and a single PVC; but otherwise, it is normal.

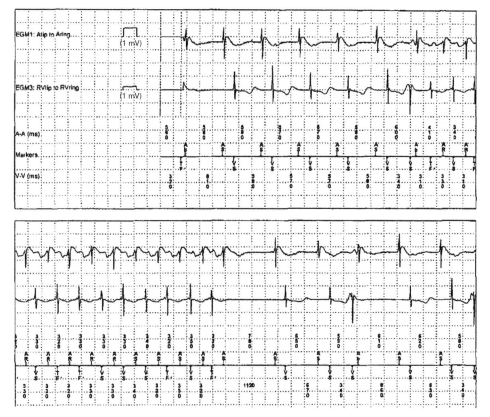

Figure 23.2 Interrogation of his ICD demonstrates frequent episodes of tachycardia that are initiated with a premature ventricular contraction and development of tachycardia with spontaneous termination with an atrial electrogram (ruling out atrial tachycardia).

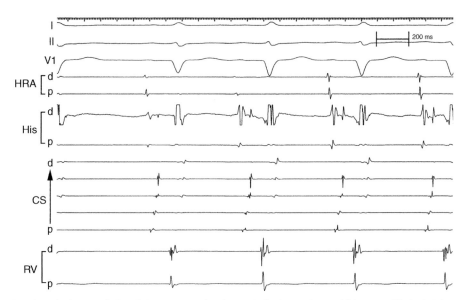

Figure 23.3 At baseline, the basic cycle length is 1090 ms and atrioventricular intervals are within normal limits (AH interval is 106 ms and the HV interval is 52 ms).

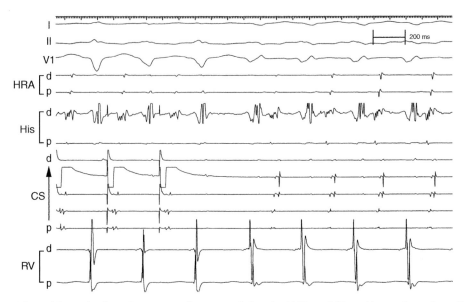

Figure 23.4 Atrial overdrive pacing from the coronary sinus at a cycle length of 320 ms yields a wide complex tachycardia of 320 ms, a QRS width of 170 ms, and a VA interval of 190 ms. On a negative note, a His bundle electrogram is not recorded during pacing.

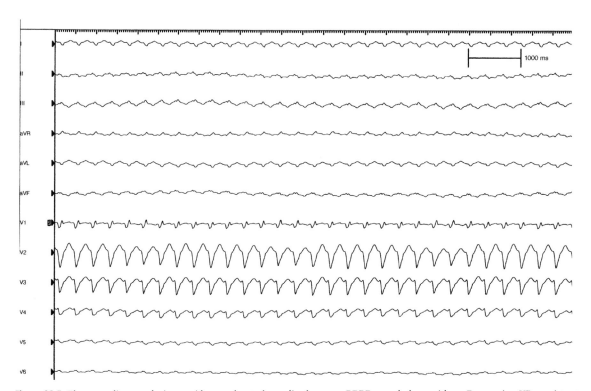

Figure 23.5 Electrocardiogram during a wide complex tachycardia shows an RBBB morphology with an R wave in aVR consistent with a right superior axis. This ECG pattern is most consistent with ventricular tachycardia.

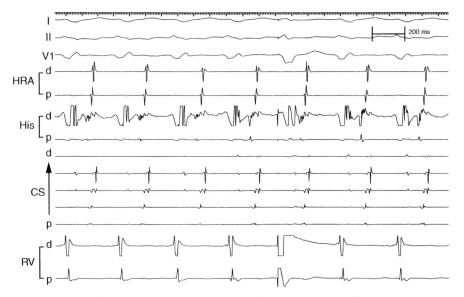

Figure 23.6 A premature ventricular contraction delivered slightly earlier than the tachycardia (343 ms) preexcites the right and left atria early and in the same pattern as tachycardia without affecting the tachycardia. This finding provides strong evidence that retrograde activation of the atria (likely due to the His bundle and AV node) does not occur in the tachycardia circuit.

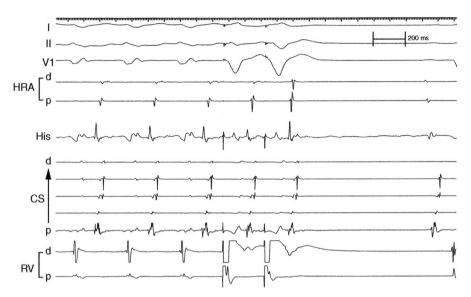

Figure 23.7 Earlier premature ventricular stimuli delivered at coupling intervals of 310 ms and 260 ms terminate the tachycardia.

has an RBBB and left axis deviation morphology (left posterior fascicle ventricular tachycardia); however, rarer forms can have RBBB and right axis deviation (left anterior fascicle ventricular tachycardia) or normal axis (upper septal fascicular ventricular tachycardia). Collectively, these tachycardias are often called idiopathic left septal ventricular tachycardias. They are due to reentry and appear to have an anterograde limb composed of abnormal Purkinje tissue with decremental properties and verapamil sensitivity and a retrograde limb that uses the normal remaining fascicles.

Mapping and ablation are very effective for eliminating these tachycardias. Careful mapping of the left ventricular septum will often reveal a series of potentials that occur during diastole (Figure 23.8). Diastolic potentials are extremely helpful for identifying

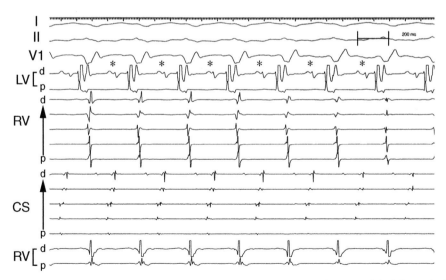

Figure 23.8 During tachycardia, a mid-diastolic potential (*) is recorded from the proximal portion of the left ventricular septum.

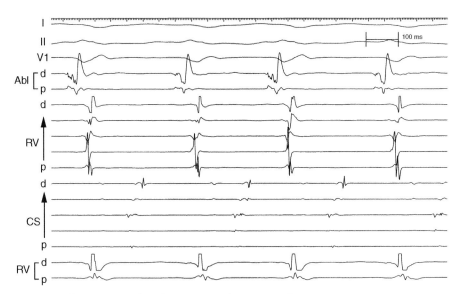

Figure 23.9 Continuation of Figure 23.8. When the mapping catheter is moved more distally along the superior portion of the left ventricular septum, a presystolic electrogram is recorded from the distal electrodes.

the successful sites for ablation. In order to reduce the likelihood of injury in the proximal portion of normal fascicular tissue, generally, more apical regions of the septum are explored, and in this case, very late diastolic potentials can be recorded (Figure 23.9). At a site in the upper portion of the distal septum, application of radiofrequency energy resulted in prompt termination of the ventricular tachycardia (Figure 23.10). During sinus rhythm after successful ablation, often a late potential will be observed due to the production of block.

After the ablation, tachycardia could not be induced despite the atrial and ventricular pacing protocols. The patient has been arrhythmia-free after 1-year follow-up.

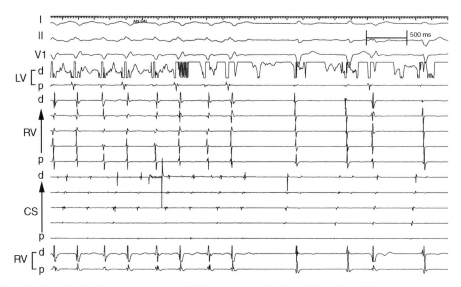

Figure 23.10 Application of radio-frequency energy results in prompt termination of the tachycardia.

The main problem that can arise during ablation of idiopathic left septal ventricular tachycardia is noninducibility due to mechanical trauma during catheter manipulation or incomplete ablation. In this case, some investigators have advocated an anatomic approach by placing a series of lesions vertically along the mid-septum. I believe the strategy will depend on patient preference. The operator must balance ablation effectiveness against the risk of collateral damage of the fascicles that could increase the likelihood of inducing ventricular dyssynchrony due to left bundle branch block or increased likelihood for the requirement of permanent pacing.

KEY POINTS

- In the absence of structural heart disease or "channelopathies" (such as Brugada syndrome or long QT syndrome), idiopathic ventricular tachycardias most commonly arise from the outflow tracts (automaticity) or the septal left ventricle (reentry).

- In left septal ventricular tachycardias, the likely exit site of the anterograde limb of the abnormal Purkinje system can be identified by the QRS axis.

- Successful ablation generally targets a diastolic potential preferably in the more apical regions of the left ventricular septum.

CHAPTER 24

Wide complex tachycardia case 5

A 67-year-old man with a prior inferior wall myocardial infarction has an ICD and a history of ventricular tachycardia has been placed on amiodarone. He comes to the hospital with a 3 h history of feeling poorly. His ECG is shown in Figure 24.1. What is the diagnosis?

Careful examination of his ECG reveals multiple criteria that are very suggestive of ventricular tachycardia. First and foremost, there is a presence of independent atrial and ventricular activity (A-V dissociation). The third, eighth, and fifteenth QRS complexes are "capture" beats that represent ventricular depolarization from a sinus beat rather than from the ventricular tachycardia. Second, the QRS complex in aVR is positive, suggesting a "northwest" axis. It would be very unusual for any form of aberrant conduction of the bundles to lead to a ventricular activation pattern that would proceed from left apex to the septal base (remember that the bundles start in the septum and extend downward). Third, the patient has broad abnormal Q waves in the inferior (II, III, and aVF) and lateral (V5 and V6) leads that represent a large inferolateral myocardial infarction. The last two findings suggest that the ventricular tachycardia is emanating from this region of scar.

Management of ventricular tachycardia in a patient with an ICD can take several forms. Options include reconsidering programming the ICD, changing medications, or ablation (Table A12). Interrogation of the device demonstrates that the ICD has already been providing antitachycardia pacing therapy for faster ventricular tachycardias that have been reasonably effective. However, the relatively slow heart rates of the ventricular tachycardia will make programming the ICD difficult because of overlap with normal heart rates. This situation is clearly worsened or perhaps even solely due to the use of amiodarone, which often leads to slowing of ventricular tachycardia rates. Catheter

ablation is a reasonable option for several reasons: the patient is relatively young and he is having frequent symptomatic arrhythmias.

The development of three-dimensional mapping technologies revolutionized catheter ablation of ventricular tachycardia. Initial attempts at catheter ablation required initiation of ventricular tachycardia (often a hemodynamically unstable arrhythmia) in an extremely ill patient often with poor left ventricular function. Mapping required careful entrainment mapping to identify critical isthmuses within the scar. Three-dimensional mapping allows the development of a comprehensive repeatable catalog of mapped sites that can define the presence and location of scar without requiring induction of arrhythmia. There are several three-dimensional mapping systems that are available that use magnetic or electrical fields to determine the position of a catheter(s) in space.

The three-dimensional map of our patient is shown in Figure 24.2. A large inferolateral scar is identified. At this point, there are several effective options for ablation. One approach is to "link" the scars and other inert regions, for example, creating an ablation line between the scar and the mitral annulus. In patients with a remote inferior wall myocardial infarction and monomorphic ventricular tachycardia, up to one-third will have ventricular tachycardias that use this isthmus. Depending on whether the tachycardia exits laterally or septally, the tachycardia will be characterized by right bundle branch block, right axis deviation or left bundle branch block, left axis deviation morphology, respectively. Approach to this type of ablation is discussed in Chapter 14 of Understanding ECGs and EGMs.

Once the scar is defined with three-dimensional mapping, in some cases, it can be very useful to induce ventricular tachycardia. Although this approach cannot be used in patients with hemodynamically unstable ventricular tachycardia, mapping during ventricular

---

Understanding Intracardiac EGMs: A Patient Centered Guide, First Edition. Fred Kusumoto.
© 2015 John Wiley & Sons, Ltd. Published 2015 by John Wiley & Sons, Ltd.

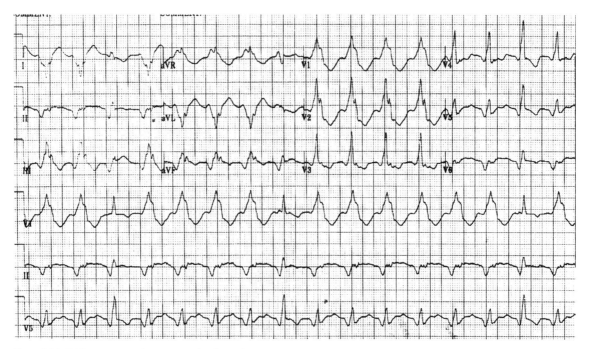

Figure 24.1 ECG on presentation. See text for discussion.

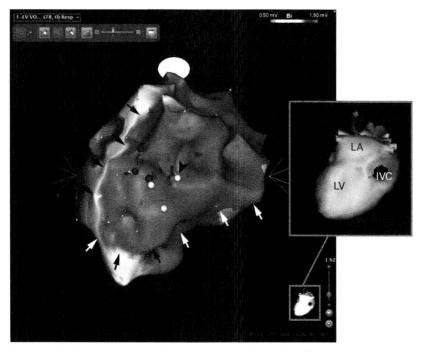

Figure 24.2 Three-dimensional voltage mapping reveals a large inferolateral scar defined by the multiple black and white arrows.

tachycardia is very helpful in the setting of stable, hemodynamically tolerated ventricular tachycardia, as in this case. Ventricular pacing is performed and a slow ventricular tachycardia is induced (Figure 24.3). Comparison of the 12-lead ECG of the induced tachycardia and the clinical tachycardia (Figure 24.1) reveals identical QRS morphologies, suggesting that the tachycardias are likely the same and at the very least use the same "exit" site. Once hemodynamic stability is confirmed, entrainment mapping can be performed. Common problems with entrainment mapping include lack of capture (often there are regions of dense scar that cannot be depolarized despite high outputs), or even if ventricular capture occurs, the tachycardia circuit is not entrained (this phenomenon is more likely if pacing is performed at a rate that is too close to the tachycardia cycle length or if pacing is not performed for a long enough period). As ventricular tachycardia uses viable tissue between the mitral valve and the inferior scar, the ablation catheter is first placed in this region. As shown in Figure 24.4, pacing is performed at a cycle length of 650 ms, 70 ms faster than the tachycardia

cycle length of 720 ms, and unfortunately only the last stimulus captures ventricular tissue and results in a change in the QRS complex. However, the stimulus apparently does not reset the tachycardia as the first QRS complex after cessation of pacing occurs at the expected time, and it is unlikely that the tachycardia circuit was entrained. Although the tachycardia was not entrained, the change in the QRS complex provides evidence that the pacing site is not within the tachycardia circuit. The paced QRS has an earlier precordial transition (multicomponent R wave in lead V1) as compared to the tachycardia, which suggests that the site is too basal (too close to the mitral annulus). As shown in Figure 24.5, the catheter is moved to the septal portion of the scar, and a premature ventricular contraction, likely catheter-induced because of the early fractionated electrogram recorded on the ablation catheter, terminates the tachycardia.

Ventricular pacing is performed again; however, the clinical ventricular tachycardia cannot be reinduced and instead more rapid ventricular tachycardias are induced that require defibrillation (Figures 24.6 and 24.7).

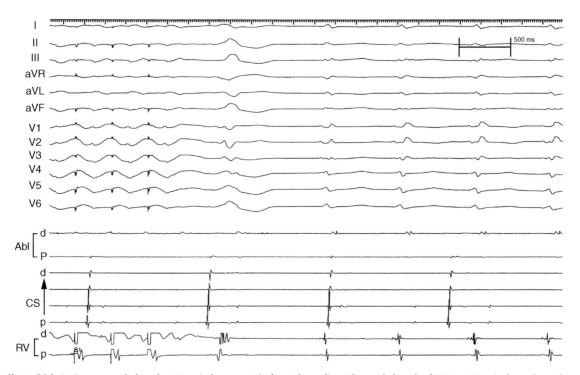

Figure 24.3 Pacing at a cycle length 650 ms induces ventricular tachycardia with a cycle length of 730 ms. Ventricular tachycardia can be confirmed quickly by the presence of AV dissociation.

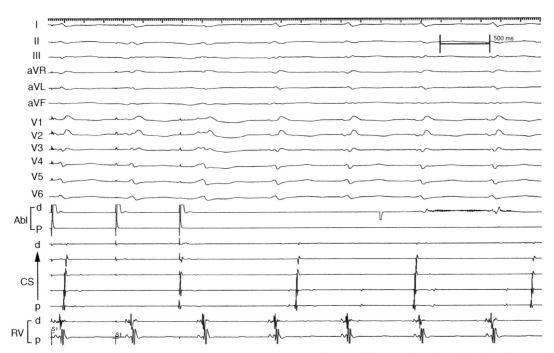

Figure 24.4 Inspection of the 12-lead ECG of the ventricular tachycardia reveals a morphology similar to that of the clinical ventricular tachycardia. For entrainment mapping, pacing from within the scar at a cycle length of 650 ms is performed. The last pacing stimulus captures the ventricle, and although the QRS complexes are similar, there are subtle differences with the paced QRS complex being more positive in leads V1 to V3.

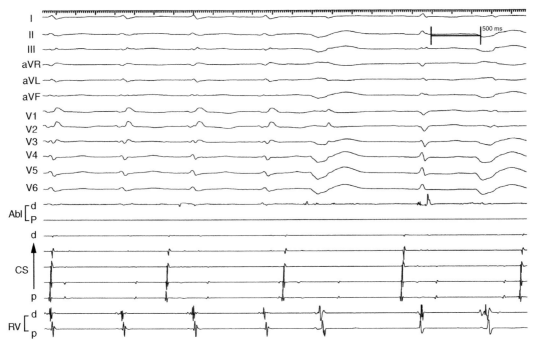

Figure 24.5 The tachycardia terminates with a spontaneous (or catheter-induced-notice the early fractionated electrogram on the distal ablation catheter) premature ventricular contraction.

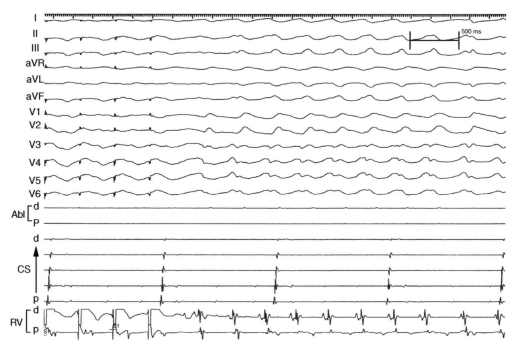

Figure 24.6 Ventricular extrastimulation protocols are performed. With ventricular overdrive pacing at a cycle length of 360 ms, a more rapid ventricular tachyarrhythmia with a cycle length of 330 ms in induced. The 12-lead ECG of the ventricular tachycardia is different from that of the clinical tachycardia.

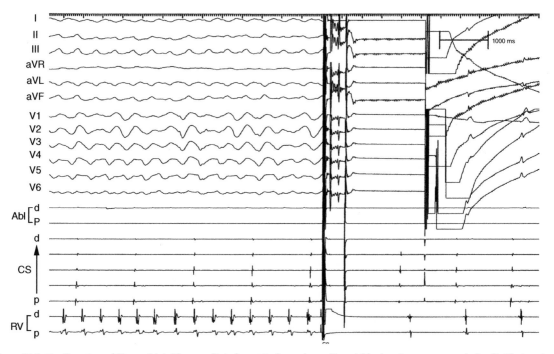

Figure 24.7 Continuation of Figure 24.6. The nonclinical ventricular tachycardia quickly deteriorates to ventricular fibrillation that requires defibrillation.

At this point, the clinician must decide whether or not to continue trying to induce the ventricular tachycardia or map the scar during sinus rhythm. This scenario is not uncommon, with large series suggesting that approximately 80% of ventricular tachycardias will not be hemodyamically tolerated during electrophysiology study and ablation.

As the patient has fragile hemodynamic status, regions within the scar are evaluated. Here, the ability to return to important sites is a critical benefit to three-dimensional mapping systems. The ablation catheter is placed at a site previously identified with very unusual electrogram properties (fluoroscopic images in Figure 24.8, arrowhead in Figure 24.2). This region

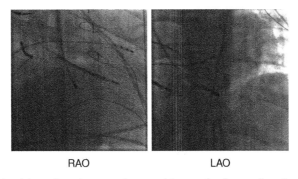

RAO   LAO

Figure 24.8 The scar is mapped and the catheter is returned to a position previously tagged on the three-dimensional map. Corresponding fluoroscopic positions are shown in the right anterior oblique (RAO) and left anterior oblique (LAO) projections.

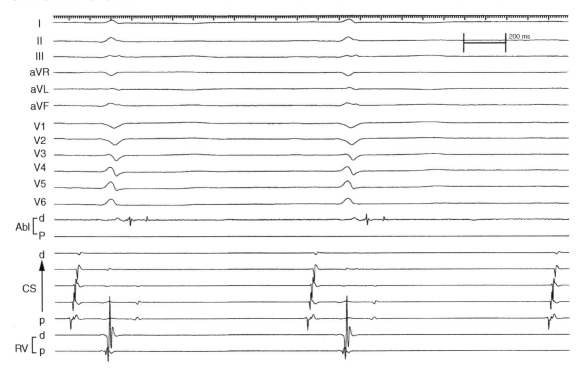

Figure 24.9 The electrograms obtained from the catheter position are shown in Figures 24.2 and 24.8. This site is characterized by very late ventricular depolarization. The multicomponent ventricular electrograms are recorded 150 ms and 240 ms after the QRS complex.

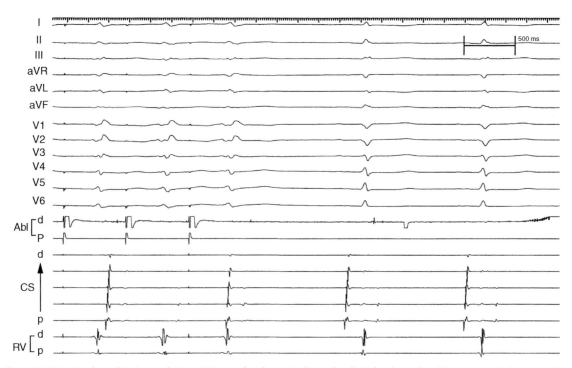

Figure 24.10 Pacing from this site results in a QRS complex that is similar to the clinical tachycardia with an extremely long stimulus to QRS interval (285 ms) suggestive of long conduction interval. Compare with Figures 24.1 and 24.4.

has fractionated multicomponent electrograms that are very delayed relative to the QRS complex (Figure 24.9). These late potentials are collectively called LAVA (local abnormal ventricular activity) and have been found to be possible targets for ablation. Pacing is performed from this site, and notice that ventricular depolarization occurs with an extremely long stimulus to QRS interval that suggests the presence of a protected zone of slow conduction (Figure 24.10). Interestingly, notice that the QRS complex produced by pacing is identical to the QRS complex of the patient's clinical tachycardia. This finding means that the exit sites from pacing and the ventricular tachycardia are the same; however, it does not necessarily mean that the putative site is critically involved in the tachycardia as the site could represent a "dead-end" within the scar. Regardless, this is a reasonable site to ablate and after application of radio-frequency energy, the site cannot be captured despite maximal outputs (10 mA), suggesting that the ablation has been effective (Figure 24.11). After several additional ablations in this region, pacing protocols

do not induce ventricular tachycardia (Figure 24.12) and follow-up device interrogation reveals no sustained ventricular tachycardia requiring ICD therapies (Figure 24.13).

Nonrandomized single-center studies have reported a wide range of acute success rates (40–90%) and long-term success rates (50–90% at 1–2-year follow-up) and high mortality rats (10–25% at 1–2-year follow-up). The sobering data clearly emphasize the complexities associated with catheter ablation in this patient population. New research has focused on procedures that alter the autonomic nervous system, catheters that can make deeper lesions in heavily scarred regions, and more accurate mapping systems that often use advanced imaging coupled with modeling algorithms to identify scars and likely isthmus sites. New strategies for ablation are evolving. Pericardial access for epicardial ablation has now become a relatively common procedure and ablation with percutaneous hemodynamic support for mapping of unstable ventricular tachycardias has been reported.

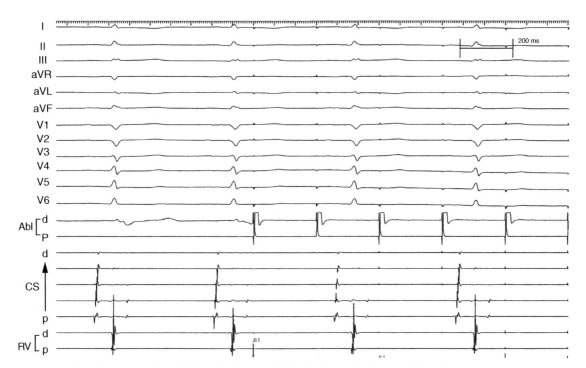

Figure 24.11 After ablation is performed, the region is nonexcitable despite maximal outputs (10 mA).

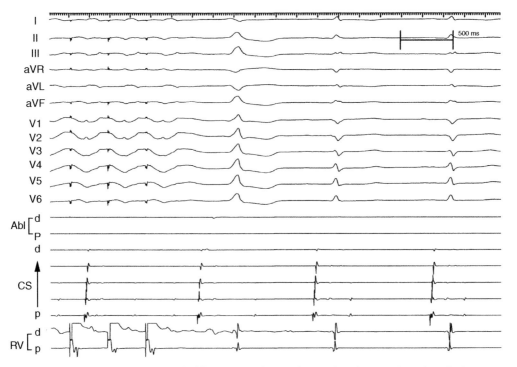

Figure 24.12 After ablation, the patient is noninducible (interestingly, even for nonclinical ventricular tachyarrhythmias).

Ventricular tachy counters	Since last reset 29 Nov 2013	Device totals
Ventricular episode counters		
Total episodes	12	451
Treated		
VF therapy	0	0
VT therapy	0	0
VT-1 therapy	0	102
Commanded therapy	0	21
Nontreated		
No therapy programmed	0	136
Nonsustained episodes	12	162
Other untreated episodes	0	30
Ventricular therapy counters		
ATP delivered	0	124
ATP % successful	0	92
Shocks delivered	0	15
First shock % successful	0	75
Shocks diverted	0	0

Figure 24.13 ICD interrogation 6 months after ablation shows no recurrent ventricular tachycardia.

KEY POINTS

- Catheter ablation is a treatment option for selected patients with ventricular tachycardia due to structural heart disease but can be extremely challenging and is associated with a high recurrence rate.

- Although entrainment mapping can be used to identify ablation targets, substrate mapping is more commonly used because it does not require the presence of tachycardia. Entrainment mapping is more effective in patients with stable hemodynamically tolerated ventricular tachycardias.

- In substrate mapping, scar is identified and regions within the scar (eliminating critical tachycardia isthmuses) or on the scar edges (eliminating exit and entrance sites) are targeted. In addition, ablation can be performed between scars or between scars and other anatomic barriers (such as the valve annuli).

CHAPTER 25

Wide complex tachycardia case 6

A 67-year-old woman is admitted for wide complex tachycardia (Figure 25.1). She undergoes cardioversion in the emergency room. Her past medical history is significant for diabetes mellitus and dilated cardiomyopathy.

As discussed in Chapter 20, wide complex tachycardia is an important reason for considering electrophysiology testing. In patients with dilated cardiomyopathy, a special type of sustained ventricular tachycardia that can be observed is bundle branch reentry. As the name suggests, bundle branch reentry uses the bundles or fascicles of the His Purkinje system as a large portion of the circuit. The most common form of bundle branch reentry is due to retrograde activation via the left bundle and anterograde conduction down the right bundle with transseptal activation of the interventricular septum completing the circuit. As the ventricles are activated via the right bundle, the QRS morphology has a typical left bundle branch block appearance. A single beat of bundle branch reentry is very commonly observed with ventricular stimulation (Figure 3.20 in Understanding Intracardiac EGMs and ECGs). Sustained bundle branch reentry is very uncommon because the fast conduction properties of the bundles lead to the advancing wavefront eventually encountering refractory tissue. However, because of disease in the bundles, patients with dilated cardiomyopathy may develop sustained bundle branch reentry. The actual incidence of bundle branch reentry in patients with dilated cardiomyopathy is somewhat controversial with some estimates as high as 30% while more recent studies suggest 10%. Although multiple forms of bundle branch reentry have been described in the literature, for example, retrograde activation via the right bundle and anterograde activation via the left bundle or perhaps one of the fascicles, these variants are generally quite rare.

Sustained bundle branch reentry is most commonly observed in patients with dilated cardiomyopathy and evidence for His Purkinje disease. The baseline ECG for our patient is shown in Figure 25.2, and it shows sinus rhythm and left bundle branch block. Figure 25.3 shows the baseline electrograms, and it is important to note the prolonged HV interval. Ventricular pacing initiates a wide QRS tachycardia associated with atrioventricular dissociation (Figure 25.4). Bundle branch reentry is suspected immediately because of the His bundle deflection preceding the QRS complex. As shown in Figure 25.5, bundle branch reentry can be confirmed because changes in the His–His interval precede the changes in the R–R intervals. In Figure 25.6, rapid ventricular pacing terminates the tachycardia. In patients in whom bundle branch reentry is suspected but cannot be induced, using a pause protocol can sometimes be effective. In a ventricular pacing pause protocol, the basic drive cycle length for ventricular pacing is relatively fast, for example, 400 ms, the first ventricular extrastimulus is delivered after a delay (600–800 ms), and the second ventricular extrastimulus is delivered at a shorter coupling interval (e.g., 350 ms) and is then brought in progressively earlier. This type of pacing can facilitate the development of reentry within the bundles by causing retrograde block in the right bundle because the refractory period of the bundles is affected most by the immediate preceding cycle length.

Ablation for bundle branch reentry generally involves ablating the right bundle or the left bundle. Figure 25.7 shows ablation of the right bundle with development of right bundle branch block within 4 s of application of radio-frequency energy. As patients usually have intrinsic disease of the His Purkinje system at baseline, development of complete heart block can be seen and is actually relatively common, affecting 20%–30% of patients. Older studies performed before widespread adoption of the ICD reported high mortality and risk for sudden cardiac death after successful ablation, highlighting the fact

Understanding Intracardiac EGMs: A Patient Centered Guide, First Edition. Fred Kusumoto.
© 2015 John Wiley & Sons, Ltd. Published 2015 by John Wiley & Sons, Ltd.

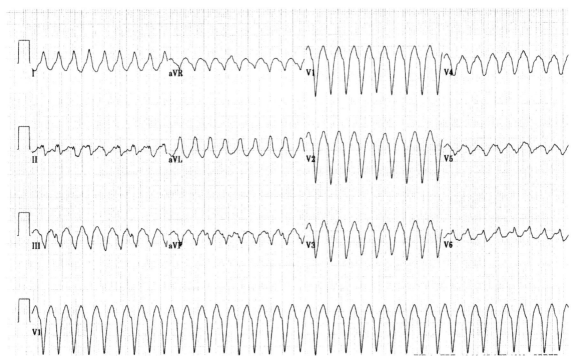

Figure 25.1 Wide complex tachycardia at a rate of 217 bpm.

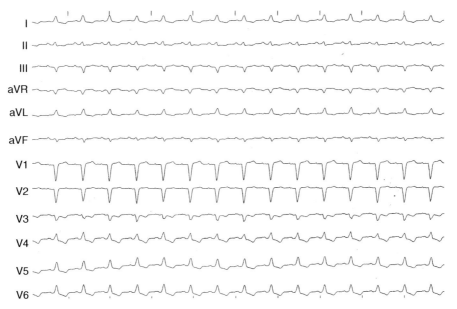

Figure 25.2 Baseline ECG shows left bundle branch block.

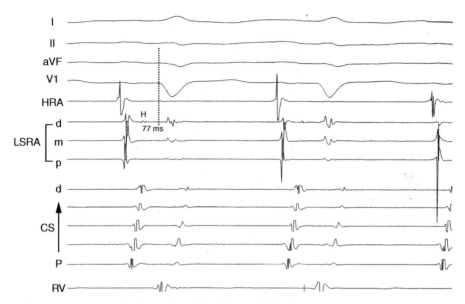

Figure 25.3 Baseline electrograms reveal prolongation of the HV interval (77 ms).

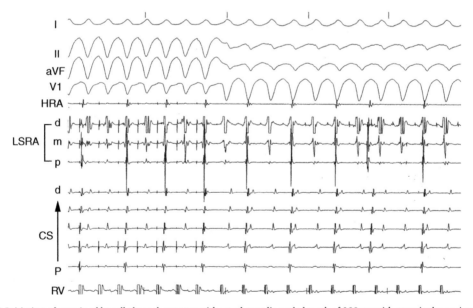

Figure 25.4 Initiation of sustained bundle branch reentry with a tachycardia cycle length of 280 ms with ventricular pacing of 250 ms.

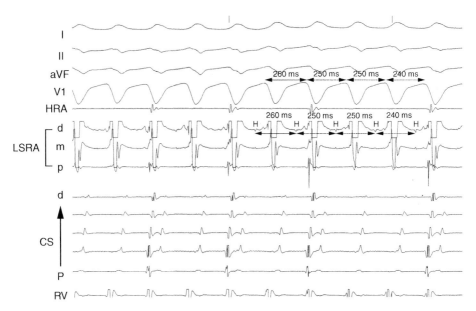

Figure 25.5 Electrograms from sustained bundle branch reentry showing a very rapid wide complex tachycardia with left bundle branch morphology with the QRS preceded by His bundle deflections. Notice that changes in the H–H intervals precede the changes in the R–R interval (double-headed arrows).

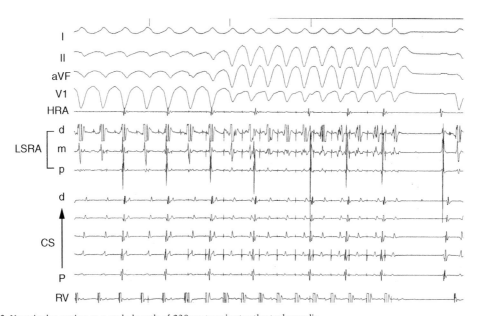

Figure 25.6 Ventricular pacing at a cycle length of 230 ms terminates the tachycardia.

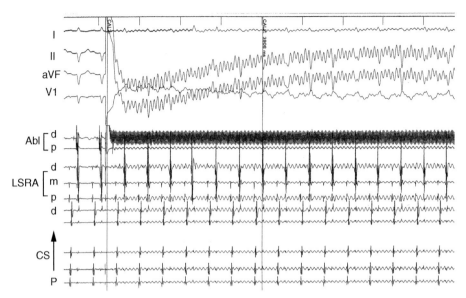

Figure 25.7 Ablation of the right bundle. Notice the right bundle potential ablation in the catheter. Application of radio-frequency energy leads to the development of right bundle branch block.

that ablation for bundle branch reentry is an adjunctive therapy to reduce ICD therapies and symptoms. Finally, even with the use of ICDs to reduce the risk of sudden cardiac death, progressive heart failure and high mortality rates are observed after successful ablation of bundle branch reentry. After the ablation the patient underwent implantation of a CRT-D device that provides both cardiac resynchronization and defibrillator back-up for ventricular arrhythmias.

- The diagnosis of bundle branch reentry should be suspected if a His bundle deflection precedes the QRS complex during tachycardia, and the diagnosis is confirmed if changes in the His–His interval precede and predict the changes in the R–R interval.

- Ablation is effective, and generally, the right bundle branch is targeted.

- Even with effective ablation, the presence of sustained bundle branch reentry is associated with a poor long-term prognosis.

KEY POINTS

- Sustained bundle branch reentry is most commonly observed in patients with dilated cardiomyopathy and accompanying His Purkinje disease.

CHAPTER 26

Syncope

A 64-year-old man had an episode of syncope while riding a bicycle several months ago. He suffered significant cervical injury but has now been referred after physical therapy and has nearly returned to full function. His baseline ECG is shown in Figure 26.1. The patient has a long history of permanent atrial fibrillation. He has known coronary artery disease and has had an inferolateral wall myocardial infarction and has a left ventricular ejection fraction of 0.40. A recent cardiac catheterization revealed an occluded obtuse marginal branch with distal filling from collaterals.

A comprehensive review of the evaluation of syncope is beyond the scope of this chapter. In addition, continuous ECG recording via an external event recorder, or an implantable loop recorder, has generally supplanted all other tests, including electrophysiology testing, as the best diagnostic tool for patients who are thought to have syncope due to arrhythmias. However, electrophysiologic testing remains a potential tool in selected patients with syncope, and recommendations from different scientific statements are summarized in Tables A10 and A11 of the Appendix.

From an arrhythmia standpoint, simplistically syncope can be due to bradycardia or tachycardia. Bradycardia can be due to sinus node dysfunction or AV block, and tachycardia can be due to supraventricular tachycardia or ventricular tachycardia. Of these causes, arguably, electrophysiology testing provides the greatest diagnostic yield when the clinician is suspicious of AV block due to infraHis disease, supraventricular tachycardia due to an accessory pathway or AVNRT, or ventricular tachycardia in the setting of prior myocardial infarction as a cause of syncope.

Bradycardia

There are several electrophysiologic tests for evaluating sinus node function. The most commonly used test is the sinus node recovery time (SNRT). To measure the SNRT, the atrium is paced at a range of cycle lengths (usually 600–350 ms), each for 30–60 s, and after cessation of pacing, the longest interval to the first sinus beat is measured (Figure 4.1 in Understanding Intracardiac EGMs and ECGs). Often, the baseline cycle length (not the pacing cycle length) is subtracted from the interval to identify the "corrected" sinus node recovery time or CSNRT. The CSNRT is more commonly used because it is useful for patients with a baseline sinus bradycardia. An abnormal SNRT and CSNRT are generally defined as 1,600 ms and 525 ms, respectively. An abnormal CSNRT or SNRT can be a useful clue to the cause of syncope and is reasonably specific but not sensitive for identifying sinus node dysfunction. In other words, the absence of sinus node dysfunction identified by electrophysiologic testing does not "rule out" sinus node dysfunction as a cause of syncope.

Identifying infraHisian block is an important factor for electrophysiologic testing. Identifying an HV interval of >100 ms with accompanying bifascicular block in a patient with syncope has been classified as an abnormal finding that provides a likely cause of syncope. Scheinman and colleagues have shown that with an HV interval >100 ms, at 4 years, 24% of patients will progress to AV block, as compared to 12% with HV intervals 70–99 ms, and <4% for patients with HV intervals <70 ms. IntraHis delay is also a specific but insensitive marker for progression to complete heart block. However, it is important to remember that simply identifying that delay within or below the His bundle is not sufficient for placement of a permanent pacemaker. As shown in Figure 26.2, a markedly prolonged HV interval of 140 ms was an incidental finding in a patient who underwent electrophysiologic testing and catheter ablation for atrial fibrillation without syncope. It is often difficult to determine whether more distally recorded potentials represent depolarization of the distal His bundle or right bundle. Regardless of the specific source

---

Understanding Intracardiac EGMs: A Patient Centered Guide, First Edition. Fred Kusumoto.
© 2015 John Wiley & Sons, Ltd. Published 2015 by John Wiley & Sons, Ltd.

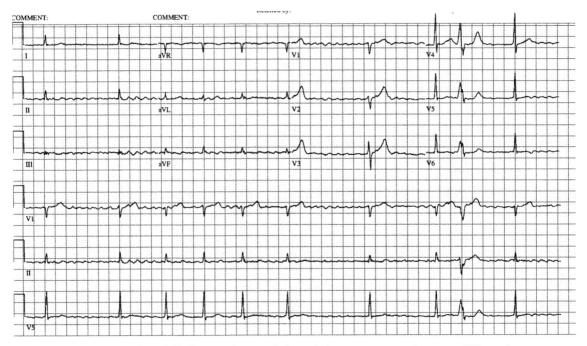

Figure 26.1 Baseline ECG with atrial fibrillation and a controlled ventricular response rate and a narrow QRS complex.

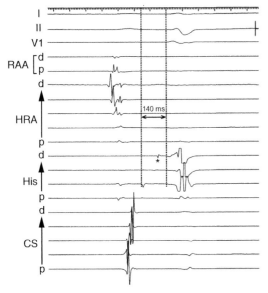

Figure 26.2 Abnormal infraHis conduction (HV 140 ms) is an incidental finding in a patient without symptoms suggestive of bradycardia. The potential recorded on the distal electrode pair of the His bundle electrode could represent depolarization of the distal His bundle or the right bundle branch.

of the distal potential, abnormal infraHis conduction is identified. However, although the patient should be warned about possible future permanent pacing requirements, in the absence of symptoms or accompanying Type II second-degree AV block, permanent pacing is not indicated.

Tachycardia

As discussed in the previous chapters, electrophysiology testing can be useful for identifying patients with supraventricular tachycardias. However, in cohorts of patients with syncope undergoing electrophysiology testing, supraventricular tachycardia is an uncommon cause, accounting for <3–5% of cases depending on the patient population.

Electrophysiology testing has been used for many years in the setting of syncope and prior myocardial infarction. Several moderately sized cohort studies have consistently shown that inducible ventricular tachyarrhythmias at electrophysiology study identify a group of patients with a higher likelihood of developing sustained ventricular arrhythmias in the future. Ventricular pacing protocols are generally performed from two sites in the right ventricle (often the right ventricular apex and the right ventricular outflow tract are chosen), using two different base cycle lengths and one, two, and three ventricular stimuli. There is significant variability in protocols used for ventricular pacing from operator to operator and institution to institution. One subgroup evaluation of a randomized trial (Electrophysiologic Study Versus Electrocardiographic Monitoring (ESVEM) Trial) found that inducible ventricular tachyarrhythmias using a protocol with up to two extrastimuli in a patient with syncope identified a group at high risk for sustained ventricular arrhythmias or sudden cardiac death. The type of ventricular tachyarrhythmia induced at electrophysiologic testing is also important. In a retrospective analysis of patients with syncope, inducible monomorphic ventricular tachycardia was associated with a significant increase in the risk of arrhythmic death; however, inducible ventricular fibrillation did not provide any prognostic information and survival was similar between the noninducible and the inducible ventricular fibrillation group. Taken collectively, the data suggest significant variability in the sensitivity and specificity of electrophysiologic testing with increased sensitivity and decreased specificity with more aggressive protocols.

The diagnostic yield of inducible ventricular arrhythmias in patients with syncope and clinical conditions other than in the setting of prior myocardial infarction is even more controversial. Inducible ventricular arrhythmias in patients with arrhythmogenic right ventricular cardiomyopathy appear to identify a group of patients who are more likely to receive appropriate ICD antitachycardia therapy. Some but not all investigators believe that inducible ventricular tachyarrhythmias provide additional prognostic information in patients with Brugada syndrome and syncope. Evaluation of inducible ventricular arrhythmias with electrophysiologic testing provides no benefit in patients with syncope and hypertrophic cardiomyopathy, dilated cardiomyopathy, or long QT syndrome. Generally the presence of syncope without symptoms suggestive of a vasovagal etiology is a poor prognostic sign in patients who have an inherited condition associated with increased risk of sudden death.

Returning to our patient, in the setting of syncope with a prior myocardial infarction and scar, electrophysiology testing is reasonable to evaluate the inducibility of ventricular tachycardia. He does not currently meet any of the three major criteria for primary prevention placement for an ICD (LVEF <0.30 due to prior MI, LVEF <0.35 with associated Class II or III heart failure symptoms, LVEF <0.40 due to prior MI, nonsustained ventricular tachycardia and inducible ventricular tachycardia at electrophysiologic testing), but an ICD would be indicated if he were inducible at EPS. Given his persistent atrial fibrillation, testing for sinus node dysfunction or evaluation of AV conduction by atrial pacing cannot be performed.

At electrophysiology study, two ventricular extrastimuli at coupling intervals of 270 ms and 240 ms induce a monomorphic ventricular tachycardia, first with a cycle length of 238 ms with positive precordial concordance and inferior axis that "settles" into a slower monomorphic ventricular tachycardia (cycle length of 315 ms) with positive concordance and a superior axis (Figures 26.3 and 26.4). Several attempts at terminating the tachycardia with ventricular tachycardia are unsuccessful and because of severe hypotension, external cardioversion is performed and the patient is converted to normal sinus rhythm (Figure 26.5) with normal conduction intervals (PR interval 180 ms, HV 50 ms). Fortunately, the procedure was performed on uninterrupted warfarin with a therapeutic INR. It is important for the clinician to anticipate all possible outcomes associated with an electrophysiology study. The patient underwent uncomplicated placement of an ICD. Evaluation of a large cohort of patients from Mayo Clinic found that cardiac device surgery with continued warfarin and an INR between 2 and 2.5 was not associated with a higher complication rate as compared to patients in whom warfarin was interrupted in preparation for surgery. Another option in this case could be the use of a wearable cardioverter defibrillator until warfarin could be safely stopped. As a final note, within 2 weeks, he developed recurrent atrial fibrillation. There was no improvement in symptoms associated with his transient period of sinus rhythm.

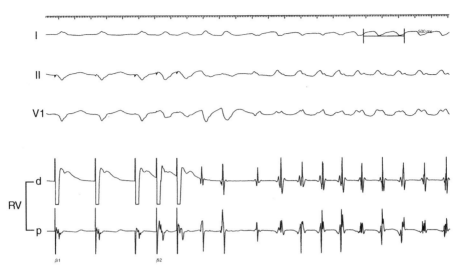

Figure 26.3 Ventricular pacing at a base cycle length of 500 ms is followed by two premature ventricular stimuli at coupling intervals of 270 ms and 240 ms inducing a rapid ventricular tachycardia at a cycle length of 238 ms.

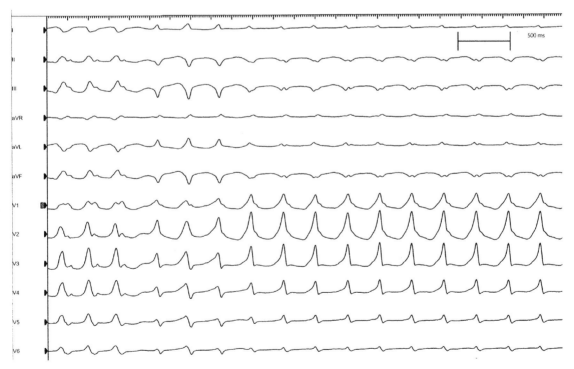

Figure 26.4 After several seconds, the ventricular tachycardia slows (315 ms) and in the frontal leads, the axis shifts completely rightward. The R wave in lead aVR is consistent with ventricular tachycardia. Despite the slower rate, the patient becomes hemodynamically compromised and cardioversion is required.

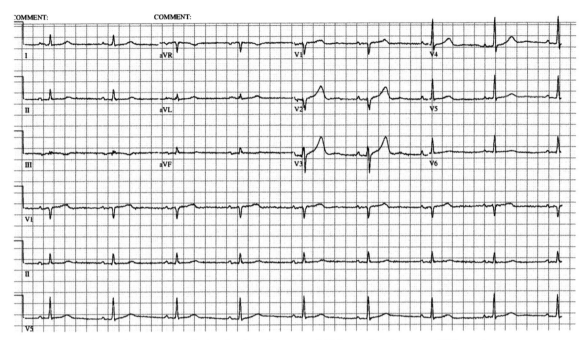

Figure 26.5 ECG after cardioversion reveals sinus bradycardia, a normal PR interval, and a narrow QRS complex.

KEY POINTS

- Electrophysiology testing may be useful in selected patients with syncope including patients with syncope and bifascicular block and patients with prior myocardial infarction with syncope who do not meet the primary prevention criteria for ICD implantation.

- Electrophysiologic testing protocols for evaluating the risk of ventricular arrhythmias vary from operator to operator and from institution to institution. As a general rule, the more aggressive the stimulation and the protocol, the less specific is the finding of inducible ventricular tachyarrhythmias.

- In patients with syncope and prior myocardial infarction, inducible monomorphic ventricular tachycardia, but not inducible ventricular fibrillation, appears to provide additional prognostic information.

CHAPTER 27

Multiple choice questions and answers

1 In a 42-year-old woman with episodes of palpitations, which arrhythmia mechanism can be excluded from consideration?

   A Atrial tachycardia

   B AVRT using a left-sided accessory pathway

   C AVRT using a right-sided accessory pathway

   D AV node reentry

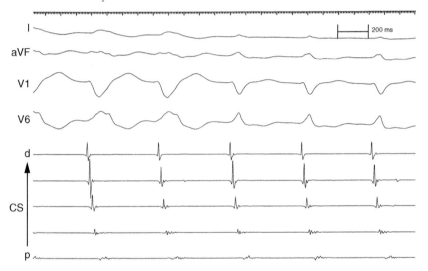

2 In a 33-year-old woman with episodes of palpitations, what is the most likely cause of supraventricular tachycardia

   A AVRT using a right-sided accessory pathway

   B AVRT using a left-sided accessory pathway

   C AVRT using a septal accessory pathway

   D AV node reentry with a bystander accessory pathway

   E Atrial tachycardia with a bystander accessory pathway

Understanding Intracardiac EGMs: A Patient Centered Guide, First Edition. Fred Kusumoto.
© 2015 John Wiley & Sons, Ltd. Published 2015 by John Wiley & Sons, Ltd.

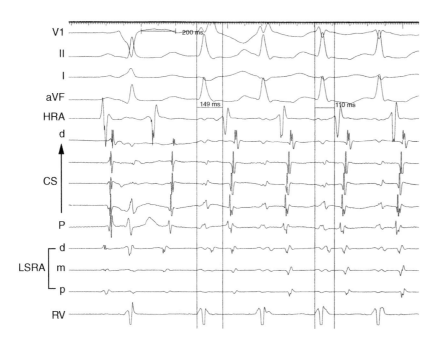

3 In a 45-year-old man with SVT, the following response establishes the diagnosis of:

   A AVNRT

   B AVRT

   C Atrial tachycardia

   D Abnormal AV conduction

   E Does not identify a specific diagnosis

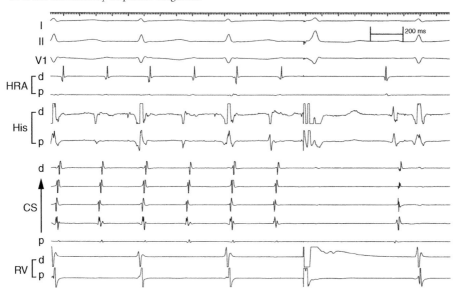

4 The following finding conclusively establishes the diagnosis of:

   A AVNRT

   B AVRT using an AV accessory pathway

   C Atrial tachycardia

   D Fascicular tachycardia

   E Does not conclusively establish a specific diagnosis

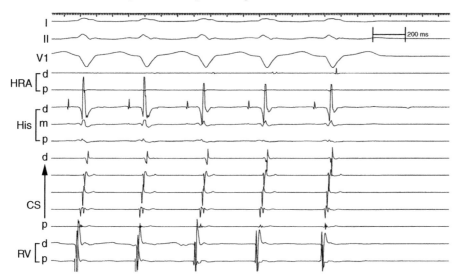

5 The following finding is observed during ablation of the slow pathway (20 watts, 40 °C). You should:

   A Increase the power

   B Decrease the power

   C Apply slight clockwise torque to establish a more septal position

   D Pull the catheter back slightly

   E Stop the ablation

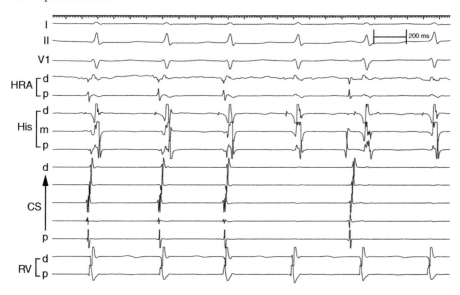

6 The following finding is characteristic of:

   A The presence of an AV accessory pathway

   B Sole activation via the AV node

C The presence of an atrioHisian accessory pathway

D The presence of a nodoventricular accessory pathway

E Inadvertant atrial capture

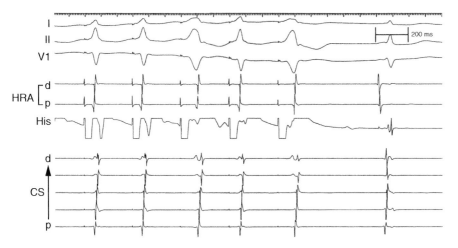

7 The mapping catheter is located near/at:

A Slowly conducting isthmus

B "Dead-end"

C Entrance site

D Exit

E A site away from the reentrant circuit

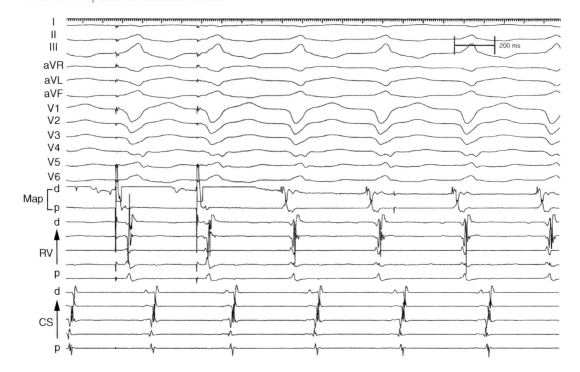

8 In a 56-year-old woman with SVT, the following response establishes the diagnosis of:

   A AVNRT

   B AVRT

   C Atrial tachycardia

   D Abnormal AV conduction

   E Does not establish anything

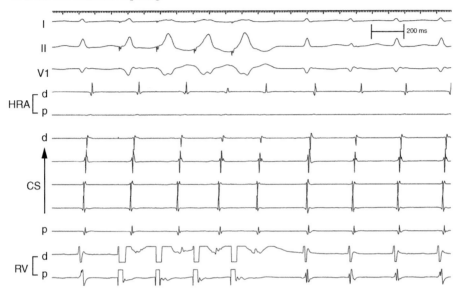

9 In a 46-year-old man with SVT, the following response establishes the diagnosis of:

   A AVNRT with a bystander left-sided accessory pathway

   B AVRT using a left-sided accessory pathway

   C Antidromic tachycardia using a Mahaim accessory pathway

   D Mitral annular atrial tachycardia

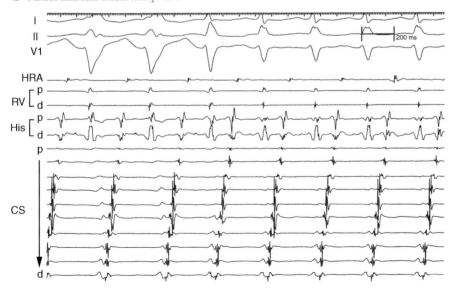

10 Which electrode position is most likely at a site that is critical for maintenance of tachycardia?

  A A
  B B
  C C
  D D
  E E

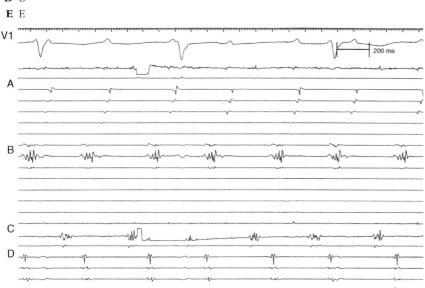

11 The following occurs after 10 s of radio-frequency energy delivery at 35 watts reaching a temperature of 45 °C, what would be the next step?

  A Stop delivery of radio-frequency energy at the current settings
  B Continue delivery of radio-frequency energy at the current settings
  C Increase power to 50 watts
  D Evaluate the fluoroscopic position of the catheter

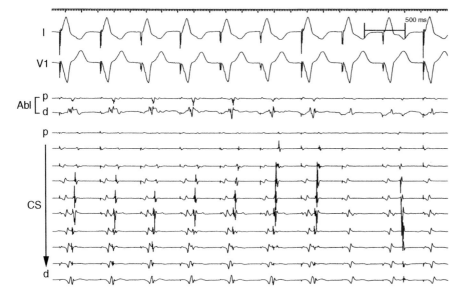

12 The following response is observed with ventricular pacing during supraventricular tachycardia. This finding confirms:

    A The patient has atrial tachycardia

    B The patient has AVNRT

    C The patient has AVRT

    D Does not confirm any specific supraventricular diagnosis

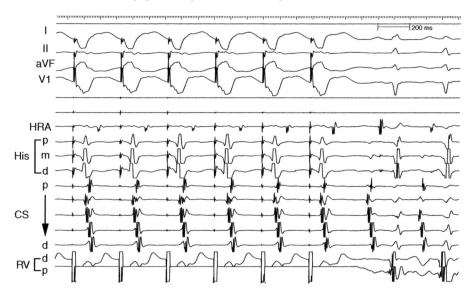

13 The same patient discussed in problem 12. This finding confirms:

    A The patient does not have atrial tachycardia

    B The patient has AVNRT

    C The patient has AVRT

    D The patient has a nodofascicular accessory pathway

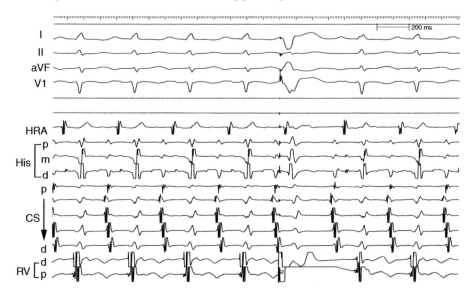

14 The same patient discussed in problems 12 and 13. The following finding is most consistent with:

   A Automatic atrial tachycardia

   B AVNRT

   C AVRT

   D Reentrant atrial flutter

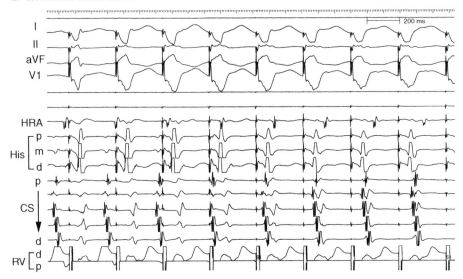

15 The following response suggests:

   A Retrograde atrial activation via the AV node

   B Retrograde activation via an AV accessory pathway

   C Retrograde activation via a His–atrial accessory pathway

   D Cannot assess retrograde activation

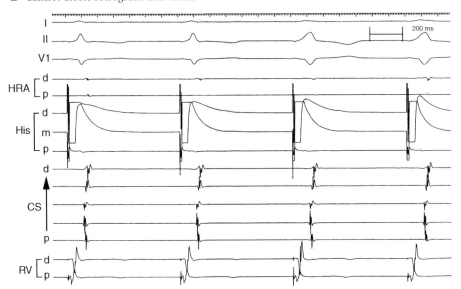

16 The following response makes the following diagnosis most likely:

    A AVRT using an AV accessory pathway

    B Automatic atrial tachycardia from a paraHisian focus

    C AVNRT

    D Automatic junctional tachycardia

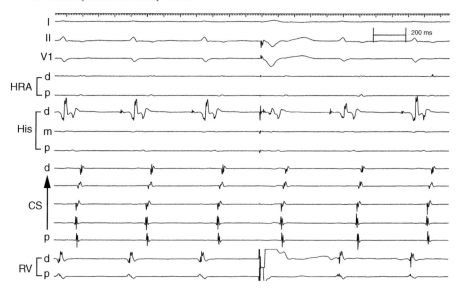

17 The following electrogram recordings definitively "rule out":

    A AVRT using an AV accessory pathway

    B AVNRT

    C Atrial tachycardia

    D Does not "rule out" any tachycardia mechanisms

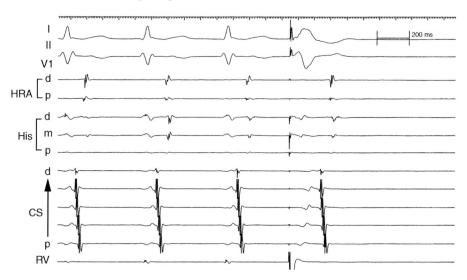

18 The following electrogram recordings are most consistent with:

    A AVNRT with bundle branch block aberrancy

    B AVNRT with bystander activation of an accessory pathway

    C Antidromic AVRT using an AV accessory pathway

    D Antidromic tachycardia using a nodoventricular accessory pathway

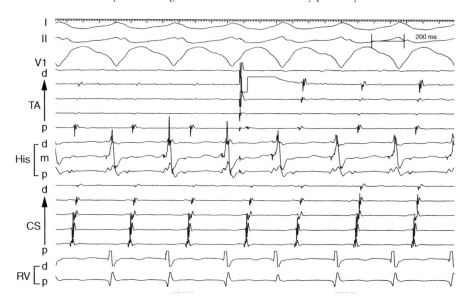

19 The ablation catheter is most likely located at:

    A Middle of the critical tachycardia isthmus

    B Entrance site

    C Nonexcitable scar

    D Exact localization not possible

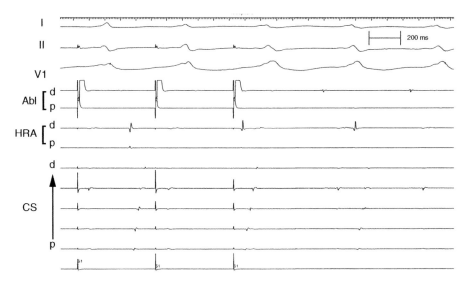

20 The electrogram recordings are most consistent with:

   A AVNRT

   B AVRT

   C Atrial tachycardia

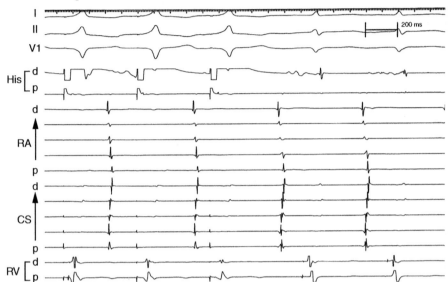

21 The electrogram recordings "rule out":

   A AVNRT

   B AVRT

   C Atrial tachycardia

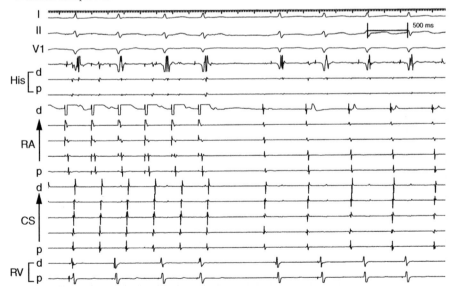

22 The electrogram recordings are most consistent with:

   A Atrial tachycardia with aberrant conduction

   B Nodofascicular tachycardia

C Antidromic AVRT

D Ventricular tachycardia

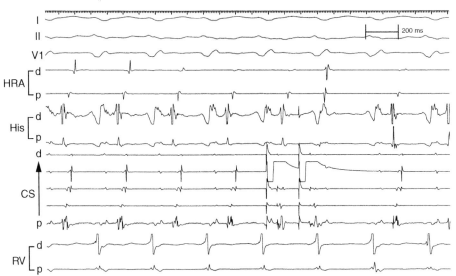

23 The following response after cessation of pacing during tachycardia makes the following diagnosis most likely:

A Rules out AVRT

B Rules in Atrial tachycardia

C Rules out AVNRT

D Does not provide diagnostic information

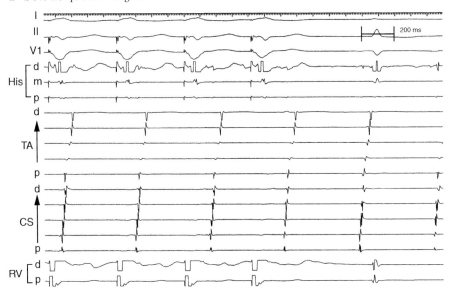

24 The ablation catheter is in a likely site for successful ablation if:

A The patient has atrial tachycardia

B The patient has AVNRT

  C The patient has atrial tachycardia or AVNRT

  D The patient has atrial tachycardia, AVNRT, or AVRT

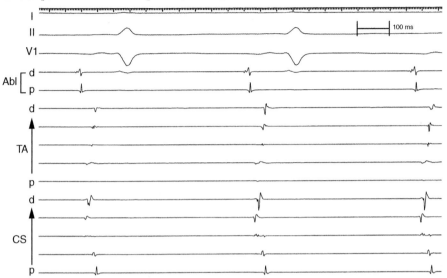

25 The electrogram recordings are most consistent with:

  A Atrial tachycardia with aberrant conduction

  B AVNRT with a bystander accessory pathway

  C Antidromic AVRT

  D Ventricular tachycardia

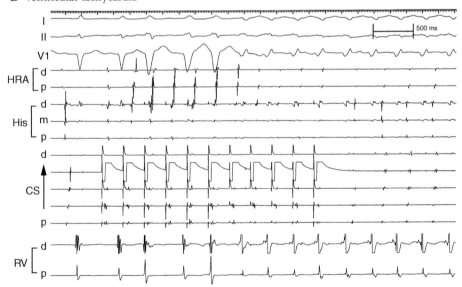

26 The pacing electrograms are consistent with:

  A Retrograde conduction via the AV node

  B Retrograde conduction via an AV accessory pathway

C No retrograde conduction

D Cannot assess retrograde conduction

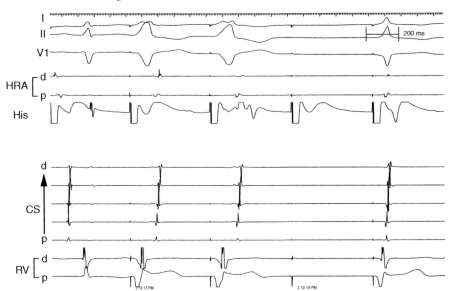

27 The beat marked by the asterisk is consistent with:

    A Conduction over an accessory pathway with normal conduction properties

    B Conduction over an accessory pathway with abnormal conduction properties

    C Conduction block in the left bundle branch

    D Induction of ventricular tachycardia

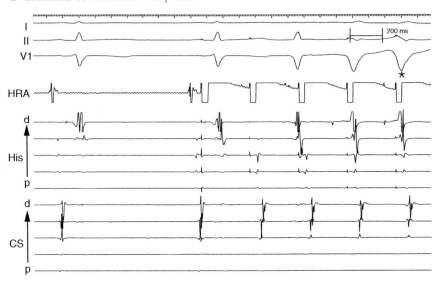

28 The beat marked by the asterisk is produced by:

    A Anterograde conduction over the right bundle

    B Anterograde conduction over an accessory pathway with abnormal conduction properties

C Dual pathway physiology within the AV node
D Anterograde conduction over a nodoventricular fiber

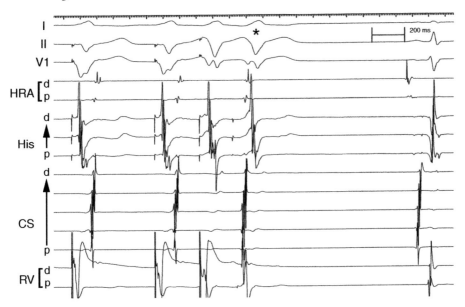

29 The ablation catheter tip is located:
    A In the left inferior pulmonary vein
    B Across a baffle in the patient who has undergone a Mustard procedure
    C In the left atrial appendage
    D In a persistent left superior vena cava

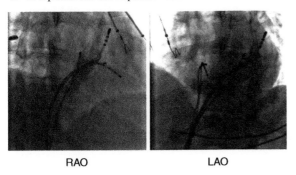

RAO   LAO

30 The lasso catheter is located in the:
    A Superior vena cava
    B Right superior pulmonary vein
    C Right inferior pulmonary vein
    D Left atrial appendage

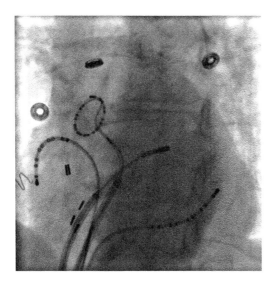

31 The following response is observed with adenosine infusion. This finding:

  A Confirms the diagnosis of atrial tachycardia

  B Confirms the presence of AVNRT

  C Confirms the presence of AVRT

  D Does not confirm the presence of an AV node dependent tachycardia

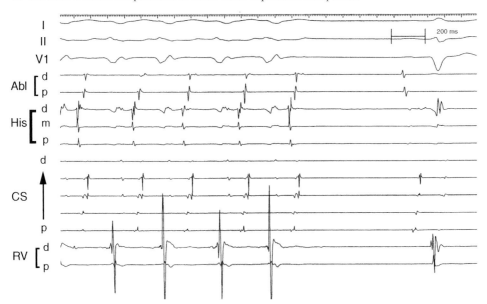

Answer

1 The correct answer is B. In this case, atrial activation in the distal coronary sinus activity precedes activation from the proximal coronary sinus, and the resolution of LBBB does not change the cycle length of tachycardia. This is a "reverse Coumel's sign" and provides important evidence that the left bundle branch is not involved in the tachycardia circuit. Although AVNRT is unlikely, given the distal-to-proximal activation of the coronary sinus, this activation pattern can be observed (Chapter); therefore, AVNRT cannot be completely "ruled out."

2 The correct answer is A. The patient has a right-sided accessory pathway with both anterograde and retrograde conduction. Initiation of SVT from a right-sided premature atrial contraction initiates a tachycardia with earliest activation in the high right atrium. The change in the ventriculoatrial conduction time with the resolution of complete right bundle branch block suggests that the right bundle is part of the tachycardia circuit.

3 The correct answer is A. PVC terminates the tachycardia without resetting the atrium. This finding rules out atrial tachycardia. The short VA interval and continuation of tachycardia in the setting of 2:1 AV block rules out AVRT using an accessory pathway. The presence of 2:1 AV block in the setting of tachycardia does not establish the diagnosis of abnormal AV conduction due to the high atrial rate.

4 The correct answer is E. The tachycardia is characterized by a very short HA interval, ruling out AVRT. The tachycardia spontaneously terminates with an atrial signal, which would generally rule out atrial tachycardia and establish the diagnosis of AVNRT. However, in this case with gradual prolongation of the AH intervals prior to termination, although very unlikely, this finding could theoretically be observed if the atrial tachycardia and AV block occurred simultaneously.

5 The correctex answer is E. During ablation, there is transient block in retrograde fast pathway conduction. At this point, it is important to immediately stop the ablation.

6 The correct answer is B. With His bundle capture, the ventriculoatrial conduction time is decreased.

7 The correct answer is D. The paced QRS complex is very similar in morphology to the QRS complex in tachycardia. The first return cycle length of tachycardia is similar to the tachycardia cycle length. Both of these findings suggest that the mapping catheter is at or near a site within the reentrant circuit. As the pacing stimulus–QRS onset and the electrogram–QRS onset intervals are very short, it is likely that the mapping catheter is near the exit site.

8 The correct answer is A. The SVT is entrained by the third ventricular paced beat and the patient has a V-A-V response. The V-A-V response in this case rules out atrial tachycardia. The short VA interval precludes involvement of an accessory pathway and AVRT.

9 The correct answer is B. Shortening of the tachycardia cycle length with the resolution of left bundle branch block confirms that the left bundle branch was a component of the tachycardia circuit using an ipsilateral (left-sided, in this case) accessory pathway.

10 The correct answer is C. Although at initial glance, variations in the tachycardia cycle length would seem to add to the complexity of mapping. In fact, identifying the region where variation in the cycle length appears to "drive" the cycle length changes at other sites can be a useful method for identifying the critical regions. In this case, the first cycle length change is identified at position C suggesting that this is an important area to focus on. In addition, notice that the fractionated signal borders (at least on one side) the areas of probable scar suggested by the absence of electrograms.

11 The correct answer is D. In this patient with a left free-wall accessory pathway, loss of accessory pathway conduction is noted with 2:1 retrograde conduction in the AV node or absence of retrograde conduction with a sinus beat (in the absence of a high right atrial catheter, these two alternatives cannot be distinguished). However, with loss of accessory pathway conduction, the annular signal with similar atrial and ventricular electrogram amplitudes recorded on the first few beats is replaced by a predominant ventricular electrogram, suggesting the catheter may have moved apically into the left ventricle. However, it is reasonable to continue application of radio-frequency energy while catheter evaluation is assessed since the likelihood of AV block or other significant problems at this site would be very low.

12 The correct answer is D. Although an apparent V-A-A-V response is observed, notice that the two atrial signals after cessation of ventricular pacing occur at the paced rate, suggesting that the last ventricular paced beat "causes" the second atrial signal due to prolonged retrograde conduction (courtesy Bob Kim, University of Florida, Jacksonville).

13 The correct answer is A. An early coupled premature ventricular contraction leads to delay of the subsequent atrial depolarization with the same atrial activation pattern. This response would not be observed in an atrial tachycardia. (courtesy Bob Kim, University of Florida, Jacksonville).

14 The correct answer is B. Ventricular pacing at a rate faster than the tachycardia rate is performed. Resetting of the tachycardia to the paced rate occurs after full capture of the ventricles (courtesy Bob Kim, University of Florida, Jacksonville).

15 The correct answer is B. ParaHisian pacing is being performed. Change in the QRS morphology with pacing from the distal His electrodes is noted. Adequate right ventricular capture is confirmed by evaluation of the ventricular electrograms, and no evidence of atrial capture is observed. The ventriculoatrial conduction interval is the same regardless of whether the His bundle is captured or not, suggesting the presence of an extranodal accessory pathway.

16 The correct answer is B. This is the tachycardia from the patient discussed in problem 15. A premature ventricular contraction is delivered when the His bundle is refractory, which leads to early atrial activation with the same atrial activation as in tachycardia.

17 The correct answer is C. The premature ventricular contraction terminates the tachycardia without an early atrial electrogram. This finding is "proof" that the tachycardia is "AV node dependent" and "rules out" atrial tachycardia. The astute observer will note that the premature ventricular contraction leads to subtle delay in the atrial electrogram, suggesting decremental properties for the retrograde ventriculoatrial conduction path. Eccentric retrograde activation makes a left free-wall accessory pathway the most likely diagnosis; however, in rare cases, AVNRT can be associated with left-sided inputs.

18 The correct answer is C. A premature atrial contraction delivered when the atrial electrogram in the His bundle region has already been depolarized preexcites the ventricle with the same QRS morphology as tachycardia and the subsequent atrial electrogram. In either AVNRT or AVRT, using a nodoventricular accessory pathway atrial depolarization after the septal atrium is committed would not affect the tachycardia. In the setting of AVNRT with a bystander accessory pathway, the premature atrial contraction would be associated with early ventricular activation but would not lead to subsequent early activation of the next atrial electrogram.

19 The correct answer is D. Pacing does not change the tachycardia cycle length although there appears to be local capture and perhaps some subtle changes in the QRS complex (making scar less likely). If local capture is present the return cycle length is suggestive that the site is near a critical isthmus. Pacing at a slightly faster rate confirmed capture and identified the site as a critical component of the tachycardia circuit.

20 The correct answer is C. Pacing from the His bundle area does not result in retrograde atrial conduction, making AVNRT or AVRT very unlikely.

21 The correct answer is B. Atrial pacing initiates tachycardia without an intervening QRS. This is initiation from the same patient as in problem 20 and rules out AVRT using an accessory pathway. AVNRT can be associated with this type of initiation because of block distal to the "turnaround point" in AVNRT but proximal to the His bundle. This patient had an atrial tachycardia from a site at the os of the coronary sinus.

22 The correct answer is D. The patient has a wide complex tachycardia with a 1:1 ventriculoatrial relationship with concentric atrial activation. Two atrial extrastimuli are delivered and do not affect the tachycardia. This finding makes atrial tachycardia or antidromic AVRT very unlikely. Although it is possible that a nodofascicular tachycardia might not be reset due to refractoriness within the AV node, this finding would be very unlikely.

23 The correct answer is A. The absence of retrograde atrial conduction during pacing rules out AVRT and makes AVNRT very unlikely.

24 The correct answer is C. The ablation catheter records a very early atrial signal relative to the P wave. This would be a reasonable site for ablation of an atrial tachycardia or an atypical AVNRT (where the slow retrogradely conducting AV node "input" would be targeted). Even with an early atrial signal, the relatively small ventricular signal suggests a nonannular site that would be less promising for ablation of a slowly conducting accessory pathway.

25 The correct answer is D. Atrial pacing initiates a wide QRS tachycardia that is associated with AV dissociation. This finding rules out antidromic AVRT. Although both atrial tachycardia and AVNRT could be associated with AV dissociation, the QRS complex should have a relationship with atrial activation.

26 The correct answer is A. ParaHisian pacing is consistent with a nodal response with a shorter ventriculoatrial conduction interval with the narrower QRS complex and His bundle capture. Ventricular rather than atrial capture is confirmed by inspection of the right ventricular electrograms.

27 The correct answer is D. Atrial pacing from the coronary sinus results in progressive prolongation of the AH interval. Although the QRS complex has an LBBB morphology and a His bundle electrogram is observed before the wide QRS beats, notice that the HV interval is progressively shortening, which is particularly evident in the last QRS complex marked by the asterisk. Notice also the progressive fusion in the QRS in the last three beats. It is possible that the beat before the asterisk represents left bundle branch block. This patient had inducible right ventricular outflow tract ventricular tachycardia.

28 The correct answer is A. The extra beat marked by the asterisk is due to a single beat of bundle branch reentry. This is a common phenomenon in the setting of right ventricular pacing. The ventricular extrastimulus resulted in retrograde block in the right bundle branch, septal activation, and retrograde depolarization of the left bundle. The wave of depolarization "turned around" at the His bundle and the right bundle was activated anterogradely producing a QRS complex with an LBBB configuration.

29 The correct answer is D. The catheter is located in a tubular structure with the tip just beyond the cardiac silhouette.

30 The correct answer is B. In this LAO projection, the circular mapping catheter has been placed in the right superior pulmonary vein. The right inferior pulmonary vein is not angled as anteriorly as the right superior pulmonary vein.

31 The correct answer is D. Termination of supraventricular tachycardia with adenosine suggests an AV node dependent mechanism. In this case the patient has a wide complex tachycardia that is actually an adenosine sensitive ventricular tachycardia. Notice that a His bundle deflection is not observed during tachycardia although unfortunately only a low amplitude signal is present at baseline. Tachycardia terminating with an atrial electrogram generally rules out the presence of an atrial tachycardia.

Appendix

Table A1 Usual initial access and catheter positions at Mayo Clinic, Florida.

Likely arrhythmia	Vascular access	Initial position: Catheter type
Supraventricular tachycardia	Four femoral vein	Superior right atrium: Quadripolar His bundle: Quadripolar Right ventricle: Quadripolar Coronary sinus: Decapolar
Typical atrial flutter	Two femoral vein	Cavotricuspid isthmus (roving): Quadripolar Coronaruy sinus: Decapolar
Atypical atrial flutter	Four femoral vein	Tricuspid annulus: Decapolar Coronary Sinus: Decapolar Mitral Annulus (LA): Decapolar or duodecapolar Roving: Quadripolar
Atrial fibrillation	Three femoral vein	Coronary sinus: Decapolar
Right-sided ventricular arrhythmias	Three femoral vein	Coronary sinus: Decapolar Right ventricle: Decapolar Roving: Quadripolar
Left-sided ventricular arrhythmias	Three femoral vein (transseptal approach) Two femoral vein and one femoral artery (retrograde approach)	Coronary sinus: Decapolar Right ventricle: Decapolar Roving: Quadripolar

Understanding Intracardiac EGMs: A Patient Centered Guide, First Edition. Fred Kusumoto.
© 2015 John Wiley & Sons, Ltd. Published 2015 by John Wiley & Sons, Ltd.

Table A2 Basic pacing protocols.

Pacing type	Method	
Atrial overdrive pacing	• Burst pace at a cycle length of 600 ms for approximately 10 stimuli • Repeat bursts at progressively shorter cycle lengths (decreasing by 50 ms at a time) • Alternatively, begin pacing at 600 ms and decrease continuously by 10 ms	• Observe the atrioventricular relationship • Identify whether there are any dramatic changes in the atrioventricular interval • Determine when atrioventricular block begins
Atrial premature stimuli	• After a constant drive cycle length (usually 600 ms, but dependent on the underlying sinus rate), deliver progressively earlier premature atrial stimuli	• Confirm atrial capture in the drive cycle and the premature atrial extrastimulus • As the stimulus is delivered at shorter coupling intervals, evaluate the AH interval, HV interval, and QRS morphology. • Identify any sudden changes in conduction intervals. • Identify blocked conduction (block in the AV node versus block in the His bundle) • Identify atrial refractoriness
Ventricular overdrive pacing	• Burst pace at a cycle length of 600 ms for approximately 10 stimuli • Repeat bursts at progressively shorter cycle lengths (decreasing by 50 ms at a time) • Alternatively, begin pacing at 600 ms and decrease continuously by 10 ms	• Observe the ventriculoatrial relationship • Identify whether there are any dramatic changes in the ventriculoatrial interval • Identify the pattern of atrial activation and identify any changes with changes in cycle length. • Determine when ventriculoatrial block occurs
Ventricular premature stimuli	• After a constant drive cycle length (usually 600 ms, but dependent on the underlying sinus rate), deliver progressively earlier premature ventricular stimuli	• Confirm ventricular capture in the drive cycle and the premature extrastimulus • As the stimulus is delivered at shorter coupling intervals, evaluate the ventriculoatrial interval • Identify any sudden changes in conduction intervals or pattern of atrial activation. • Identify blocked conduction and the site of block. • Identify ventricular refractoriness

Table A3 Helpful electrophysiologic responses in SVT.

"Rules in" AVRT	• Bundle branch block is associated with changes in the tachycardia cycle length
	• PVC on His:
	○ Resets the tachycardia with the same retrograde activation (either early or late)
	○ Terminates the tachycardia without a subsequent atrial electrogram
"Rules out" Atrial tachycardia *(Proves AV node dependence)*	• Spontaneous termination on an atrial electrogram without preceding AV block
	• PVC:
	○ Terminates the tachycardia without resetting the atrial electrogram
	○ Terminates the tachycardia without an atrial signal
	• Ventricular pacing yields a V-A-V response

Table A4 Approximate risks for different types of ablations.

	SVT	AF	VT (SHD)	VT (idiopathic)
Death	nil	0.1%	<0.5%	nil
Vascular	0–3%	0–13%	3–7%	0–2%
Thromboembolism	0–1%	0–7%	0.8–2.7	0.4%
Tamponade	1%	0.2–2.4%	2.7%	0–1%
Major	1–3%	6%	5–8%	1–3%

Table A5 Approximate additional risks for specific ablations.

AF ablation
PV stenosis: 0–38%
Phrenic nerve injury (balloon): 5–8%
Esophageal atrial fistula: 0.1–0.25%
Gastric problems: 1%

AVNRT
AV block: < 1%

AVRT
AV block: 0–8% depending on location

Table A6 Recommendations for catheter ablation for different supraventricular tachycardias: From ACC/AHA/ESC guidelines for the management of patients with supraventricular arrhythmias – executive summary: a report of the American College of Cardiology/American Heart Association Task Force on Practice Guidelines and the European Society of Cardiology Committee for Practice Guidelines (writing committee to develop guidelines for the management of patients with supraventricular arrhythmias) developed in collaboration with NASPE-Heart Rhythm Society.

AVNRT

Class I

Poorly tolerated AVNRT with hemodynamic intolerance

Recurrent symptomatic AVNRT

AVNRT with infrequent or single episode in patients who desire complete control of arrhythmia

Documented PSVT with only dual AV-nodal pathways or single echo beats demonstrated during electrophysiological study and no other identified cause of arrhythmia

Infrequent, well-tolerated AVNRT

Focal and nonparoxysmal junctional tachycardia

Class IIa

Focal junctional tachycardia

Accessory pathway mediated arrhythmias

Class I

WPW syndrome (pre-excitation and symptomatic arrhythmias), well tolerated

WPW syndrome (with AF and rapid-conduction or poorly tolerated AVRT)

AVRT, poorly tolerated (no pre-excitation)

Class IIa

Single or infrequent AVRT episode(s) (no pre-excitation)

Class IIb

Pre-excitation, asymptomatic

Focal atrial tachycardia

Class I

Recurrent symptomatic AT

Asymptomatic or symptomatic incessant AT

Class III

Nonsustained and asymptomatic AT

Atrial flutter

Class I

Recurrent and well-tolerated atrial flutter

Poorly tolerated atrial flutter

Atrial flutter appearing after use of class Ic agents or amiodarone for treatment of AF

Class IIa

First episode and well-tolerated atrial flutter

Symptomatic non-CTI-dependent flutter after failed antiarrhythmic drug therapy

Blomstrom Lundqvist C, Scheinman MM, Aliot EM *et al.* J Am Coll Cardiol. 2003 Oct 15;42(8):1493–531.

Table A7 2012 HRS/EHRA/ECAS expert consensus statement on catheter and surgical ablation of atrial fibrillation: recommendations for patient selection, procedural techniques, patient management and follow-up, definitions, endpoints, and research trial design.

Is recommended

Symptomatic AF refractory or intolerant to at least one Class 1 or 3 antiarrhythmic medication (paroxysmal)

Is reasonable

Symptomatic AF refractory or intolerant to at least one Class 1 or 3 antiarrhythmic medication (persistent)
Symptomatic AF before initiation of antiarrhythmic drug therapy with a Class 1 or 3 antiarrhythmic agent (paroxysmal)

May be considered

Symptomatic AF refractory or intolerant to at least one Class 1 or 3 antiarrhythmic medication (long-standing persistent)
Symptomatic AF before initiation of antiarrhythmic drug therapy with a Class 1 or 3 antiarrhythmic agent (persistent or long-standing persistent)

Calkins H, Kuck KH, Cappato R, Heart Rhythm. 2012 Apr;9(4):632–696.

Table A8 2014 AHA/ACC/HRS Guideline for the management of patients with atrial fibrillation: a report of the American College of Cardiology/American Heart Association Task Force on Practice Guidelines and the Heart Rhythm Society.

Class I

AF catheter ablation is useful for symptomatic paroxysmal AF refractory or intolerant to at least one Class I or III antiarrhythmic medication when a rhythm control strategy is desired

Class IIa

AF catheter ablation is reasonable for selected patients with symptomatic persistent AF refractory or intolerant to at least one Class I or III antiarrhythmic medication
In patients with recurrent symptomatic paroxysmal AF, catheter ablation is a reasonable initial rhythm control strategy before therapeutic trials of antiarrhythmic drug therapy, after weighing the risks and outcomes of drug and ablation therapy

Class IIb

AF catheter ablation may be considered for symptomatic long-standing (> 12 months) persistent AF refractory or intolerant to at least one Class I or III antiarrhythmic medication, when a rhythm control strategy is desired
AF catheter ablation may be considered before initiation of antiarrhythmic drug therapy with a Class I or III antiarrhythmic medication for symptomatic persistent AF, when a rhythm control strategy is desired.

January CT, Wann LS, Alpert JS *et al.*, J Am Coll Cardiol. 2014 Mar 28. S0735-1097(14)01740-9.

Table A9 Electrophysiology testing: From ACC/AHA/ESC 2006 guidelines for management of patients with ventricular arrhythmias and the prevention of sudden cardiac death: a report of the American College of Cardiology/American Heart Association Task Force and the European Society of Cardiology Committee for Practice Guidelines (writing committee to develop guidelines for management of patients with ventricular arrhythmias and the prevention of sudden cardiac death).

Coronary artery disease
Class I

EP testing is recommended for diagnostic evaluation of patients with remote MI with symptoms suggestive of ventricular tachyarrhythmias, including palpitations, presyncope, and syncope

EP testing is recommended in patients with CHD to guide and assess the efficacy of VT ablation

EP testing is useful in patients with CHD for the diagnostic evaluation of wide-QRS-complex tachycardias of unclear mechanism.

Class IIa

EP testing is reasonable for risk stratification in patients with remote MI, NSVT, and LVEF equal to or less than 40%

Syncope
Class I

EP testing is recommended in patients with syncope of unknown cause with impaired LV function or structural heart disease

Class IIa

EP testing can be useful in patients with syncope when bradyarrhythmias or tachyarrhythmias are suspected and in whom noninvasive diagnostic studies are not conclusive

CHD, coronary heart disease; MI, myocardial infarction; EP, electrophysiology; NSVT, nonsustained ventricular tachycardia; LVEF, left ventricular ejection fraction.
Zipes DP, Camm AJ, Borgreffe M, *et al.*, J Am Coll Cardiol. 2006 Sep 5;48(5):e247–346.

Table A10 Electrophysiology testing in patients with syncope: Recommendations from Guidelines for the diagnosis and management of syncope (version 2009). Task Force for the Diagnosis and Management of Syncope; European Society of Cardiology (ESC); European Heart Rhythm Association (EHRA); Heart Failure Association (HFA); Heart Rhythm Society (HRS).

Class I

In patients with ischemic heart disease, EPS is indicated when initial evaluation suggests an arrhythmic cause of syncope unless there is already an established indication for ICD

Class IIa

In patients with bundle branch block, EPS should be considered when noninvasive tests have failed to make the diagnosis

Class IIb

In patients with syncope preceded by sudden and brief palpitations, EPS may be performed when other noninvasive tests have failed to make the diagnosis

In patients with Brugada syndrome, ARVC, and hypertrophic cardiomyopathy, an EPS may be performed in selected cases.

Class III

EPS is not recommended in patients with normal ECG, no heart disease, and no palpitations

Moya A, Sutton R, Ammirati F, *et al.* Eur Heart J. 2009 Nov;30(21):2631–71.

Table A11 Ablation for Ventricular Tachycardia: Recommendations from the EHRA/HRS Expert Consensus on Catheter Ablation of Ventricular Arrhythmias: developed in a partnership with the European Heart Rhythm Association (EHRA), a Registered Branch of the European Society of Cardiology (ESC), and the Heart Rhythm Society (HRS); in collaboration with the American College of Cardiology (ACC) and the American Heart Association (AHA).

Patients with structural heart disease

Catheter Ablation is recommended

for symptomatic sustained monomorphic VT (SMVT), including VT terminated by an ICD, that recurs despite antiarrhythmic drug therapy or when antiarrhythmic drugs are not tolerated or not desired

for control of incessant SMVT or VT storm that is not due to a transient reversible cause

for patients with frequent PVCs, NSVTs, or VT that is presumed to cause ventricular dysfunction

for bundle branch reentrant or interfascicular VTs

for recurrent sustained polymorphic VT and VF that is refractory to antiarrhythmic therapy when there is a suspected trigger that can be targeted for ablation

Catheter ablation should be considered

in patients who have one or more episodes of SMVT despite therapy with one of more Class I or III antiarrhythmic drugs

in patients with recurrent SMVT due to prior MI who have LV ejection fraction > 0.30 and expectation for 1 year of survival, and it is an acceptable alternative to amiodarone therapy

in patients with haemodynamically tolerated SMVT due to prior MI who have reasonably preserved LV ejection fraction (> 0.35) even if they have not failed antiarrhythmic drug therapy

Patients without structural heart disease

Catheter ablation of VT is recommended for

for monomorphic VT that causes severe symptoms

for monomorphic VT when antiarrhythmic drugs are not effective, not tolerated, or not desired

for recurrent sustained polymorphic VT and VF (electrical storm) that is refractory to antiarrhythmic therapy when there is a suspected trigger that can be targeted for ablation

VT catheter ablation is contraindicated

in the presence of a mobile ventricular thrombus (epicardial ablation may be considered);

for asymptomatic PVCs and/or NSVT that are not suspected of causing or contributing to ventricular dysfunction

for VT due to transient, reversible causes, such as acute ischemia, hyperkalemia, or drug-induced torsade de pointes

Aliot EM, Stevenson WG, Almendral-Garrote *et al.*, Heart Rhythm. 2009 Jun;6(6):886–933.

Table A12 Recommendations for EPS and ablation in idiopathic ventricular tachycardia: From ACC/AHA/ESC 2006 guidelines for management of patients with ventricular arrhythmias and the prevention of sudden cardiac death: a report of the American College of Cardiology/American Heart Association Task Force and the European Society of Cardiology Committee for Practice Guidelines (writing committee to develop guidelines for management of patients with ventricular arrhythmias and the prevention of sudden cardiac death).

Class I

Catheter ablation is useful in patients with structurally normal hearts with symptomatic, drug-refractory VT arising from the RV or LV or in those who are drug intolerant or who do not desire long-term drug therapy

Class IIa

EP testing is reasonable for diagnostic evaluation in patients with structurally normal hearts with palpitations or suspected outflow tract VT.

Drug therapy with beta-blockers and/or calcium channel blockers (and/or IC agents in RVOT VT) can be useful in patients with structurally normal hearts with symptomatic VT arising from the RV

Zipes DP, Camm AJ, Borgreffe M, *et al.*, J Am Coll Cardiol. 2006 Sep 5;48(5):e247–346.

Index

Chapter organization by arrhythmia type.

Chapter 1: Basic EP

Short RP tachycardias
Chapter 2: AVNRT; short HA
Chapter 3: Slow AVNRT; short HA
Chapter 4: AVNRT; longer HA with concentric atrial activation

Eccentric atrial activation/accessory pathways
Chapter 5: Eccentric activation (distal coronary sinus first) due to AVRT and an atrioventricular accessory pathway with normal properties
Chapter 6: Eccentric activation (distal coronary sinus first) due to AVRT and a slowly conducting accessory pathway
Chapter 7: Baseline pre-excitation: Wolff–Parkinson–White Syndrome
Chapter 8: Baseline pre-excitation (Mahaim)
Chapter 9: Eccentric activation (distal coronary sinus first) due to AVNRT

Atrial tachycardias/Atrial flutters
Chapter 10: Atrial tachycardia
Chapter 11: Pulmonary vein atrial tachycardia
Chapter 12: Typical atrial flutter
Chapter 13: Atrial flutter with prior atrial surgery

Atrial fibrillation/Atrial arrhythmias after AF ablation
Chapter 14: Atrial fibrillation
Chapter 15: Pulmonary vein atrial flutter after AF ablation
Chapter 16: Mitral annular flutter after AF ablation
Chapter 17: Atrial flutter from the LA roof after AF ablation
Chapter 18: Atrial flutter from a cavotricuspid isthmus pouch
Chapter 19: Atrial tachycardia from a paraHisian focus

Wide Complex Tachycardias
Chapter 20: Antidromic tachycardia
Chapter 21: Ventricular tachycardia from the right ventricular outflow tract
Chapter 22: Premature ventricular contractions from the left ventricular outflow tract
Chapter 23: Left septal ventricular tachycardia
Chapter 24: Ventricular tachycardia after myocardial infarction
Chapter 25: Bundle branch reentry
Chapter 26: Syncope (inducible ventricular tachycardia)

Extras
Chapter 27: Multiple Choice Questions and Answers
Chapter 28: Appendix

Understanding Intracardiac EGMs: A Patient Centered Guide, First Edition. Fred Kusumoto.
© 2015 John Wiley & Sons, Ltd. Published 2015 by John Wiley & Sons, Ltd.

Printed and bound by CPI Group (UK) Ltd, Croydon, CR0 4YY

27/10/2024

14580357-0002